Practices of Freedom

A series edited by Michèle Aina Barale,

Jonathan Goldberg, Michael Moon,

and Eve Kosofsky Sedgwick

Practices of Freedom

SELECTED WRITINGS ON HIV / AIDS

by Simon Watney

DUKE UNIVERSITY PRESS   *Durham 1994*

First published in 1994 by Rivers Oram Press
144 Hemingford Road, London, N1 1DE
First U.S. edition, Duke University Press, 1994
Copyright © Simon Peter Watney 1994
Printed in the United States of America on acid-free paper ∞
Typeset by Tseng Information Systems in Berkeley Medium
Library of Congress Cataloging-in-Publication Data
appear on the last printed page of this book.

for John-Paul Philippé,
with gratitude and love

Contents

Acknowledgements

Throughout the better part of the last decade I have had the great good fortune to be able to work with a large number of remarkable people, united in our various responses to HIV/AIDS. My own work has been constantly informed by ongoing national and international dialogue with friends and colleagues in Britain, Europe, North America, Australia, and elsewhere. Indeed, I am keenly aware that my work is part of a far wider international project, aiming to sustain close contact between non-government AIDS service organisations around the world. Such exchange is of vital importance in order to stay up to date with the latest developments in HIV education, care and service provision, treatment issues, cultural and political analysis, and so on. Such an encyclopedic project is necessarily collective, both in spirit and in practice.

In this respect I feel very much part of what Dennis Altman has dubbed 'the AIDS community', meaning that largely informal network of people thrown together in the urgent community-based struggle to save lives in an emergency which sadly remains subject to widespread misunderstanding, prejudice, and discrimination. In such circumstances personal support takes on a very special significance, as our work continually intersects with our personal lives. For example, many of those whose help I wish to acknowledge are now dead, including friends and lovers I knew long before this nightmare began, as well as friends I made in the course of my work. I would therefore like to thank the following individuals, who have been especially kind, reliable, supportive and helpful:

Peter Aggleton, Keith Alcorn, Will Anderson, Dennis Altman; Charles Barber, Allan Barnett, David Barr, Phyllida Brown, André Bongers, Beverley Brown, Michael Budd, Michael Bronski, Greg Bordowitz, Tessa

Boffin, Tina Bird; Angela Carter, Erica Carter, George Cant, Kay Cheese, Roger Cheese, Michael Callen, Douglas Crimp, Emmanuel Cooper; Gary Dowsett; Kristen Engberg; Garance Franke-Rute, Ann Guidici Fettner, Jean Fraser, Mark Finch; Robin Gorna, Peter Gordon, Richard Goldstein, Jonathan Grimshaw, Caroline Guiness, Sunil Gupta, John Greyson, Gregg Gonsalvez, Sue Golding, Jan Zita Grover; Stuart Hall, Simon Hall, Mark Harrington, Adam Hassuk, Martin Hazell, Benny Henryksson, Derek Hodel, Meurig Horton, Robert Huff, Cerri Hutton; Hugo Irwin, Gary Indiana; Derek Jarman, Isaac Julien; Larry Kramer, Marie-Clare Koralek, Tom Kalin, Peter Keogh, Edward King, Robert Kemp; Frankie Lynch; Josef Marie, Neil McKenna, Simon Mansfield, Paul Morris, Stuart Marshall, Donald Moffett, Alfredo Monferre, Huw Morgan, Rita O'Brien, Sue O'Sullivan, Craig Owens, Sean O'Connor; Cindy Patton, Nick Partridge, Laura Pinsky, David Rampton, Vito Russo, Michael Rooney, Chris Reed; Peter Scott, Rebecca Smith, Eve Kosofsky Sedgwick, Jo Spence, Riek Stienstra, Andreas Salmen, Joseph Sonnabend, Wieland Speck, Hazel Slavin, George Sved, Jimmy Somerville; Paula Treichler, Lynne Tillman, Peter Tatchell, Helen Thomas; Mathieu Verboud, Peter van Rooyen; Neil Wallace, Ian Warwick, Judith Williamson, Chris Woods, Tony Whitehead, Stuart Watson, Kaye Wellings, Jeffrey Weeks and Lynne Yaeger.

I would also like to thank Liz Fidlon and the Rivers Oram Press, without whose enthusiasm and practical help this book could not have been produced. In conclusion, I want to thank my partner, John-Paul Philippé, who has seen me through these harrowing years with grace and patience.

Simon Watney
London, October 1993

Preface: My project

One can resist only in the terms of the identity that is under attack.—Hannah Arendt, *Men in Dark Times*

At the time I wrote the first article in this book I was still a full-time teacher, working in the field of cultural studies, with a special commitment to photographic education. I had been teaching for more than a decade, and was the author of a couple of books and many academic articles. I had also written extensively in the British gay press for many years; my professional life had always been closely interwoven with my involvement in lesbian and gay politics. In 1971 I had helped establish a Gay Liberation Front group in Brighton, where I had been an undergraduate. Moving to London a few years later, I became a volunteer with the newly formed Lesbian and Gay Switchboard, a twenty-four hour advice and information service, which many years later organised the first British conference about AIDS. In 1977 I joined the *Gay Left* collective, a small group which met weekly for several years to discuss sexual politics. We also published a regular magazine.[1] *Gay Left* questioned traditional Marxist and socialist assumptions concerning the nature and social significance of sexuality, and was an influential voice in the emergent sexual politics of the period. Our discussions, readings and writings were increasingly influenced by Freud, Gramsci, and Foucault, as opposed to Marx and Lenin.

In my late teens and early twenties, I had been a frequent visitor to both Paris and Amsterdam. Like many other British gay men of my generation, Amsterdam in particular provided me with a strong awareness of just how socially and culturally different Britain was from other northern European countries, not least in relation to the situation of lesbians and gay men. The supposedly 'swinging' sixties certainly had comparatively little to offer us back home again in Britain. It was my involvement in gay politics that led me to the United States for the first time in 1976, and I have subsequently returned at least once annually ever since. To someone who was weaned on *I Love Lucy,* the films of Bette Davis and Katharine Hepburn, and the music of Billie Holiday, Otis Redding and Aretha Franklin, the vehemence of European anti-Americanism from the Left or the Right always struck me as absurdly crude and parochial.

In the late 1970s I also joined the editorial board of *Screen* magazine, and wrote widely as both an art critic and a photographic historian, working with others such as Victor Burgin and the late Jo Spence in order to try to enlarge the scope of photographic education. In other words, I was just the type of younger British gay man who became more Anglo-American than Anglo-European in those years, more through historical accident than design. At a time when British gay politics were largely dominated by the far Left, American gay politics seemed more interesting, and pleasurable, with a deeper sense of democratic principles, firmly rooted in the Civil Rights movements. Like many other European gay men of my generation, I was alerted to the impending AIDS crisis quite early on, as a direct consequence of close personal and professional connections with the United States in the 1970s.

Yet I was not in any way involved in the early stages of setting up the Terrence Higgins Trust, the first non-government AIDS service organisation established early in 1983, although Tony Whitehead, one of its founders, was a friend of many years. Indeed, I didn't really get involved in serious AIDS work until 1984, though I tried to keep up with the latest information. Like many other people, then as now, I think I simply assumed that the necessary work was being done, somewhere, by other people who knew what they were doing. Looking back, I think I was also doing my own homework as it were, prior to any actual direct involvement in an area where I felt no self-confidence. After all, this was seemingly a world of medical information and research, about which I knew very little, or of the institutions regulating British medicine. This would also involve questions of housing, social security, the insurance industry, the workings of the Department of Health, and so on. Did I have any skills that might be of practical benefit? The first time I spoke in public about AIDS was at the *Sexual Difference* conference in Southampton in the summer of 1985. A year later I helped set up the first UK conference on the subject of AIDS and the role of the mass media at the Watershed Arts Centre in Bristol. In 1986 I also spoke at the first 'Social

Aspects of AIDS' conference, also in Bristol. It is with the paper from this significant conference that this book begins. In the spring of 1987 I was invited to speak in New York at a symposium on 'AIDS and the Future', organised by the *Village Voice,* just before the publication of my first book on AIDS, *Policing Desire: Pornography AIDS and the Media.*[2]

This had been based on a course about the representation of AIDS that I had taught at the Polytechnic of Central London in the autumn of 1985, in what proved to be my final year as a full-time lecturer. For it was becoming increasingly obvious to me that I could no longer manage to combine the responsibilities of teaching with the growing demands of the AIDS crisis. It was on the basis of my teaching that I published my first major article on AIDS, which appeared in *Screen* in January 1986.[3] Such early writings were attempts on my part to situate the epidemic in the fullest possible historical and cultural setting in order to understand its scale and complexity, and the responses to it around the world. This included the history of discrimination against homosexuality, and the field of popular culture in which legislation and prejudice find sanction and support. It also included the history of medicine, and the workings of local government, the civil service, and the National Health Service. Above all I was trying to demonstrate the significance of the complex intersections between debates and legislation concerning public health policies, sexuality, gender, pornography, and so on, and the role played by the mass media in all of this. Certainly it would be difficult to exaggerate the impact of media sensationalism, stupidity, and malicious inhumanity, in drawing gay men together in those early years of the epidemic, as the targets of repeated insult and vilification, long before most of us had any direct experience of HIV or AIDS in our everyday lives. We saw the sick pilloried, and the worst abuse reserved for the most severely devastated communities. This situation has been modified subsequently but not, I think, substantially changed. As the *New Yorker* recently pointed out:

> much of the press today has come to see itself only peripherally engaged with democracy. It is as if the press were like the Post Office—a semi-official arm of government delivering a product, and with no more responsibility for what that product contains than the postman has for what's in the envelope.[4]

It is also perhaps difficult today to imagine or recall quite how helpless and beleaguered many people felt in the early years of the epidemic. There was no readily available blueprint concerning how to set up charities, or how to design health education campaigns. We knew that large numbers of our fellow gay men, and many others, had been infected at a time when nobody had the faintest idea that a new, sexually transmitted pathogen was in our midst. Yet the government showed no interest. How do you talk to government departments which steadfastly deny your very existence, or your right to exist as a social constituency? What was most urgently needed? In 1984 I had undertaken a brief two-day training session in AIDS education with Gay Men's Health Crisis (GMHC) in New York. This was before the announcement of the discovery of the human immuno-deficiency virus, HIV. Back in London I became at first informally and then officially involved in the voluntary sector, with the work of the Health Education Group of the Terrence Higgins Trust, which I subsequently chaired for a couple of years. I also chaired the Policy Group at the THT for several years, and was jointly responsible for defining the Trust's policies on such matters as HIV antibody testing, the insurance industry, health education, and so on. Unfortunately it became increasingly difficult to ensure the implementation of such policies, and for several years I have only been involved with the THT as a volunteer member of the Gay Men's Health Education Group.

From very early on in my involvement with the epidemic, I decided that I wanted my principal role to be within the gay community, where I felt at home, rather than in the world of academia or the statutory sector. At the same time I certainly didn't want to be employed by any of the fast emerging AIDS service organisations since I intended, as far as possible, to preserve my independence. I have never claimed to represent anyone but myself; my aim was to work with and for organisations such as the THT, Body Positive, The London Lighthouse, and so on, but not to be of them. Thus in late 1987 and early 1988 I worked for several months with Peter Aggleton and his colleagues at Bristol Polytechnic on the 'Learning about AIDS' project, which was jointly funded by the Local Authority, the Health Education Authority, and a small independent charity, AVERT. Subsequent attempts by the Department of Health to censor this important educational resource, together with the HEA's largely supine response, were to me a tremendous eye-opener.[5]

Early in 1988 I also began writing a regular column on HIV/AIDS issues in the leading national monthly magazine for gay men, *Gay Times*. I was also writing quite frequently in other gay magazines and newspapers such as *Capital Gay* and the *Pink Paper*. My *Gay Times* column remains extremely important to me, for it provides the most direct contact I could possibly make with an extremely wide, national gay readership.

The gay press is an invaluable resource in this epidemic, functioning as a parish-pump for reliable information, and ongoing debate and discussion. I learned early on that it is sometimes necessary to throw petrol onto bonfires (as it were) in order to attract attention to vitally important issues. I wanted to influence the complex circuitry of gossip and conversation which is the basic ground on which perceptions of the significance of HIV in our lives are established and contested. I wanted to make people think about issues, and sometimes I wanted to make people angry about the injustice and plain stupidity surrounding so many aspects of the epidemic.

It was in this context that I gradually came to a more or less coherent sense of what I might indeed be able to do, usefully—a sense of my work as a project in its own right. This has involved three distinct, yet at times closely overlapping, areas of work. First, HIV education amongst gay men. Second, questions of treatment, together with the conduct and directions of biomedical research, and the complex relations between government institutions such as the Medical Research Council and the private sector multi-national pharmaceutical industry. Third, to develop a cultural analysis of the epidemic, which can monitor and even perhaps have an effect upon ongoing television, film and press representations of the epidemic, with all their significant and constantly changing contradictions, omissions, repetitions, associations, policy prescriptions, and so on.

This third area of my HIV/AIDS work relates most obviously to the person I was before the epidemic. As I have argued elsewhere:

> In a modern media culture, you don't know who you are if you don't know how you are represented, by whom, and for what purposes.[6]

I therefore thought it important to try to analyse the complex and frequently contradictory messages about HIV/AIDS generated by the mass media, since television and the press have been the principal source of information to which most people have regular access. I have been highly critical of the Anglo-American media response to the epidemic; I have written a great deal on this vexed topic, and taken part in numerous television and radio programmes on the subject. I have also been more directly involved in the makng of other television programmes, including the BBC2 'Late Show' edition about cultural and political responses to AIDS in New York, and the 'Red Hot & Blue' project, which manages to combine the usually distinct domains of HIV education and fund raising.[7] I do quite a lot of radio work, and have spoken at seemingly innumerable conferences in Britain and around the world. For many years I have also organised and introduced screenings of American AIDS activist videos in London and elsewhere, and have helped set up numerous exhibitions of health education materials, as well as AIDS-related photography and graphics. My aim in such work is always to try to constructively compare international experience, and to encourage the production of better imagery than that produced by the mass media. And for many years I have lectured with slides at universities, colleges, art galleries, community bookshops, and so on, from San Francisco to Sydney, by way of Stockholm, Helsinki, Paris, Berlin, Boston, Edinburgh, Montreal, etc.

This book thus stands as a somewhat fragmentary record of a diverse project, which has involved the continual development of ideas and analysis in relation to many different aspects of the epidemic as it has unfolded over time. Most of this work has been very much against the grain of dominant AIDS commentary. Like many of my friends, I have frequently felt extremely isolated, and at times hopeless. This will doubtless be apparent from the tone of several of the articles collected here, as much as from their subject matter. Indeed, one of the main reasons for producing this book, at this state in the history of the epidemic, is to try to show how gay men have consistently attempted to develop rational and humane policies for HIV/AIDS education and care, in a climate of widely legitimated bigotry and discrimination. As Douglas Crimp has pointed out:

> Seldom has a society so savaged people during their hour of loss. . . .
> The violence we encounter is relentless, the violence of silence
> and omission almost as impossible to endure as the violence of
> unleashed hatred and outright murder. Because this violence also
> desecrates the memories of our dead, we rise in anger to vindicate
> them. For many of us, mourning *became* militancy.[8]

In Britain it is still possible for widely read and respected journalists writing for national newspapers to reject the possibility of heterosexual HIV transmission. To the best of my knowledge only one British journalist in the heterosexual press has ever grasped the unconscious, if not conscious logic of most British media commentary about AIDS, namely, that all gay men and junkies *deserve* to die.[9]

From the beginning, my interest in AIDS was closely connected to American experience.[10] In any case, my personal history made it very likely that I would identify strongly with the plight of those living with

HIV or AIDS in cities such as New York where I had many close friends, and where some 50 per cent of gay men are generally thought to be HIV positive. The experience of seeing American friends go blind for the lack of treatment drugs available on routine prescription in the UK has a somewhat galvanising effect on one's sense of moral and political priorities. In a personal sense, my slight involvement with American community-based AIDS activism has been the most inspiring political experience in my life. Indeed, it is impossible for me to adequately express my admiration and gratitude to American activists who have consistently kept us in Europe fully informed on the latest developments in the conduct and developments of HIV/AIDS-related medical research in the US. The extent and quality of information provided by groups such as the Treatment and Data (T&D) committee of ACT UP New York, and more recently the Treatment Action Group (TAG), has been one of the most remarkable aspects of the community-based US response to HIV/ AIDS. Moreover, by making treatment drugs available to large numbers of people, such work has also helped prolong many lives.

I have now published almost half a million words on AIDS in many different languages and publications. I have written for the gay press around the world, because that has always been my primary constituency. I have also given seemingly countless interviews—a most convenient and strategically useful way of summarising issues. This book contains a sequence of writings, many of which synthesise ideas and arguments that I have previously tried out, as it were, in my talks and my journalism. It is not strictly representative of my shorter writings however, insofar as it brings together a disproportionate amount of work done for inclusion in books. Such writing has of course been important to me, not least because it may possibly reach and influence those who design and conduct research, on the basis of which policies and practices are instituted. There are repetitions which I have retained in order to demonstrate how I have attempted to address different audiences with similar arguments. Insofar as I have aimed to make interventions in both the actual management of the epidemic and its cultural representations far beyond its lived, day-to-day reality, I have been at least as glad and grateful to have been published in *Elle* and *Vanity Fair,* as in august academic anthologies.[11] Indeed, it is especially important, and especially difficult, to intervene precisely at the level of national popular culture.

Since I am very frequently invited to speak in other countries, I have felt it my responsibility to try to translate the significance of the epidemic for gay men in those countries to us in Britain, and also to explain what is going on in Europe to people on other continents. Yet it has proved increasingly difficult for me to try to live the entire US epidemic concurrently with the epidemics at home and elsewhere in Europe. It is simply too emotionally stressful to be constantly travelling to and fro between London and New York, living both the US and the UK epidemics, the latter running at least four years behind the former. I've lost too many friends from New York now, and only one or two survive who knew me as I was in my twenties and early thirties. Moreover, younger friends are also infected, and with little evidence for optimism concerning the possible discovery and availability of effective anti-HIV drugs, it is sometimes necessary to consider just how many people one will be able to fully support to the extent that they might need and reasonably expect it. Such calculations also have a central relation to my work, which proceeds from the simple principle that it is our primary responsibility to try our best to devise ever more effective HIV education, and to campaign ceaselessly for more and better biomedical research.

The history of AIDS is, in many respects, a story of criminal neglect and stupidity, as well as of astonishing courage and resourcefulness on the part of individuals and their affected communities. It is all but intolerable for me to think, sitting here in London in the Spring of 1992, that there are still no official needle-exchange facilities in either France or the United States. It is equally painful and infuriating to think about the scandalous under-funding of gay men's HIV education throughout Europe, at a time when we are so much more affected by the epidemic than any other social constituency in most countries in the developed world. All along my aim has been to contribute what I could to the design and implementation of rational, humane and demonstrably effective social policies in relation to AIDS. On the cultural level however, we shall only truly understand the epidemic if we can relate it meaningfully to such other contemporary issues as abortion, reproductive sexual technology, adoption rights, child abuse, 'the family', 'the nation' and so on.

In conclusion, I would like to emphasise the extremely provisional nature of much of my written work. This is my third book, in what now feels like an informal trilogy, dealing with the epidemic. In the first, written in 1986, I tried to analyse and interpret the immediate consequences of debates about 'pornography' and obscenity legislation, to the need for sexually explicit safer sex materials. It was an extremely angry book, and in Britain it was almost entirely ignored, save by a few HIV/AIDS workers. By contrast, it was extremely successful in the US, and has subsequently gone into a second edition.[12] As far as I'm aware it is still the only basic available introduction to questions concerned with the cultural representations of the epidemic. In 1989 I co-edited a collection of essays with Erica Carter entitled *Taking Liberties: AIDS and Cultural Politics*.[13] This brought together a wide range of British and American HIV/AIDS workers who had spoken the previous year at a conference that Erica and I had organised at the ICA in London. Yet why produce books in an epidemic? Some would argue that it is much more important to be able to provide information in a different updateable way, in the form of magazines and journal articles and loose-leaf manuals. All these are of course admirable, and indeed necessary. Nonetheless, books *do* matter, since rightly or wrongly they tend to be taken more seriously than other forms of publication. So many bad and misleading and inadequate books have been published about HIV/AIDS, often by the politically motivated, and religious bigots, that it is important to record and pay attention to community-based experience, which is all too frequently forgotten, ignored, or otherwise marginalised.

The articles contained in this book were mostly written in some haste, under difficult and frequently distracting circumstances. Some were commissioned for books, some were written up from lectures, and some were written and never published. At the same time I am aware that there were many talks and lectures which I never found time to write up, other articles I'd intended or at least hoped to be able to write, which survive only as sheets of notes in manilla files. The route into audibility in an epidemic is by no means obvious, or consistent.

Many of the articles in this book were written as attempts to draw attention to issues where policies were either lacking or misguided. Other articles were more immediately reactive, responding to issues of the day as they arose. There are changes of mind, and of emphasis. This is inevitable, given the constantly changing nature of the epidemic. For most policies have unintended as well as intended consequences, and a strategy which is correct at one stage of the epidemic, or in relation to one type of epidemic, may well become redundant at another stage, or in a different type of epidemic. For example, criticism of the epidemiological category of 'risk groups' in the mid-1980s reflected widespread anxiety amongst many gay men, and others, that this might increase public misunderstanding about HIV transmission. Such anxieties were a reaction to routine misreporting in the mass media, and I for one shared them. It quickly became apparent however that unless one could speak clearly and confidently about named 'risk groups', those at greatest risk from HIV could simply be made to disappear. Thus a strategy which had been developed to counter homophobia all too soon became widely taken up and accepted as a way of distracting attention away from the very constituencies which were by far the worst affected by HIV in the UK, as in the rest of the developed world. Always one is trying to connect the past to the present, the short-term to the mid-term, the detail to the whole. Always one is trying to develop effective policies in constantly changing circumstances, and to anticipate future needs. This is what contingency means.

Whilst our experience of HIV/AIDS is always local, it is always important to be able to frame it in relation to the wider national picture, which includes the great and powerful institutions that determine its course, from elected governments, to churches, political parties, drug companies, university research departments, banks, cinemas, hospitals, television channels, newspapers, and so on. These in turn sometimes need to be viewed in a still-wider international context if we are to understand how and where we need to apply pressure for improvements and change when necessary. The articles in this book are thus part of a broadly international response to the epidemic on the part of many individuals like myself who have tried to communicate what we regard as urgent messages, at the height of an emergency which governments continue to routinely mismanage all around the world, with tragic and terrible consequences. It is not a book of witness, but of direct participation. I hope it will help people understand something of the difficulties faced by community-based AIDS service organisations in the epidemic, as well as something of our achievements.

I could not finish without saying something about the role of friendship in these new bad times. In Britain, the US, Canada, Australia and Europe, I have had the privilege to work alongside people whom I already knew and loved, together with people I have met through my AIDS work. Many of them are now ill, some already dead. So many people who should have lived long, creative and influential lives in our communities are no longer alive. The richness and diversity of our culture has been relentlessly scythed, not least in relation to our awareness of our own history. Entire groups and networks of friends have died, and with them the wealth of accumulated memory, taste, and hard-won practical wisdom they shared. In such tragic circumstances I am acutely aware of the significance of Neil Bartlett's observation that:

> We suggest that a gay culture is something to be struggled for, not dreamt or bought. At this point, our rewriting of history becomes

a truly dangerous activity. . . . In any formation of my desires, my sense of history has a very particular role to play. We are, in many obvious ways, written out of history. At the same time, we are acutely conscious of the shifting history of our own traditions, our heritage.[14]

We can hardly begin to imagine the personal consequences of the long-term scale of loss which still lies ahead of us, whatever we may have achieved in the field of safer sex education and improved treatments. Already terms such as 'anger', 'numbing' or 'depression' seem pathetically inadequate to the range and depth of human suffering that they are called on to describe.

In this context it is most important to recognise that the most efficient and effective responses to the epidemic have almost invariably arisen from community-based organisations set up in the first place by groups of friends, often stretching across national boundaries, and generations, from those far-off days before the epidemic began. For those of us who 'came out' before the early 1980s, the past often seems like a prelapsarian dream, impossibly distant. This in turn makes many of us feel far older than our natural years. Old photographs take on a new poignancy, not simply of nostalgia, but in relation to our awareness of what our lives might have been like if this catastrophe had not happened, and if it had not been tacitly aided and abetted by governments, newspapers, religions and political parties all around the world.

Yet our friendships are never only matters of private intimacy and affection. Whatever else it may also be, gay identity is always political. For gay identity has given us the ability to speak and act openly in the wider world of public affairs and institutions, which is politics. In our gay friendships we recognise our ethical and political responsibilities to and for one another in the public world to which our shared identity gives us access, however little we may be wanted there. Besides, how could our friendships not be of political relevance, especially in times of crisis, which are all we have ever known? This affirmation of the political and ethical dimensions of gay friendship strikes me as a quality which is quite distinct from the shared, and essentially negative experience of being hated, despised, feared, and systematically marginalised.

I am in touch with my friends morning, noon and night. We are constantly exchanging ideas, bibliographies, policy proposals, medical data, recipes, the latest epidemiology, haircut advice, boyfriend gossip, news of friends in other countries, Morrissey tapes, clinical trial protocols, worries about one another's health, pornography, the minutes from last week's meetings, jokes, and so on. There is a process of mutual care which carries us through, more or less, to the uncertainties of the future. It is a formation I think, of great mutual love and respect, which recognises and attempts to respond to the impossible situation in which we find ourselves. Someone is terribly depressed by the death of an ex-lover and needs comfort. Someone just can't cope with someone else's recent diagnosis. Someone is struggling at midnight to finish writing an article. Someone is just back from New York. Someone is just back from a new club. Someone is just back from a hospital visit. Someone is waiting for his own HIV antibody test result. Someone got mugged. Someone has fallen in love. This is the immediate, day-to-day world of gay friendship in this epidemic, and it is sustained with courage, wit, and great candour. In all of this I can only conclude that there is no way of predicting how individuals may respond to any single aspect of the AIDS crisis, or how such responses may change over time. At the best of times most people are reliably and often endearingly contradictory. AIDS does not change this. So I should like to end this Preface simply by thanking my friends, the people whom I care for, and who have cared for me, and helped me in more ways than I could possibly enumerate, save perhaps in the more distanced objectivity of fiction. I think we may fairly say that we've done what we could.

A note on the texts

Whilst I have done varying amounts of editing on all the texts included in this book, I have not attempted to remove or change arguments or emphases with which I no longer agree. I have edited according to the principle of redundancy, taking out repetitions, and some digressions. The most important editing has lain in the choice of texts. Many of these have been published in slightly different versions, in different publications, as indicated. I also hope in the near future to publish a further selection of my writings about HIV/AIDS, with a particular focus on questions of sexual identity and lesbian and gay politics.

How with this rage shall beauty hold a plea,
Whose action is no stronger than a flower
—Shakespeare, *Sonnet no. 65*

1986 ——————

1. AIDS, 'Moral Panic' Theory, and Homophobia

> *Pleasure is the only thing worth having a theory about.*
> —Oscar Wilde, *The Picture of Dorian Gray*

After five years of reporting on the AIDS epidemic British television and press coverage is locked into an agenda which blocks out any approach to the subject which does not conform to the values and language of a homophobic culture—that is, a culture which does not regard gay men as fully or properly human. There are few differences in this agenda between the 'quality' or 'tabloid' newspapers, or between 'popular' and 'serious' television. The *People* is still able to report that 'AIDS is not just a gay disease, victims now include a rocketing number of heterosexual men, women and children'.[1] But note the use of the word 'just' in this context. Its report goes on to describe how 'One respectable, middle-aged housewife died recently aged 53, a victim of her husband's promiscuity.' He had 'slept with an AIDS-infested prostitute during a business trip to Africa'. The piece concludes that 'experts agree the AIDS plague is heading for crisis proportions in Britain', a verdict reached in the larger context of a private doctor calling for the mass quarantine of all people with AIDS.

Addressing a more upwardly mobile readership, The *Mail on Sunday* recently argued that 'The greatest danger facing Britain is not unemployment. It is not poverty. It is not even nuclear war. The greatest danger today is the growing epidemic of the killer disease AIDS.'[2] Jeff Ferry reports from New York that:

> The US has 25,000 cases. And, according to an official US government estimate, in five years that will have increased to 270,000 cases (that is five times as many people in America lost in the Vietnam war). No wonder the word plague is heard with increasing

frequency in the States. In New York alone there are half a million people carrying the AIDS virus—including 40,000 women. That is 10 per cent of the population. Of these 7700 have active symptoms and know they are dying. The others are simply waiting on a length of fusewire.

The article ends with the question, 'Will a country that is indifferent to the threat listen? I hope so because I have just seen the future if we don't.'

My last example comes from a recent edition of the avowedly Conservative *Daily Telegraph*. At the top of the 'Tuesday Matters' page, a statistical chart shows numbers of cases since 1982 projected through to 1990. Two large arrows sweep upwards from behind a pair of drastically feminised men, the first to the figure of '20,000 projected total of all AIDS cases by 1990', the second to the figure of '800 projected total of heterosexual victims by 1990 at today's rate of increase, which may well be conservative'.[3] The text states that 'Between 10,000 and 14,000 people in Britain could be carrying the AIDS virus'. Discussion stems from the situation of Karen and Jane, who are described as 'two young women desperately trying to face the numbing emotional consequences of their early sexual encounters. Both are infected by the AIDS virus'. Unless Britain does something now 'we will inexorably follow America, where public health officers describe "rivulets of heterosexual infection" snaking out beyond the risk groups'. The article dismisses notions of risk from casual contact with people with AIDS, and also argues against calls for mass quarantine on the grounds that sheer numbers make it unrealistic, smacking 'more of the concentration camp than of rational public health'. Professor Michael Adler is quoted, calling for a publicity campaign on radio and television, pointing out that 'Everyone should know that the AIDS virus cannot cross a condom'. Of the syndrome itself, the report states that 'Like an individual disease time-bomb, the virus exerts a remote-control effect. Infections and cancers, reflecting a breakdown in the immune system, may take from weeks to years to erupt'. We also learn from an American psychologist that 'The British public is in a state of "AIDS phobia" or generalised fear, based on lack of knowledge of the disease'. Addresses and telephone numbers are provided for the College of Health AIDS Healthline, the Haemophilia Society, and the Health Education Council, but not, significantly, for The Terrence Higgins Trust, which is the vector of information for gay men who are clearly the constituency most directly vulnerable to infection, and most in need of information.

All three of these reports create profound problems for our understanding of AIDS, and issues of social policy surrounding it. Thus the *People* divides up people with AIDS into two categories in a discourse of victims, the majority of whom are 'guilty' and a minority 'innocent'. Its report also colludes with an underlying racism and misogyny which contrasts the 'respectable' housewife with AIDS to the 'infested' African prostitute. The crucial term here is 'promiscuity', which effectively cordons off married women from independent non-monogamous female sexuality, drawing on a deep reservoir of retributive judgement which is a major characteristic of Western AIDS commentary. The *Mail on Sunday* carries this approach over into its use of statistics, by wilfully confusing the numbers of people infected by HIV with those who have gone on to develop AIDS. This is a fundamental point. If we do not distinguish between those who have contracted HIV (a disease of the blood, transmitted via direct blood-to-blood or blood-to-sexual contact) from the various opportunistic infections which result from damage to the body's immune system, we will have a highly misleading picture both of AIDS and of the epidemic. Such a telescoping of HIV infection with AIDS, exemplified by lazy talk of there being an 'AIDS virus', as it is described in both the *Mail on Sunday* and the *Daily Telegraph,* actively obscures understanding of the central issues involved. The 70 per cent, or so, of HIV-infected individuals who present no symptoms at all are hardly likely to be reassured by the information that they are 'simply waiting on the end of a fusewire', whilst the 10 to 30 per cent who have developed opportunistic infections are simply shamed into being regarded as responsible for their own illnesses, or else regarded as tragically 'innocent' victims, at least if they are white, middle-class and heterosexual.

AIDS and discourses about sexuality

It is a commonplace of medical history that every major epidemic initially appears in a specific localised population. When the *People* reports that AIDS is not 'just a gay disease', and the *Daily Telegraph* conjures up the spectacle of 'rivulets of heterosexual infection snaking out beyond the risk groups', it should be apparent that something very strange and significant is going on. AIDS is being used to articulate modern theories of sexuality, or what Freud called object-choice, as if the virus itself is intrinsically attracted to particular sexual constituencies and not others. We need to establish once and for all that like any other virus, HIV is not a property or respecter of persons or of groups of persons. It is a viral disease, against which relatively simple precautions are highly effective. That public information campaigns are unable to address this fact needs explanation together with the tendency to either stigmatise or ignore the situation of the vast majority of people with AIDS. Recent British figures describe some 533 gay men with AIDS, and seventeen (presumably heterosexual) women.[4] The enormity of the displacement of attention to the situation of non-gay people with AIDS speaks volumes in itself. As Richard Goldstein has pointed out:

> For gay men sex, that most powerful implement of attachment, and arousal, is also an agent of communion, replacing an often hostile family and even shaping politics. It represents an ecstatic break with years of glances and guises, the furtive past we left behind. Straight people have no comparable experience, though it may seem so in memory. They are never called upon to deny desire, only to defer its consummation.[5]

He concludes that 'for heterosexuals to act as if AIDS were a threat to everyone demeans the anxiety of gay men who really are at risk, and for gay men to act as if we're all going to die demeans the anguish of those who are actually ill'. A media communications industry which can only acknowledge the existence of gay men as a target for contempt and thinly veiled hatred is unlikely to be able to address itself to the issues of sexual diversity which the AIDS epidemic requires us to face as the *sine qua non* of any effective preventative strategies which alone may prevent the spread of HIV infection, or adequate support measures for the two million gay men in the UK who live from day to day through these terrible times with varying degrees of courage and fear, anger and grief.

The limits of panic

Many lesbian and gay commentators on such attitudes have favoured the influential British Sociological theory of 'moral panics' for the purposes of explanation and analysis. Drawing on the 'new' criminology developed in the late 1960s, Stanley Cohen described how societies:

> appear to be subject, every now and then, to periods of moral panic. A condition, episode or person emerges to become defined as a threat to societal values and interests; its nature is presented in a stylised and stereotypical fashion by the mass media; the moral barricades are manned by editors, bishops, politicians and other right-thinking people; . . . Sometimes the panic passes over and is forgotten, except in folk-lore and collective memory; at other times it

has more serious and long-lasting repercussions and might produce such changes as those in legal and social policy or even in the way the society perceives itself.[6]

Subsequent writers, of whom Stuart Hall is perhaps the most notable, have developed this general picture to embrace the process by which popular consent is won for measures which require a 'more than usual' exercise of regulation. This is especially the case in relation to domains which are traditionally understood in liberal philosophy to be private, and especially the home. Hall's work has encouraged a 'stages' view of moral panics, leading to increasingly punitive state control, although it is important to stress that moral panics do not necessarily stem from the state itself, or any of its immediate avatars. On the contrary, what is at stake is the relationship between governments and other uneven and conflicting institutions addressing a supposedly unified 'general public' through the mass media. This is particularly important to bear in mind for anyone approaching the question of the representation of homosexuality in this culture, since the subject is already historically preconstituted as 'scandal'. Indeed, one of the major reasons why lesbian and gay critics were attracted to 'moral panic' theory in the first place was because it offered a corrective alternative to the (then) dominant school of orthodox sociological 'deviance' theory which holds, as Jeffrey Weeks has pointed out, that sexual unorthodoxy 'is somehow a quality inherent in . . . individuals, to which the social then has to respond'.[8] For 'deviance' theorists homosexuality is itself a problem, whereas 'moral panic' theory allows us to examine some of the conditions and means whereby homosexuality is problematised.

In his recent book *Sexuality,* Weeks describes how 'one of the most striking features of the AIDS crisis is that, unlike most illnesses, its chief victims were blamed for causing the disease, whether because of their social attitudes or sexual practices'. He goes on to explain how, 'In the normal course of a moral panic there is a characteristic stereotyping of the main actors as peculiar types of monsters, leading to an escalating level of fear and perceived threat, the taking up of panic stations and absolutist positions, and a search for symbolic, and usually imaginary solutions to the dramatised problem'.[9] Gayle Rubin has also described moral panics as:

> the 'political moment' of sex, in which diffuse attitudes are channelled into political action and from there into social change. The white slavery hysteria of the 1950s, and the child pornography panic of the late 1970s were typical moral panics. Because sexuality

in Western societies is so mystified, the wars over it are often fought at oblique angles, aimed at phony targets, conducted with misplaced passions, and are highly, intensely symbolic. Sexual activities often function as signifiers for personal and social apprehensions to which they have no intrinsic connection. During a moral panic, such fears attach to some unfortunate sexual activity or population. The media become ablaze with indignation, the public behaves like a rabid mob, the police are activated, and the state enacts new laws and regulations. When the furore has passed, some innocent erotic group has been decimated, and the state has extended its power into new areas of erotic behaviour. Moral panics rarely alleviate any real problem, because they are aimed at chimeras and signifiers. They draw on the pre-existing discursive structure which invents victims in order to justify treating 'vices' as crimes.[10]

However, the very longevity and continuity of AIDS commentary already presents a problem for 'moral panic' theory, in so far as this is evidently a panic which refuses to go away—a *permanent panic,* as it were—rather than a 'political moment'. Whilst we may find a certain initial descriptive likeness to familiar events in their description as moral panics, this does not help us to understand the constant nature of ideological supervision and non-state regulation of sexuality throughout the modern period, especially in matters concerning representation. To begin with, the idea of a moral panic may be employed to characterise *all* conflicts in the public domain where stigmatisation takes place. It cannot however discriminate between different orders or different degrees of moral panic. Nor can it explain why certain types of event should be especially privileged in this way. Above all, it obscures the endless 'overhead' narrative of such phenomena as one panic gives way to another, and different panics overlap and reinforce one another. We need to understand how some moral panics may condense a host of anxieties, focusing them on a single-target object, whilst others work in tandem to produce a unified effect which is only partially present and articulated in any one of its component elements. Thus, for example, AIDS commentary tends to draw on a wide range of concerns about childhood sexuality, homosexuality, prostitution, pornography, drug use, and so on, which heavily overdetermine all discussion of the virus. At the same time, the continual reporting of sexual assaults, murders, debates on sex education in schools, all orchestrate the larger question of sexuality itself, as if it were something intrinsically dangerous.

Moral panic theory directs our attention to sites of visible intervention concerning, for example, pornography, immigration policy or abortion, which have strong public profiles. In this respect we might think of a moral panic around AIDS in terms of stories concerning the forcible detention of people with AIDS, or the presence of gay men (by now practically synonymous with the rhetorical figure, 'AIDS carrier') on the Royal Yacht Britannia, and so on and so forth. But this encouragement to think of AIDS commentary primarily if not exclusively in terms of excess does not help us make sense of government inaction, or the hysterical modesty of politicians from Mrs Thatcher downwards who have been against the provision of explicit safer sex advice on television or in newspaper 'public information' campaigns. Their actions are far more damaging and dangerous in the long run than all the ravings of Fleet Street, since they effectively condemn thousands of people to ignorance about the very strategies by which lives may be saved. Just as the Centers for Disease Control in the United States have consistently refused to fund sexually explicit educational materials, so until recently the British government has effectively sentenced countless gay to men to death. As Ann Guidici Fettner concludes, 'AIDS education should have been started the moment it was realised that the disease is sexually transmitted'.[11] In this situation it is difficult but vitally important to recognise, that from the perspective of the state, gay men are regarded as a disposable population.

Classical moral panic theory interprets representations of specific 'scandals' as events which appear and then disappear, having run their ideological course. Such a view makes it difficult to theorise representation as a site of permanent ideological struggle and contestation between rival pictures of the world. We do not watch the unfolding of discontinuous and discrete 'moral panics', but rather the mobility of ideological confrontations across the entire field of industrialised communications. This is most markedly the case in relation to those images which handle and evaluate the meanings of the human body, where rival and incompatible institutions and values are involved in a ceaseless and remorseless struggle to discover and disclose its supposedly universal 'human' truth. Hence the intensity of struggle to define the meanings of AIDS, with the virus being used by all and sundry as a kind of glove puppet from the mouth of which different interest groups speak their values. AIDS, however, has no single 'truth' of its own, but becomes a powerful condenser for a great range of social, sexual and psychic anxieties. This is why it is better to think in terms of AIDS commentary, rather than assuming the existence of a coherent uni-vocal 'moral panic' on the subject. We are here considering the circulation of symbols, of the raw materials from which human subjectivity is constructed. AIDS has been mobilised to embody a variety of perceived threats to individual and social stability, organised around the spectacle of illicit sex and physical corruption. It has been used to stabilise the figure of the heterosexual family unit which remains the central image in our society with which individuals are endlessly invited to identify their collective interests and their very core of being.

The instrumental family

As Foucault and others have argued, we need to recognise that the image of the threatened and vulnerable family is a central motif in a society like ours for which the family is not simply a given object, but is rather an instrument of social policy.[12] What AIDS commentary reveals is the ongoing crisis surrounding the representation of the family in a culture in which only a minority of citizens actually occupy its conventional space at any given moment. Familial ideology is thus obliged to fight a continual rearguard action in order to disavow the social and sexual diversity of a culture which can never be adequately pictured in the traditional guise of the family. Those who threaten to expose the ideological operations of familialism will inevitably be castigated as 'enemies' of the family, which is pictured as under constant threat. Thus Sir Rhodes Boyson, the Minister for Local Government, recently grouped together feminists, single-parent families, and 'the fashion of the flaunting and propagation of homosexuality and lesbianism as anti-family and anti-life'.[13] In such a view, lesbians and gay men cannot be regarded as constituencies within a pluralist society. Rather, they are to be identified as prime agents of anti-social, and even extra-human danger. It is clear that the categories which hold together the public profile of familialism—notions of 'decency', 'respectability', 'manliness' 'innocence', and so on—are primarily defensive, in so far as they work to protect individuals from the partially acknowledged fact of diversity. Hence the repetitive nature of moral panics, their fundamentally serial nature, and the wide range of tones and postures which they can assume 'on behalf' of the national family unit. The organisation of desire in all its forms into the narrow channels of modern sexual identities ensures that the presence of 'enemies' is felt everywhere, within the self, and from without. This is why there is such a dramatic disparity between the lived experience of people with AIDS, and the model of contagion which they are made to embody. We are not living through a distinct, coherent 'moral panic' concerning AIDS, a panic with a linear narrative and the prospect of closure. On the contrary, we are witnessing the ideological manoeu-vres which unconsciously 'make sense' of this accidental triangulation of disease, sexuality, and homophobia. Hence the obsession of AIDS commentary with the distinction between supposedly 'innocent' and 'guilty' victims, and the total inability to distinguish between infectious and contagious illness. AIDS commentary rarely troubles to separate the question of HIV infection from individual opportunistic infection, pre-ferring to talk of 'AIDS carriers' and an 'AIDS virus'. What we should recognise is that such telescoping of medical terms indicates a collapsing together of ideological concerns, which transform AIDS into a *malade imaginaire*—the viral personification of unorthodox deregulative desire, dressed up in the ghoulish likeness of degeneracy.

Hence, in the popular imagination of AIDS, we come close to the core of modern familial identities and social policy for which the perverse maps out the boundaries of the legitimate social order. This is why we need to be able to analyse the relations of contingency, analogy and sub-stitution between phenomena which moral panic theory obliges us to think of as discrete and unconnected. Sociology invites us to think of individual 'moral panics' around drugs, video films, football hooligan-ism, and so on, because it regards the family as 'a point of departure' rather than a product of complex negotiation between different institu-tional and discursive formations. Moral panics do not 'reflect' something we should think of as 'the social': on the contrary, they constitute the ground on which 'the social' emerges, in the words of Jacques Donzelot, as 'a concrete space of intelligibility of the family' in which 'it is the social that suddenly looms as a strange abstraction'.[14]

It is thus particularly unhelpful to think of AIDS commentary as a moral panic which somehow makes gay men into monsters, since that is an intrinsic effect of the medicalisation of morality which accompanied the emergence of the modern categories of sexuality in the course of the last 200 years. What AIDS commentary does is to elide the virus and its presenting symptoms with the dominant cultural meanings of those constituencies in which it has emerged—black Africans, injecting drug users, prostitutes and, of course, gay men. In this manner 'the social' is ever more narrowly confined within familial definitions and values, with the family being scrutinised ever more closely for physical symp-toms of moral dissent. The sheer range and variety of AIDS commentary should alert us to the danger of any attempt to explain it in terms of any single, primary and all determining cause. This however is precisely the tendency of the many lesbian and gay commentators who rely upon the notion of 'homophobia' as if this were an adequate, sufficient, and self-evident explanatory category. The term itself was first defined by George Weinberg in the immediate wake of Gay Liberationist politics in the early 1970s as a 'disease' and 'an attitude held by many nonhomosexuals and perhaps by the majority of homosexuals in countries where there is discrimination against homosexuality'.[15] From its inception, it uncomfortably straddled both the situation of all social and psychic aspects of attitudes towards homosexuality, as well as both homosexual and heterosexual identities. In effect the notion simply reversed the sociological and psychiatric tendencies to pathologise all forms of homosexual identity and desire as symptoms of either 'deviance' or 'perversion'.

Conclusion

Elsewhere, I have attempted to separate out some of the central strands within the hysterical dimensions of homosexual stigmatisation.[16] In this context though, I would like to return to the question of *systematic misinformation* concerning medical aspects of AIDS with which I began this chapter. Journalists, like doctors, tend to come from professional backgrounds which massively privilege the family as the central term of social intelligibility. That doctors should be in the vanguard of calls for the mass quarantine of people with AIDS is not in the least surprising, given the 'protective' identity which they are taught in medical school and in medical practice. Medicine remains perhaps the most difficult profession in which to 'come out' in the UK, and young doctors have been ostracised and held back in their careers for no other reason. Indeed, the National Health Service itself addresses a 'national' population which signally and conspicuously fails to recognise the existence of lesbians and gay men as a fundamental constituency within the nation, let alone our specific medical needs. Effectively, 'national' medicine thereby becomes 'heterosexual' medicine, as is evident from the dramatic under-funding of hospitals and clinics as the AIDS epidemic proceeds to escalate. This is equally apparent from the inability of a medically constituted, public information campaign to directly address the actual diversity of sexual practice of the 'public' which they are supposedly addressing. Whilst the avoidance of a forbidden object is certainly a sign of phobia, we should remember that phobic avoidance is focused not on what it is unconsciously afraid of, but on displaced symbols of the terrifying object. Some degrees of phobic response to homosexuality would seem to be the inevitable result of the psychic violence involved in the process which attempts to homogenise all children into the 'correct' identities of adult heterosexuality. But the notion of homophobia precisely avoids the whole question of how desire operates to motivate particular sexual behaviours. At the same time it serves to further regulate and reinforce the workings of modern sexual categories by seemingly forcing together all the varieties of homosexual desire and identity into a monolithic totality, faced by an equally monolithic heterosexuality. Whatever else might be said to characterise homophobia, the fact remains that its signs are understood to be expulsive and aggressive, rather than aversive and defensive.

Thus any approach to AIDS commentary rooted in a theory of homophobia is unlikely to be able to come to grips with subtle questions of metaphor, displacement, repetition, substitutions or absences, privileging instead the most violent physical and verbal abuse of people with AIDS, which in any case is relatively transparent in terms of ordinary liberal 'civil rights' analysis. The question of why HIV continues to be treated as if it were contagious and transmissible by casual contact, proves stubbornly resistant to the explanatory schemes provided either by 'moral panic' theory, or notions of a unified homophobia. Both in effect offer little more than 'false-consciousness' accounts of how different desiring constituencies perceive and evaluate one another, together with a latent functionalism which glimpses either a unified purposive state or a coherent collectivity of 'heterosexuality' at work behind social and psychic attitudes to AIDS.

Nonetheless, it is probably more helpful than not at this time to retain the notion of homophobia at least as a collective term, referring to the entire range of interacting institutions, discourses and psychic processes which align AIDS with homosexuality as if by essence. This argument is supported by the probability that much hostility towards homosexuality is indeed phobic in origin, insofar as it stems from the threatening return to consciousness of desires and fantasies concerning the human body which can never be completely contained and successfully repressed within the narrow compass of heterosexual identities which defensively equate sexuality with sexual reproduction. The real 'threat' comes not from lesbians or gay men, but from the destabilisation of conscious heterosexual identities from within themselves.

In this respect we can recognise that the most frequently encountered characteristic of AIDS commentary is projection, defined by Leo Bersani as 'a frantic defence against the return of dangerous images and sensations to the surface of consciousness; therefore, the individual urgently needs to maintain that certain representations or affects belong to the world and not to the self.[17] In this manner we can begin to account for the ways in which AIDS is invariably made to carry a supplement of fantasy which both precedes and exceeds any actual medical issues. In the same way we can chart the compulsive displacements which add up to the public meanings of AIDS, the scattering of themes and motifs across the entire field of public representation. To fail to notice the systematic connections between contemporary campaigns around sex education, procreation, children's sexuality and AIDS, by classifying them as separate and autonomous 'moral panics' is as dangerous today as any temptation to regard them all as no more than epiphenomena related to a unified and totally recalcitrant homophobia.

1987 ———————

2. Visual AIDS: Advertising ignorance

On the last Sunday of 1986, the *Observer* informed its readers with a bracing mixture of ignorance and insensitivity that '1987 will be the Second Year of AIDS for Britain'. It had evidently not occurred to journalist Nicholas Wapshott that ever since HIV was identified in 1983, *every* year has been a 'Year of AIDS'—as he so crassly put it—for the gay population. That is, for the one to two million gay men who have been living through these terrible times with varying degrees of anxiety and fear, courage and dignity.

Wapshott may observe that 'AIDS is not a gay plague, nor ever was,' but his words ring hollow in the context of his metaphor of unexploded bombs for those infected by the virus, and sickeningly hypocritical cant about the need for 'sympathy and understanding for those trapped by their own proclivities.' Such euphemistically stilted language makes it painfully clear that AIDS is still being handled right across the media with all the most up-to-date medical, psychiatric and sociological resources of the late nineteenth century.

According to Wapshott's standardised version of recent events, '[Health Minister] Norman Fowler emerges as an unlikely hero in this miserable story.' It is certainly a miserable tale, but if Fowler has been heroic it is only in forcing the present government to recognise something of the full enormity of an epidemic which the rest of Europe faced up to some years ago. The official campaign that Fowler has launched suggests that government understanding of AIDS remains lamentably defective. 1986 was undoubtedly the first 'Year of AIDS' as far as British politicians of all persuasions were concerned. What this means in simple terms is that thousands will now inevitably die as the direct result of Tory prudery, moralism and an exaggerated faith in the medical profession's ability to find a cure or vaccine for HIV infection, aided and abetted by the resounding silence of the entire British party political system.

In Britain the number of newly reported AIDS cases doubled between October and November 1986, bringing the total to 599, of whom 296 are now dead. This total includes 17 women, 2 babies, 11 patients infected by blood transfusions, and 22 haemophiliacs. The Center for Disease Control reported a total of 27,773 cases in the United States as of November, of whom 15,597 are dead. This is the grim backdrop against which the British government has launched a 'forceful' propaganda campaign 'to alert the public to the risk of AIDS'.

What remains so particularly shocking about the British response to AIDS is the way in which the social group most devastated has had its legitimate needs almost entirely ignored.

Official neglect

Thus the Terrence Higgins Trust, until recently the only voluntary organisation providing information and counselling services to gay men and the rest of the population, has had to struggle through each year with a mere £100,000 per annum of public assistance. The Trust needs a minimum of £250,000 per annum for its educational work and support services, and the shortfall has had to be met by intensive fund raising among gay men themselves. And all along the line its activities have been hampered by doctors and politicians holding the purse strings, who have refused to support the production and distribution of explicit safer sex materials for gay men.

Safer sex videos, like the New York Gay Men's Health Crisis's *Chance of a Lifetime,* are banned over here by our ludicrous censorship laws. And until Her Majesty's Customs dropped their charges against London's *Gay's the Word* bookshop in the summer of 1985, none of the leading American or European gay newspapers (containing the most up-to-date information and debate about AIDS) were available here—they could not be safely imported. Hence the all but incredible story of how the government's own Chief Medical Officer had to have copies of the *Advocate* and *New York Native* smuggled into England in diplomatic bags to avoid the possibility of their seizure as the AIDS campaign was first being drawn up!

As long ago as August 1983, the British *Medical News* recommended gay men start using condoms as a matter of routine sexual practice and, more recently the respected American medical correspondent Ann

Guidici Fettner has pointed out that 'AIDS education should have been started the moment it was realised that the disease is sexually transmitted.' Which is precisely what the Terrence Higgins Trust has been saying all along. But as long as AIDS was perceived as a 'gay plague' the entire problem was calculated only in terms of the possible 'leakage' from affected groups to the 'general public'—from which gay men are evidently excluded.

The belated recognition that it is not 'just' prostitutes, drug-users and 'queers' who are at risk, but even people in the Tory counties, explains much of the energy behind the current campaign. Thus an advertisement appeared in many magazines at Christmas, spelling out the words 'AIDS' in seasonal wrapping paper, with the accompanying question: 'How many people will get it for Christmas?' Another conveys the message 'Your next sexual partner could be that very special person', framed inside a heart-like Valentine card, beneath which we read: 'The one that gives you AIDS.' The official line is clearly *anti-sex,* drawing on an assumed rhetoric concerning 'promiscuity' as the supposed 'cause' of AIDS, in order to terrorise people into monogamy. But monogamy is no more intrinsically safe than any other kind of sex, unless precautions are taken. Mortal fears are being whipped up, as if sexuality were entirely within the control of rational consciousness, and as if sexual desire were a tap with just two simple positions—on and off.

Education or homophobia?

Still more problematic is the ubiquitous series of posters which have recently appeared all over Britain, their messages seemingly carved into granite-like tombstones. Thus we read the solemn injunction 'AIDS: DON'T DIE OF IGNORANCE', with the secondary advice that 'Anyone can get it, gay or straight, male or female. Already 30,000 people are infected. At the moment the infection is *mainly confined to relatively small groups of people* in this country. But it is spreading.'

Something extraordinary is going on here. On the one hand the government appears to acknowledge the actual diversity of sexual identities in the modern world—yet this is evidently not the case since we are intended to dismiss the majority of people with AIDS as members of 'relatively small groups of people.' At the same time the poster peddles a mischievous implication of responsibility onto people with AIDS as if they'd somehow set out to contract it by ignoring advice and information which has never been widely available. It also cynically looks entirely over the heads of everyone most immediately affected by the epidemic. Apart from lesbians and gay men, what other social group with almost 600 dead and dying could be so casually erased from all public consideration?

'AIDS IS NOT PREJUDICED: IT CAN KILL ANYONE' screams another poster, this time with the subheading: 'It's true more men than women have AIDS. But this does not mean it is a homosexual disease. It isn't.' Here the implication is either that there are viruses which consciously select their victims, motivated by sexual desire, or that some diseases are the intrinsic properties of gay men. There is of course no such thing as a virus which only affects men *or* women, but medical facts are irrelevant here, since what the poster is actually saying is that it doesn't matter if you *are* prejudiced, as long as you don't make the mistake of thinking that AIDS is 'only' killing off the queers!

Yet another poster proclaims that 'THE LONGER YOU BELIEVE AIDS ONLY INFECTS OTHERS, THE FASTER IT'LL SPREAD'. While the 'you' addressed here is at least open to all readers to identify with, there is still no information and advice—beyond the totally incorrect implication that AIDS is itself infectious. The inability to distinguish between AIDS and HIV is typical of a campaign which is evidently not educational in any useful sense, but which aims only to frighten and alarm as many people as possible.

The worst poster simply asks: 'AIDS: HOW MUCH BIGGER DOES IT HAVE TO GET BEFORE YOU TAKE NOTICE?' It is, however, far from clear what we are expected to take notice of, beyond the poster itself, which again suggests that the campaign is largely diversionary, giving the impression that the government is doing something about AIDS and that the epidemic is in hand. The question which we should be asking some five years into the epidemic is, how big did it have to get before *they* took any notice? The folly of the entire campaign is its failure to talk to people in any but the most abstract and over-generalised terms. We thus still face the nightmarish situation of an epidemic running out of control, under a government and opposition totally unable to acknowledge or assess the actual social and sexual diversity of the society they purport to represent!

The same funereal graphics are used on the front of the leaflet distributed recently to every household. Like the posters, it was drawn up without consultation with the Terrence Higgins Trust or any other organisation with direct experience of AIDS educational work. To add insult to injury, the Trust's telephone number was placed on the leaflet without permission, and in belated recognition of the fact that it was swamped with calls the government has agreed to install a number of extra telephone lines. While the leaflet offers a lot of straightforward and helpful information, it nonetheless proceeds from the statement that AIDS is 'not just a homosexual disease'. This is a shocking statement, and if anyone still doubts that gay men are officially regarded *in our entirety* as a disposable community, they need look no further.

Taking AIDS seriously

In 1983, when there were fewer than 3000 recorded cases of AIDS in the United States, Richard Goldstein wrote that 'for heterosexuals to act as if AIDS were a threat to everyone demeans the anxiety of gay men who really are at risk, and for gay men to act as if we're all going to die demeans the anguish of those who are actually ill.' His message is as timely as ever. Millions of pounds have been squandered in a facesaving exercise which directs its crude, loud-hailing machinery at nobody in particular, least of all towards those who are in most need of a positive health education programme. How could this be otherwise from a government which is profoundly hostile to sex education as such, and which in all other circumstances regards gay men only as the target for punitive legislation, prosecution, and surveillance?

The AIDS initiative is no more than an extension of the familiar public agenda which has proved so stubbornly resistant to the actual complexity of issues raised by the epidemic. It is a discourse whose words are sticky with blood-lust, hatred and thinly-veiled contempt for the thousands of sick and dying, offering a heady brew of racism, misogyny and homophobia, which speaks volumes about the real moral condition of contemporary Britain. That socialists and feminists alike have so totally failed to grasp the implications of AIDS for the future politics of Britain is particularly regrettable. We are living through a catastrophe that has systematically been denied the status of a natural disaster, let alone a tragedy.

This terrible epidemic should teach us once and for all that if our species has any worth or beauty it lies in its diversity, and in our capacity to embrace and celebrate all our variously consenting states of desire. And if in these dreadful times we should wish somewhat to alleviate the pain of our losses—of freedoms and friends—then we might possibly think of AIDS as a monstrously ironic means to that end.

3. The Subject of AIDS

The subject of AIDS is produced and reproduced in a punitive discourse of garrulous morbidity. It has been massively amplified by the powerful institutionalised voices of racism, familialism, nationalism, and a range of deeply-seated anxieties concerning sexual behaviour in general, and homosexual behaviour in particular. In this context, the advent of modern cultural 'theory', with its emphasis on signification, sexuality, 'difference', the unconscious, power, voyeurism, narrative, and so on, seems as fortuitous in its own way as those developments in the fields of virology and immunology which permitted the isolation and identification of HIV in 1983. Indeed, it could be said that contemporary debates in cultural studies, women's studies, psychoanalytic criticism, textual analysis, the theory of ideology, and so on, have been preparing us for a better understanding of what is now being done—and what is not being done in the name of AIDS. Yet so far, little by way of deconstructionist analysis has entered the public arena of AIDS commentary. Nor has liberalism yet addressed itself to the question of AIDS with anything like the concern which it has shown for other examples of gross social injustice.

In *The Birth of the Clinic,* Michel Foucault noted that 'the morbid authorises a subtle perception of the way in which life finds in death its most differentiated figure'.[1] Within this context it is important to recognise that academics and liberal intellectuals possess no more natural immunity to the effects of 'the morbid' than they have to HIV infection. I will therefore consider here some of the ways in which the subject of AIDS sheds light on the political role of modern cultural theory. I will also examine the cultural agenda of AIDS insofar as it fixes and reinforces a rigid network of heavily medicalised perceptions concerning the gravest matters of potential individual and collective risk. Finally, I will seek to identify the 'other' subject of AIDS, central yet systematically marginalised, the discursively absented Person with Acquired Immune Deficiency Syndrome (PWA).

It is towards the corrective transformation of the dominant cultural agenda concerning AIDS that the analysis here is directed. For this agenda informs *all* our perceptions of AIDS, no matter how they may be mediated by factors such as class, race, gender and sexuality. No single issue in the modern world is currently more politically loaded than AIDS, and in this arena social policy decisions which will affect and determine all our lives are being proposed, summarily debated, and enacted daily. Gayle Rubin has nicely observed that 'for over a century, no tactic for stirring up erotic hysteria has been as reliable as the appeal to protect children.'[2] How much more reliable the construction of AIDS as a supposed threat to the entire family structure will be depends on our capacity to intervene and interrupt an agenda which is now being actively challenged and resisted by those whom it already functions most efficiently to de-legitimate—namely, people with AIDS.

The cultural agenda of AIDS

The cultural agenda of AIDS relies upon a limited set of heavily overdetermined words and images, any one of which can stand in isolation for the logic of the total structure. It imposes a domino theory of AIDS which proceeds from the initial notion of 'the AIDS virus'—a phenomenon which it is crucial to recognise as an ideological condensation rather than a medical construction. In making sense of this cultural agenda, we must also distinguish between an infectious disease of the blood (HIV infection), which may be transmitted sexually as well as via direct blood-to-blood contact with an infected person, and the many consequences that this may have. First, HIV may simply lie dormant. Second, it may attack and damage the central nervous system, leading to progressive neurological damage and behavioural change. Third, it may weaken the body's immunological defences, rendering the individual vulnerable to a wide range of AIDS-Related Conditions (ARCs), which are often fatal. Fourth, HIV may so impair the immune system that the body becomes vulnerable to those specific infections and malignancies that result in the diagnosis of AIDS.

The simple distinction between a virus and a syndrome is entirely obscured as soon as the phrase 'the AIDS virus' is used. At the same time, however, this phrase establishes a basis from which the equally inaccurate notion of 'the AIDS carrier' can be advanced. Thereafter, a discourse comes into being which draws on a rich historical legacy which summons up the all too familiar imagery of contagion and plague. By this time, however, a second condensation has occurred. This collapses together the crucial distinction between infectious and contagious diseases. AIDS is thus presented as if it were indeed a miasmatic condition, with the implication that it can be 'caught' by casual contact.

It is therefore not surprising that 17 per cent of Britons recently polled believe that AIDS can be caught from the seat of a lavatory. But what we should also recognise is that the terms in which such polls are conducted tend only to reinforce prevailing misconceptions. Thus it was recently reported in *Newsday* that 40 per cent of those asked thought that AIDS can be caught by giving blood.[3] What is at stake here is not simply a rational distinction between 'ignorance' and 'knowledge', but the ways in which a specific cultural agenda imposes its values via the very questions it asks. Responses in the *Newsday* poll were triggered by a single question: 'To the best of your 'knowledge, can a person catch AIDS by giving blood or not?' Readers were then reliably informed that 'the correct answer is no'. The only 'correct' answer to this question would in fact require a challenge to inbuilt implication that AIDS can be caught at all. AIDS is a syndrome of at least thirty distinct life-threatening conditions. Of itself it is neither contagious nor infectious. Thus AIDS commentary effects a remarkable and sinister reversal. Instead of being regarded as threatened, people with AIDS become threatening.

From the notions of 'the AIDS virus' and 'the AIDS carrier' it is a relatively easy syntagmatic slippage to talk of an 'AIDS test'. However, the test referred to here only reveals the presence, or absence, of antibodies produced in response to HIV. Given that these may not be produced until many months after infection, results from an HIV-antibody test— as it should always be described—are highly ambiguous. For even when an individual tests positive and is found to have seroconverted, this does not reveal whether or not she or he will go on to develop neurological damage, ARC or AIDS. Nor does it offer a prognosis concerning which symptoms might appear first. Given that we now know so much about the transmission of HIV, and the ways to prevent it from spreading, it remains to be explained why the cultural agenda of AIDS remains so exhaustively—and exhaustingly—taken up with the issue of testing. By far the most important news in recent months has concerned the seroconversion rate among gay men, which has now fallen to below 1 per cent of those taking the HIV antibody test in San Francisco and New

York.[4] This signals one of the most astonishing achievements in modern US history. Yet, wherever one looks in the American press—in *The New York Times* or the *Village Voice*, in the *New York Post* or *The Advocate*, the cultural agenda continues to exercise absolute authority. The spectacular success of safer sex campaigning in the gay communities of North America, and the sheer enormity of this achievement as it has been lived through in hundreds of thousands of individual lives, continues to be all but obliterated by an agenda which calls relentlessly for mass testing and/or the quarantine of all those infected.

To understand the force of this forward slippage from the notion of 'the AIDS virus' to the supposed 'remedy' of 'the AIDS test', we need to return to the ways in which the cultural agenda surrounding AIDS has consistently presented the syndrome as if it were an intrinsic property of particular social groups. In this respect, AIDS commentary merely amplifies lay perceptions of health and disease: equating the *source* of an epidemic with its *cause*. According to this view, and following the crudest of retributory logic, the context in which a virus emerges and those first affected are held to be directly responsible for its emergence. Calls for compulsory HIV-antibody testing from general practitioners and other medical professionals thereby demonstrate the profound discontinuity at work between the 'knowledge' generated by epidemiology, and that endemic in other medical institutions.

AIDS is predominantly associated with some supposed 'essence' of those social groups in which it first appeared both in Britain and in the United States. That it should still be so widely regarded as a retributive condition, speaks volumes about the extent to which pre-modern beliefs about disease causation can continue to co-exist with other more scientific understandings. Hence the notion of the 'high-risk group' (which functions as an avatar for 'the AIDS carrier') operates to suggest that certain social groups may of their essence present a risk to others. Admittedly, some commentators have preferred to think in terms of 'high-risk behaviours', and while this term does indeed re-emphasise modes of transmission, it only partially interrupts the relentlessly retributive logic of the overall agenda. Instead of 'risk', we should be talking of 'vulnerability'. Instead of high-risk groups, we should be talking of 'highly vulnerable groups'. Instead of 'AIDS victims', a term which carries connotations of terrorism, we should be talking of people with AIDS. Instead of 'AIDS carriers' we should be talking of people with HIV infection. Instead of 'the AIDS virus', we should be talking of HIV. And, most importantly, instead of talking about 'compulsory' testing—or as President

Reagan put it in 1987, 'routine' testing—we should be talking of punitive testing.

The dominant cultural agenda clearly invites us to regard AIDS as both a well-deserved punishment and a justification for further punitive actions—the latter rationalised as defence mechanisms against its 'spread'. This is the primary motivation at work within an agenda which endlessly sides *with* HIV in what we are positioned to regard as its purposive mission, to purge the entire planet of the regrettable existence of black Africans, injecting drug users, workers in the sex industry, the 'promiscuous', and, above all gay men. Beyond this identification with the virus, however, lies a still-larger unconscious ambition to erase all evidence of the mobility of sexual desire, together with any variation of sexual object-choice beyond the ideal goal of a purely reproductive heterosexuality. If the cultural agenda of AIDS resembles the traditional domino theory of external threat, then this is its internal solution.

AIDS and the politics of 'theory'

The generating force behind AIDS commentary is, of course, the highly competitive market place of the multinational, mass media industry, for which AIDS is always 'good news' insofar as it promises to increase sales, audience ratings and profit margins. AIDS is thus mobilised to the purposes of an industry which habitually regards its audience as an ideal national family unit, united by child-raising and consumption above all the divisions and complexities of existing social relations. In this manner, the media industry is able to picture itself actively 'serving' and 'satisfying' an audience which it has constricted through modes of address which systematically (mis)represent the entire panorama of the social in the likeness of consumer-spectators who recognise themselves with pleasure in the fantasy space of national family unity. It is in this context that we should recognise the full significance of Foucault's argument that 'the family' is not the *a priori* object of social policy, but is on the contrary its central and indispensable *instrument*.[5]

Little of the above could have been thought or written when HIV was first thought to have emerged in the United States, at some time in the early 1970s. Since then we have worked our way, with difficulty, through an extraordinary cross-fertilisation of ideas to arrive at a mode of theoretical practice which has been alerted by cultural theory to 'what cannot be spoken in what is actually being said'.[6] As Jacqueline Rose has explained, this mode of analysis proceeds from the assumption 'that there is a difficulty in language, that in speaking to others we might be speaking against ourselves, or at least against that part of ourselves which would rather remain unspoken'.[7] Hence we may arrive at the unconscious of AIDS commentary, operating in systematic reversals, in disavowal, and in the most aggressive modes of self-defence. AIDS commentary suggests that throughout contemporary British and American culture, large sections of the population are calmly and routinely regarded in their entirety as disposable constituencies.[8] Thus, while a recent British survey suggests that over 90 per cent of the population is in favour of compulsory sex education in schools, another survey reports that a similar percentage of parents is altogether opposed to any kind of teaching about homosexuality. It is from such contradictions that we may learn much about the nature and scale of sexual anxieties and boundaries in both our societies. AIDS evidently threatens the fragile stability of the most fundamental organising categories for both individual and collective identities, insofar as it raises the reality of sexual diversity.

It seems that both cultures will stop at nothing to prevent the dreadful possibility of sympathetic identification across the chasm of sexual object-choice. Here we may recognise the role of sexuality as the *sine qua non* of modern social organisation and control, operating beneath all other levels of gender, class, race and nationality. The political challenge of AIDS lies in the sheer range of issues which it finally obliges us to acknowledge—the sickening ease with which hundreds of thousands of sick and dying people can be cynically dismissed as the supposed agents of their own destruction; the barbarous lengths to which 'modern' and supposedly 'civilised' societies will enthusiastically go to persecute and deny all responsibility for those who are held to threaten 'the family'— an institution and ideological construct from which they are themselves most vigorously and venomously excluded; the sheer volume of hatred and contempt for the marginalised and the oppressed; the question of whether health care is finally a right or a privilege. The degree to which Anglo-American Society treats people with AIDS as if they were less than human is the exact and terrifying index of the extent to which both cultures have already been systematically dehumanised. This is not to subscribe to some 'humanist' thoughtcrime, but merely to observe the bizarre contradictions of a period in which the theoretical diversity of race and sexual object-choice is so endlessly celebrated, while political organisations working on behalf of lesbians and gay men are so lightly dismissed as jejune, or 'essentialist', or merely 'confessional'.[9] It should not therefore come as any surprise to discover that the most eloquent analysts of disavowal should themselves ultimately draw attention so clearly to their own psychic defences. The silence of 'theory' on the subject of AIDS speaks volumes for its own resistances.

The 'other' subject of AIDS

The 'other' subject of AIDS is the person with AIDS, bound, gagged and hidden away behind the antiseptic screens and curtains of AIDS commentary, which are occasionally pulled to one side in order to reveal the elaborately stage-managed spectacle of the monstrous. This is the *ne plus ultra* of the cultural agenda of AIDS, the moment at which we are permitted to 'identify' AIDS, and simultaneously denied the possibility of identifying with its sufferers. The 'look' of AIDS thus guarantees that it is made visible (and remembered and dreamed of and dreaded) as if it were indeed a unitary phenomenon, stamping its 'victims' with the un-mistakable and irrefutable signs of the innately degenerate. We thus 'see' AIDS under two guises. First, as 'the AIDS virus', materialised by the technologies of computer graphics and electron microscopy, floating like some alien spacecraft in a dense space of violently saturated colour. Sec-ond, we 'see' AIDS in living bodies which have been all but stripped of the sensual luxury of flesh, and in faces which are blistered and swollen beyond human recognition. Such images are calculated to appeal to the sadistic. They embody the entire cultural agenda of AIDS at its most concentrated, efficient and revealing. They tell us unambiguously: 'This is what AIDS looks like.' They forbid any further enquiry.[10]

Yet the vast majority of people with AIDS wear no visible stigmata of disease. They go about their lives like everybody else, but with the added burden of a cultural agenda which makes employment, housing, insur-ance, health care and ordinary social life into a continual and neverend-ing nightmare. They have been totally leperised. We can only understand the magnitude and significance of this terrible and unrelenting perse-cution in relation to the position of gay men—who make up by far the majority of people with AIDS—before the epidemic began. Nor are we helped in this situation by the available concepts of 'moral panics' and 'homophobia'. The widespread tendency to regard AIDS commentary as a species of moral panic overlooks the fact that homosexual desire is regarded as scandalous in its totality, and presents moral panic, highly misleadingly, as a discrete and unitary phenomenon.[11] Similarly, the con-cept of 'homophobia' merely encourages us either to psychologise all aspects of homosexual stigmatisation, or else to pathologise cultural and historical factors. It is highly unlikely that we shall ever be able to 'explain' the complex domain of attitudes to homosexuality by recourse to a single psychic mechanism. Above all, we must avoid the danger of collapsing together the workings of the social and the psychic. An understanding of the kinds of germ theory that underpin lay perceptions of health and disease can hardly be clarified if we attribute them to the agency of the unconscious, though it should be said that we will not be able to understand how and why they are so widely taken up as sexualised metaphors without the aid of psychoanalysis.

It is precisely in relation to lay perceptions of health that we should begin to develop strategies of resistance to the cultural agenda of AIDS. The simple distinction between infection and contagion, once firmly established, is already a significant block to the internal logic of AIDS commentary. Nor can the facts of the HIV antibody test be easily digested by those who advocate compulsory (punitive) 'AIDS testing'. In this manner, the 'rhetoric of AIDS' can be forced to speak new meanings. At present it detracts from the security which should come from our knowledge about HIV's modes of transmission and the ways in which infection can be prevented. AIDS rhetoric is therefore a device used by those who would seemingly prefer to see all gay men annihilated rather than contemplate any changes whatsoever in their own sexual behaviour. For although the much-discussed topic of a 'possible' epidemic among 'ordinary' heterosexuals is invariably presented on behalf of women and children, it is in fact straight men who are the most threatened—not by HIV infection or AIDS—but by the simple use of condoms. At the same time, the rhetoric speaks on behalf of those who would seemingly prefer to see their children die of AIDS rather than let them be 'defiled' by prophylactic education. For there can be no mistake here: AIDS education is sex education, and those like Congressman Dannemeyer who oppose safer sex campaigning in America are directly and immediately responsible for the spread of HIV infection and its many consequences. HIV has not yet proved itself to be a respecter of persons. Heterosexual culture can only afford to turn its back on the experience and wisdom of the gay community, achieved from so much pain and suffering, at a truly terrible cost in potential loss of life.

Experience strongly suggests that people cannot be frightened into celibacy, and that monogamy is no defence against HIV. It is therefore particularly tragic and regrettable that 1980s America seems to be steadfastly opposed to recognising that the only way in which it truly leads the world these days is in the example of safer sex campaigns amongst its gay citizens. In Britain, drugs are currently being denied to people with AIDS on the grounds of cost, for the first time in the history of the National Health Service. In America, people with AIDS are being expected to pay to be used as guinea pigs for drug corporations which already make a 300 per cent higher profit on AIDS drugs than on any of their other products.[12] It is therefore hardly surprising to find people with AIDS organising politically in groups such as ACT UP and the 'People with AIDS Coalition' in order to collectively resist the consequences of the cultural agenda of AIDS which I have outlined. If anything can ever teach us about the need to construct new political alliances and identities within and between marginalised groups, it is AIDS. Yet at this moment in time, the entire burden of resisting both the intermediate consequences of ongoing social policy concerning AIDS, as well as the cultural agenda of AIDS, falls on the shoulders of those who already have more than enough to deal with in staying well and taking care of their health and refusing to be destroyed by the deafening chorus of hatred all around them, or on those whose lives are spent taking care of them.

Finally it is the image of fatality itself which people with AIDS have done most to challenge. The social identity they have created will be a lasting one, forged in relation to the structures of sexuality, medicine and the state, and demanding both the right to adequate health care and to adequate cultural and political representation. In the long run, people with AIDS' heroic assertion of the intrinsically unremarkable diversity and complexity of human sexuality can only make our cultures stronger and more flexible, insofar as it obliges us all to think more seriously than ever before about the meaning and value of human life. Sooner rather than later we must wake up to the uncomfortable fact that it is only the example of gay men which will ultimately save everyone else's lives. In the meantime we move like Auden's expressive lover,

> To further griefs and greater
> And the defeat of grief.

4. The Politics of AIDS

Two articles which make major contributions to our understanding of the politics of AIDS have recently been published in the United States, written by Larry Kramer, who was an original cofounder of Gay Men's Health Crisis (GMHC) which is the largest voluntary organisation involved in the fight against AIDS in New York City. He is best known in Britain as the author of the novel *Faggots*, and *The Normal Heart*, a play which dramatised his own role in the formation of GMHC back in 1982, and which enjoyed a huge success on the London stage last year. Until recently his most celebrated contribution to the American debate on AIDS was his 1983 article *1,112 And Counting*, published in *New York Native*, Issue 59. There he began with the now famous words 'If this article doesn't scare the shit out of you we're in real trouble. If this article doesn't rouse you to anger, fury, rage, and action, gay men may have no future on this earth. Our continued existence depends on just how angry you can get'. At that time the United States was in almost exactly the same statistical situation that we are in right now. His message, in five words, 'we must fight to live', is as timely as ever, as the newspaper industries in both our nations compete with their calls for mass quarantine and compulsory HIV testing.

Kramer's latest excursion onto the front page of *New York Native* was in Issue 197, and takes the form of an open letter to Richard Dunne, the current executive director of GMHC. It is written in the context of the 274 AIDS deaths each week in America, and argues passionately that 'as presently constituted, organised and managed, Gay Men's Health Crisis is simply not equipped or prepared or able to deal with an emergency of this magnitude'. His words matter, because so much of what he has to say about GMHC could equally be addressed to the Terrence Higgins

Trust in London, and to the British gay community, which is so much more atomised and divided than its American counterpart.

He writes: 'I cannot for the life of me understand how the organisation I helped to form has become such a bastion of conservatism and such a bureaucratic mess. The bigger you get, the more cowardly you become; the more money you receive, the more self-satisfied. No longer do you fight for the living. You have become a funeral home.' And he goes on to accuse GMHC of colluding with the effective privatisation of the social and medical treatment of people with AIDS, and refusing to get involved in the scandal surrounding the limited availability of AZT, the drug which may prevent the HIV virus from duplicating and reproducing itself, which is only on offer to a very limited number of PWAs, and nobody with ARC, or who is 'merely' HIV antibody-positive, whom the drug might help.

Whilst I think his attacks on GMHC's services to the terminally ill, instead of to the well, are fundamentally mistaken, there is a much larger issue at stake concerning the politics of AIDS, and it lies in his assertion that: 'There is nothing in this whole AIDS mess that is not political', from questions of medical research funding, to the financing and services offered by voluntary sector organisations, to the general attitude of affected communities—above all in the sense of risk perception amongst gay men, to whom for example the British Government has yet to direct a single supportive word. As he points out, GMHC, is 'now in thrall to forces other than its board'—professional doctors, psychologists, social workers, and government agencies—which have no sense whatsoever of the sexual politics of AIDS. It is certainly the case that many people work as volunteers for the Terrence Higgins Trust, and support it financially, in the belief that it is a kind of Trojan Horse, working on behalf of gay men (who make up over 80 per cent of AIDS cases in the UK) in a profoundly homophobic society, presided over by a Government which would gladly see us all dead anyway. It turns out however that it is the Trust which has been invaded, as a result of its continued attempts to try to please institutions and lobbies which—to put it mildly—do not have the interests of gay men at heart. Hence the Trust's extraordinary new official policy of not distributing condoms, on the advice of doctors who seem to lack any idea whatsoever of contemporary health education needs for different communities, let alone the social and political consequences for women and gays of colluding with an official campaign which simply equates sex with death.

Kramer argues that GMHC has become weaker as it has 'tried to take care of everyone' and that it should concentrate its services on gay men: 'There is nothing wrong with becoming a special-interest group. Indeed, that is what you were established to be.' Recent statements from Norman Fowler, and the re-constitution of a new Health Education Authority, make clear what he learned from GMHC and San Francisco's SHANTI Project: the need to take power and control away from special-interest groups (including gays) and to treat AIDS as if it were a purely medical crisis, with no civil rights dimensions or political implications. The Trust has been increasingly marginalised by the DHSS, especially in respect of its pioneering work on behalf of drug users and women; though even there, the THT's only leaflet for women is dismally anti-sex in tone. It is obvious that the Government is only concerned with the 'threat' of AIDS in the heterosexual community, and with further policing of gay sex in all its forms. How else can one possibly explain the three years of total inactivity until 1986, when AIDS began to be perceived as other than a 'gay plague'? Gay men have been consistently regarded and treated as a disposable constituency. Which is why Kramer's Open Letter, though written in very different circumstances, and full of problems, is so timely and relevant to the British situation. We should all bear in mind the moving 'Statement of Purpose of the National Association of People with AIDS', published in San Francisco last September:

> We do not see ourselves as victims. We will not be victimised. We have the right to be treated with respect, dignity, compassion and understanding. We have the right to live fulfilling productive lives—to live and die with dignity and compassion. . . . We are born of and inextricably bound to the historical struggle for rights—civil, feminist, disability, lesbian, gay and human. We will not be denied our rights!

One can scrutinise the entire literature produced by the Terrence Higgins Trust in vain for the remotest glimmer of sympathy with those brave and absolutely fundamental assertions.

Kramer's second, and equally important recent article appeared in the February issue of Andy Warhol's *Interview* magazine. It takes the form of an extended conversation with Dr Mathilde Krim, the national Co-Chairperson of the American Foundation for AIDS Research. She describes how she recognised as early as 1981:

> the potential for social disruption and cruelties associated with a condition that was of unknown origin, progressive, irreversible,

transmissible, and which occurred in a minority group. The potential for catastrophe at the social level, let alone the health problem, was enormous.

Krim is relentlessly critical of under-funding for research purposes since the early 1980s as well as the moral hypocrisy of media-informed popular attitudes on AIDS:

> I am angry at the straight world, I find it so hypocritical when we, the straight scientists, say to gay men, 'You'd better behave yourselves and leave these lascivious ways and establish stable, monogamous relationships'. But do we make it possible? The answer is no.

But above all she criticises 'the arrogance of many people in the biochemical community', especially in relation to AZT: 'To me it is cold-blooded and totally morally unacceptable to deny experimental treatment to people who have no time to wait until the end of a trial experiement.' We should remember that AZT, which is manufactured here in England, had been available to more than 3000 people in the USA, but only 12 in the whole of the UK, although it is soon to be more widely available on the National Health Service, though not thanks to any campaigning from the *Trust*.

Krim also points out that the American insurance industry does not exist for the public good, but for private profit, and that the USA is going 'to end up with millions of people who are uninsured and who are going to need medical services. The question of a national health service will come up again, and the sooner the better'. She has equally sharp things to say about the consequences of the criminalisation of drugs in relation to crime. Her description of how her work has changed her whole attitude to sexuality and civil rights, and established a deep sense of solidarity with gay patients in particular is something else we can learn from. There is still a whole world of difference between the social attitudes of doctors who work in the real world of sexual diversity and complexity, and those whose training has only prepared them for a completely heterosexualised notion of 'family practice'. In the long run AIDS will oblige the British and American medical professions to acknowledge the social as well as the scientific advances and changes of the twentieth century. In the meantime it is up to the rest of us to push them energetically in that direction. As rare and courageous doctors like Mathilde Krim suggest, AIDS is already leading to the establishment of a far more patient-oriented medicine than of old. But socialised medicine, of itself, does not guarantee such changes, which will never come about if we passively accept the absolute authority of professional medicine, and continue to collude with the wholesale medicalisation of debate about AIDS.

1988 ————————

5. Talking to the Future: Gay rights in Britain and the USA

Margaret Thatcher has governed Britain for the past eight years on the basis of a popular consensus which has little to do with any of her actual economic policies, failed or successful. Her authority lies in the degree to which she has convinced voters that she and she alone is vigilantly on the side of what she presents as the most threatened and vulnerable institution in contemporary Britain—'the family'. Clause 28 should come as no surprise to anyone who noted the deafening ovation which accompanied the Prime Minister's words at the 1987 Conservative Party conference in Blackpool, when she stated unambiguously that 'Children who need to be taught traditional moral values are being taught that they have an inalienable right to be gay.' Three weeks previously her Education Secretary, Kenneth Baker, issued a circular to all state schools forbidding teachers from 'advocating homosexual behaviour'. Behind this is a theory that lesbians and gay men do not have 'inalienable rights' because we are calculating perverts who have chosen our sexuality, rejecting 'family values', and at the same time threatening them. Clearly we are perceived as threatening, but the question remains what exactly it is that we threaten.

This is the context in which Tory MP David Wilshire introduced his now notorious Clause 27 (later Clause 28) to the ongoing Local Government Bill in early December 1987, taking up almost exactly the same wording as had been used earlier in the year by Dame Jill Knight in a parliamentary move which only failed because of the general election. Since Wilshire's amendment constitutes much the most serious threat to the civil liberties of lesbians and gay men throughout the UK since the Labouchere amendment of 1885, it is critically important that we consider its wording very closely in order to develop strategies of resistance which are not just so much hot air. The clause states that:

A local authority shall not (a) 'promote homosexuality or publish material for the promotion of homosexuality', or (b) 'promote the teaching in any maintained school of the acceptability of homosexuality as a pretended family relationship by the publication of such material or otherwise; (c) give financial support or other assistance to any person for either of the purposes referred to in paragraphs (a) and (b) above.'

At the same time none of this 'shall be taken to prohibit the doing of anything for the purpose of treating or preventing the spread of disease'. Two closely related assumptions stand out here. First, the idea that homosexuality may be 'promoted', with the implication that children stand in particular risk from gay people. Second, there is a significant distinction between supposedly real, and 'pretended' families. Unless we understand that this image of 'real families' is an immensely powerful fantasy underpinning much of contemporary British culture, we will be radically disabled from effectively resisting the legal and parliamentary manoeuvres which are bound to follow in the years ahead. This fantasy has four major characteristics.

First, it defends individuals from acknowledging the actual complexity and diversity of British society. For example, the *Guardian* reported on 13 January that 13 per cent of children are now raised in single-parent families, the same single-parent families which ex-minister Dr Rhodes Boyson stridently denounced as immoral to another ovation at last year's Tory conference. Second, the fantasy protects people from recognising the actual and inescapable diversity of human sexuality— even in Britain. It pretends that lesbians and gay men are not themselves members of families, either as parents or as children, and sometimes as both. It imagines all families as 100 per cent heterosexual. Third, it depicts lesbians and gays as the most serious threat imaginable to this grotesquely over-simplified and insultingly idealised picture of 'family' life. The fact that children are most at risk in their own homes from their own parents must evidently be denied at all costs. The *Independent* recently reported that antenatal child care has 'stagnated for 30 years in many areas',[1] and the extent to which British society really cares about its children is clear from a decade of relentless cuts in nursery provision, education at all levels, welfare benefits, and the NHS, together with massive youth unemployment. We have apparently been selected to distract attention away from the dismal picture.

Last, but far from least, Clause 28 categorically denies the validity of lesbian and gay relationships. It denies us the right to love. In its own terms the Clause tells us far more than its authors intend, or probably even realise, about their actual beliefs and motives. Its careful targeting of our communities cannot disguise the fact that the only sexual 'promotion' going on in schools, and elsewhere, is that of heterosexuality. It is chilling to remember that the rights of lesbian and gay children are never considered because their very existence is so totally denied. Clause 28 simply means that heterosexuality is henceforth to be imposed with the full force of law as the only acceptable form of social or sexual relationship. At the same time its miserably meanspirited and impoverished view of human sexuality serves ultimately to draw attention more clearly to the point that it is a neurotic fantasy of 'family life' and 'traditional values' which is actually being pretended right across the political spectrum in contemporary Britain. Nor should the sickening hypocrisy with which the Clause excludes anything 'preventing the spread of disease' be permitted to obscure our recognition that behind all this brutal cant there lies a single word, which is all the more powerful for not being stated directly, AIDS.

The history of the AIDS epidemic in Britain has reached a critical moment. Large sections of the mass media are still vainly insisting that HIV offers no real threat to heterosexuals. At the same time those who do address the wider reality of AIDS persist in regarding the first groups affected by AIDS as if they were somehow its cause. Whilst the rest of Europe, together with Australasia and South America, has recognised that we are dealing with a virus with known modes of transmission, Britain, the USA and Canada persist in persecuting people with AIDS, together with the communities they come from. British lesbians and gay men are just waking up to the extent to which the pathological hatred and fear of homosexuality which is such a major characteristic of Anglo-American culture has been intensified and focused by AIDS.

It is in this context that we can learn vital lessons from the experience of lesbian and gay communities in the United States. They are approximately five years ahead of us in the history of AIDS, and we thus have a real opportunity to 'talk to the future' with them, and to prepare ourselves for the kinds of onslaught which American AIDS organisations are already facing and resisting. It is sometimes tempting to assume that because the USA has a Constitution and a Bill of Rights it is automatically more democratic than Britain, especially for sexual and racial minorities. We should, however, recall that in the case of Michael Hardwick's appeal against the anti-sodomy statutes in the state of Georgia, the US Supreme Court decided in June 1986 that the Constitution does not protect gay relationships between consenting adults, even in the privacy of the home. But at least the Constitution is there, and its crucial importance has rarely been more clearly demonstrated than in relation to the recent amendment passed with massive support in both the Senate and the House of Representatives, banning all federal funding for safer sex education for gay people in the USA proposed by the veteran arch-homophobe Senator Jesse Helms. It requires that 'no federal funds shall be used to promote or encourage homosexual activity. It further requires that AIDS education emphasise sexual abstinence outside a sexually monogamous marriage, and abstinence from drugs as well'.[2] Helms successfully argued that Safer Sex materials produced by the New York-based AIDS organisation Gay Men's Health Crisis are pornographic and that anyone voting against the amendment would be seen to be voting for pornography. In an election year in the United States this proved to be a clinching blackmail manoeuvre.

Helms's amendment is based on the straightforward assertion that 'the virus turned plague has only one source—sodomy'. AIDS is 'explained' in the familiar paranoid terms of the old American 'domino-theory' concerning the supposed international 'threat' of communism, which was used to justify the Vietnam war, and current incursions into Nicaragua and elsewhere. 'Heterosexuals are infected only from homosexuals, or from heterosexuals infected by bisexuals'.[3] Helms shares the British Tory attitude that lesbians and gay men are basically outside the boundaries of ordinary national identity, but he pushes it to a murderous extreme which has now led to the prevention of any state funding for safer sex materials or counselling which addresses the real world of contemporary America, whereas one of the only two Senators to vote against the amendment pointed out, by the age of fifteen, '16 per cent of boys and 5 per cent of girls have had heterosexual intercourse at least once' and by the age of nineteen, 'three-quarters of all boys and almost two-thirds of all girls have been sexually active'. The amendment has now passed out from its subsequent committee stage and awaits Presidential approval, with only one word removed, but a rider added to it that: 'the language in the Bill should not be construed to prohibit descriptions of methods to reduce the risk of HIV infection, to limit eligibility for federal funds of a general or particular practice because of its non-federal activities, nor shall it be construed to limit counselling or referrals to agencies that are not Federally funded'. Whilst this is not part of the Bill itself, Helms's amendment will have to be interpreted in relation to it. Some latitude has thus been restored to the Centers for Disease Control to finance safer sex education which doesn't simply advocate heterosexual monogamous marriage as the only valid form of sexual behaviour. As a spokesperson from Gay Men's Health Crisis told me 'the damage is political. It's going to be harder for everyone now to get funding'. It is hard not to conclude that campaigners like Helms would like to see all gay men dead. That is the only explanation of his attack on safer sex information which addresses the actual lived experience of our communities. We have no right to exist, and if Helms can't wipe us out himself he can do the next best thing and make sure that HIV does it for him. His strategy has already been taken up in California, where the right-wing Republican Senator John Doolittle has successfully lobbied the state Republican Party to call for the criminal prosecution of both the San Francisco Department of Public Health and the San Francisco AIDS Foundation for allegedly 'distributing obscene material'.[4] We need only consider the example of President Reagan's own family—a divorced man, not on speaking terms with his son Ron Jr, and who calls his wife 'Mommy' in private—to gauge the ruthless sentimentality and emotional dishonesty of Reaganite rhetoric concerning 'the family'. Those who would seemingly prefer to see their own children die of AIDS rather than allow them to receive information about the modes of transmission of HIV are hardly suited to be parents, let alone legislators of other people's morality. Both the Helms amendment and the 'Jill Knight' Clause demonstrate the ease with which AIDS can be used to justify massive punitive discrimination against lesbians and gay men. Large and powerful sections of contemporary American and British society are evidently determined not to acknowledge the actual and intrinsically unremarkable diversity of sexual behaviour and identity in both nations. We must seriously consider the relationship between the frankly hate-filled outpourings of one of President Reagan's ex-speech writers, claiming recently that 'There is one, only one, cause of the AIDS crisis, the wilful refusal of homosexuals to cease indulging in the immoral, unnatural, unsanitary, unhealthy and suicidal practice of anal intercourse',[5] and the more 'moderate' but equally dangerous assumption that 'Those of us who entered adulthood in the now distinctly unfashionable late 1960s and early 1970s grew up in what is likely to be the only brief period this century when there was widespread tolerance towards homosexuality'.[6]

Whilst many share the pessimistic assumption that we will not live to see Britain transformed into the kind of genuinely democratic society that we would like to live in, we surely cannot afford to take it for granted that all is already lost. There seem to me to be five substantial lessons to be learned from the Helms and Wilshire affairs. First, we must always challenge any notion of 'tradition' or 'traditional values' which seek to exclude our role as lesbians and gay men in British history and culture. The so-called 'traditional moral values' peddled by Mrs Thatcher and politicians from all the political parties these days are, in fact, of recent origin indeed. The fact that we have been persecuted for centuries only demonstrates that we have been here for centuries, and that we have the same rights to 'the pursuit of happiness' as any other British citizen. Second, we need to challenge the mindbogglingly foolish notion that homosexuality is, or can be, 'promoted'. If we allow politicians and moralists to get away with the idea that heterosexuality is the only 'natural' form of human emotional and erotic expression then we are colluding with the possible extinction of our entire culture. Third, we need to insist that any notion of 'the family' which denies the existence and rights of lesbians and gay teenagers as an ordinary and unremarkable fact of everyday life, actively condemns a significant proportion of the young people of Britain to utter misery and isolation with no love or support whatsoever. In this respect we have to expose 'the family' as a murderous myth, which is responsible for incalculable emotional and psychological damage for everyone involved. It is the diversity and richness of our various ways of living and loving which we must constantly affirm and celebrate, for *everybody's* sake.

Fourth, we must be alert to the ease with which our entire cultures may be summarily dismissed as 'pornographic' and legislated against as such. New proposals to increase sexual censorship still further in Britain in the name of attacking 'pornography' are forthcoming in Britain from both the Labour and Conservative parties. It is therefore of the utmost importance that we ally ourselves with progressive feminists, and organisations such as the national Campaign for Press and Broadcasting Freedom in order to collectively resist such moves. For it is the entire network of our various lesbian and gay communities which such laws threaten, and only a concerted community-based response will be able to challenge them. We must all be prepared, organised and articulate on this vital issue because our entire culture in all its richness and complexity is at stake. Fifth, we should recognise that we only find ourselves in this terrible situation because of the basic institutional failings of our supposedly democratic societies. In the short term we have little choice but to lobby and organise on behalf of changes in the law and greater Parliamentary political representation. But in the longer term we must refuse to accept a system of party politics which claims the right to legislate over matters of basic and fundamental human rights. Without a written Constitution or Bill of Rights we will never be able to establish a culture which is secure from just the kinds of pathological hatred and fear which are currently in the political ascendent.

6. The Spectacle of AIDS

And now what shall become of us without any barbarians?
Those people were a kind of solution.—C.P. Cavafy, *Expecting*
the Barbarians

The question of identity—how it is constituted and maintained—is there-
fore the central issue through which psychoanalysis enters the political field.
—Jacqueline Rose, 'Feminism and the Psychic'

As I write, there have been 'about' a thousand cases of AIDS in the United Kingdom. Writing on the subject of statistics, the great Polish poet Zbigniew Herbert describes the fundamentally shameful nature of the word 'about' when used in circumstances of disaster. For, in such matters:

> accuracy is essential
> we must not be wrong
> even by a single one
>
> we are despite everything
> the guardians of our brothers
>
> ignorance about those who have disappeared
> undermines the reality of the world.[1]

Five years have passed since the isolation of the retrovirus responsible for AIDS. Millions of pounds have been spent by the British government on public information campaigns. AIDS education workers have been appointed by local authorities throughout Britain. Tens if not hundreds of thousands of lives have been directly affected by the consequences of HIV. Yet even the most fundamental medical facts concerning HIV and

AIDS remain all but universally misunderstood. The entire subject continues to be framed by a cultural agenda that is as medically misinformed as it is socially misleading and politically motivated.[2] For those of us living and working in the various constituencies most devastated by HIV it seems, as Richard Goldstein has pointed out, as if the rest of the population were tourists, casually wandering through at the very height of a blitz of which they are totally unaware. This is hardly surprising at a time when the only sources of AIDS information are themselves so profoundly polluted and unreliable. Thus in England recently the *Guardian* noted that 'by the end of August 1,013 cases had been reported, of whom 572 had died'; while on the same day the *Star* informed its readers that 'AIDS has now killed more than 1,000 people in Britain'.[3]

Misreporting on such a scale has been regular and systematic since the earliest days of the epidemic, and is indicative of the values and priorities of an international information industry that continues to oscillate daily between meretricious gloating over the fate of those deemed responsible for their own misfortune, and the supposed 'threat' of a 'real' epidemic. Currently in the United States, someone dies of AIDS every half hour. An estimated six per cent of all Africans have been infected by HIV, including nearly a quarter of the entire populations of Malawi and Uganda.[4] If statistics teach us anything, it is the sheer scale and efficiency of the cultural censorship within and between different countries and continents, which guarantees that the actual situation of the vast majority of people with HIV and/or AIDS is rarely if ever discussed. Moreover, this disappearance is strategic, and faithfully duplicates the positions the social groups most vulnerable to HIV found themselves in even before the epidemic began. Thus the Latino population of the two continents of America, IV drug users, workers in the sex industry, black Africans, and gay men are carefully confined in the penal category of the 'high-risk group' from which position their experience and achievements may be safely ignored. In this manner a terrible ongoing human catastrophe has been ruthlessly denied the status of tragedy, or even natural disaster.

The British government's AIDS information campaign, which has been widely admired overseas, dutifully exhorted the 'general public' not to die of ignorance.[5] Yet this campaign has still found itself unable to address one single word to British gay men, who constitute almost ninety per cent of people with AIDS in Britain. At every level of 'public' address and readership, ignorance is sustained on a massively institutionalised scale by British and American media commentary. The modes of address of such commentary reveal much about the ways in which the state and the media industry 'think' the question of population. Indeed, the relentless monotony and sadism of AIDS commentary in the West only serve to manifest a sense of profound cultural uneasiness concerning the fragility of the nationalistic fantasy of an undifferentiated 'general public', supposedly united above all divisions of class, religion, and gender, yet totally excluding everyone who stands outside the institution of marriage. Popular perceptions of all aspects of AIDS thus remain all but exclusively informed by a cultural agenda that seriously and culpably impedes any attempt to understand the complex history of the epidemic, or to plan effectively against its future. In this context it is impossible to separate individual perceptions of risk, and endlessly amplified fears concerning the 'threat' of 'spread', from the drastically miniaturised 'truth' of AIDS, which has remained impervious to challenge or correction since the syndrome was first identified in the ideologically constitutive and immensely significant name GRID (gay-related immunodeficiency) in 1981.[6]

In this manner a 'knowledge' of AIDS has been uniformly constituted across the boundaries of formal and informal information, accurately duplicating the contours of other, previous 'knowledges' that speak confidently on behalf of the 'general public', viewed as a homogenous entity organised into discrete family units over and above all the fissures and conflicts of both the social and the psychic. This 'truth' of AIDS also resolutely insists that the point of emergence of the virus should be identified as its *cause*. Epidemiology is thus replaced by a moral etiology of disease that can only conceive homosexual desire within a medicalised metaphor of contagion. Reading AIDS as the outward and visible sign of an imagined depravity of will, AIDS commentary deftly returns us to a premodern vision of the body, according to which heresy and sin are held to be scored in the features of their voluntary subjects by punitive and admonitory manifestations of disease. Moreover, this rhetoric of AIDS incites a violent siege mentality in the 'morally well', a mentality that locks only too easily into other rhetorics of 'preemptive defense'.[7] Thus an essentially modern universalising discourse of 'family values', 'standards of decency', and so on, recruits subjects to an ever more disciplinary 'knowledge' of themselves and 'their' world. This 'knowledge' is effortlessly stitched in the likeness of an already-familiar *broderie Anglaise* picture of seemingly timeless 'national values' and the 'national past'.[8] At the same time, secular institutions appropriate and refashion an equally sober discourse of 'promiscuity', which drifts out across the Mediterranean to incorporate the entire African subcontinent and beyond, re-charging 'the Orient' with a deadly cargo of exoticism that reminds 'us' that negritude has always been, for whites, a sign of sexual excess and death.

The government of the home

All discussion of AIDS should proceed from the known facts concerning the modes of transmission of HIV in relation to lay perceptions of health and disease that mediate and 'handle' this information. That this is far from the case in contemporary AIDS commentary remains in urgent need of explanation. To begin with, an overly rational model of health education continues to ignore all questions of cultural and psychic resistance. Similarly, the study of risk perception lacks a theory of the subject, even in its explicitly anti-economistic 'culturalist' modes.[9] Both disciplines recognise that the localisation of HIV infection in particular communities is no more intrinsically remarkable than the localisation of any other infectious agent in any other specific constituencies. Yet the heavily concentrated and disseminated image of AIDS as a species of 'gay plague' cannot be adequately explained by available sociological theories of scapegoating, boundary protection, or 'moral panics'. What is at stake here is the capacity of particular ideological configurations to activate deep psychic anxieties that run far beneath the tangible divisions of the social formation. In particular, we should consider the active legacy of eugenic theory, which is as much at work within the sociobiological dogmatics of contemporary familialism as it was in the biomedical politics of National Socialism. This is not to posit a crude parallel of objectives or identities between Thatcherite Britain and Nazi Germany, but merely to observe that whenever history is biologised with recourse to the authority of seemingly unquestionable and innate laws, 'the perception of a natural order of social structure and stratification' is always 'thought to be readily available in the evidence of the human body'.[10] It is the sense of a *totalised* threat to a biologised identification of self with nation that characterises both Nazi medical politics and modern familialism. Thus Jews, antifascists, gypsies, and 'degenerates' (including, of course, large numbers of lesbians and gay men) were postulated as intrinsic and self-evident threats to the perceived unity and the very existence of the German *Volk,* and the policy of killing them all 'as a therapeutic imperative' only emerged in relation to the deeply felt danger of *Volkstod,* or 'death of the people' (or 'nation', or 'race').[11] It is in precisely this sense that people with HIV infection, usually misdescribed as 'AIDS carriers', are widely understood to threaten the equally spurious unity of 'the family', 'the nation', and even the 'species'.[12] Hence the overriding need to return to the pressing question of the contemporary government of the home, especially in the light of Foucault's argument that in the modern period:

> the family becomes an instrument rather than a model: the privileged instrument for the government of the population and not the chimerical model for good government: this shift from the level of the model to that of the instrument is, I believe, absolutely fundamental, and it is from the middle of the eighteenth century that the family appears in this dimension of instrumentality with respect to the population: hence the campaigns on morality, marriage, vaccinations, etc.[13]

This is why it is so important to avoid any temptation to think of the ongoing AIDS crisis as a form of 'moral panic', which carries the implication that it is an entirely discrete phenomenon, distinct from other elements and dramas in the perpetual moral management of the home. On the contrary, homosexuality, understood by AIDS commentary as the 'cause' of AIDS, is always available as a coercive and menacing category to entrench the institutions of family life and to prop up the profoundly unstable identities those institutions generate. The felt 'problem' of sexual diversity is not established and imposed externally by the state, but rather internally, by the categorical imperatives of the modern organisation of sexuality. The state, of course, responds to this situation, but it is not its originator. This, after all, is what sexuality means. Thus, consent to social policy is grafted from desire itself, as political prescriptions are understood to 'protect' heterosexual identities, which are stabilised by an ever proliferating sense of permanent personal threat, with corresponding emotional responses ranging from 'outrage' to actual violence against imaginary adversaries. Hence, as I have written elsewhere:

> We can begin to understand the seeming obsession with homosexuality in contemporary Britain, whether it is presented as a threat within the home, in the form of deviant members of the family who must be expelled, or as deviant images invading the 'innocent' space of domesticity via TV or video; or as a supposedly external threat in the form of explicit sex education in schools, the (homo)sexuality of public figures, and above all, now, in the guise of AIDS.[14]

Homosexuality has lately come to occupy a most peculiar and centrally privileged position in the government of the home—homosexuality ideologically constructed as a regulative admonitory sign throughout the field of 'popular' culture in the likeness of the ruthless pervert, justifying any amount of state intervention in the cause of 'family values' and so on. Yet at the same time, the male homosexual becomes an impossible object, a monster that can only be engendered by a process of corruption through seduction, which is itself inexplicable, since familialism lacks any theory of desire beyond the supposed 'needs' of reproduction. It is this rigorously anti-Freudian scenario that actively encourages the forward slippage from corruption theories of homosexuality to contagion theories of AIDS. In this manner the axiomatic identification of AIDS as a sign and symptom of homosexual behaviour reconfirms the passionately held view of 'the family' as a uniquely vulnerable institution. It also sanctions the strongest calls for 'protectionist' measures, of an ever intensified censorship that will obliterate the evidently unbearable cultural evidence of that sexual diversity which stalks the *terra incognita* beyond the home.

Hence the incomparably strange reincarnation of the cultural figure of the male homosexual as a predatory, determined invert, wrapped in a Grand Guignol cloak of degeneracy theory, and casting his lascivious eyes and hands out from the pages of Victorian sexology manuals and onto 'our' children, and above all onto 'our' sons. Undoubtedly there is a real threat in the above scenario, which only serves to reveal the full extent to which the home is always a site of intense sexual fantasy. But the unspeakable that lurks in the very bosom of 'the family' is not so much the real danger of child-molestation from outside, but the more radical possibility of acknowledging that the child's body is invariably an object of parental desire, and further, that the child itself is not only desirable but desiring. Calls for the quarantining of people infected with HIV, or the compulsory HIV testing of all gay men, immigrants, and other extra-familial categories, clearly derive from this prior, unconscious compulsion to censor and expel the signs of sexual diversity from the domestic field of vision, which is always equated with the child's point of view. Identifying with the child, the 'good' parent is thus protected from troubling disturbances of adult identities, taking refuge in a projective fantasy of childhood 'innocence' that significantly desexualises all the actors involved. The utter violence of AIDS commentary suggests much about the force with which these repressed sexual materials return, and the forms of hysteria and hysterical identification that are responsible for successfully paralysing the family ensemble into the rigidly stereotyped routines of 'respectable' domesticity.

It is from this perspective that we may glimpse something of the political unconscious of the visual register of AIDS commentary, which assumes the form of a diptych. On one panel we are shown the HIV retrovirus (repeatedly misdescribed as the 'AIDS virus') made to appear, by means of electron microscopy or reconstructive computer graphics, like a huge technicolour asteroid. On the other panel we witness the 'AIDS victim', usually hospitalised and physically debilitated, 'withered, wrinkled, and loathsome of visage'—the authentic cadaver of Dorian Gray.[15] This is the spectacle of AIDS, constituted in a regime of massively overdetermined images, which are sensitive only to the values of the dominant familial 'truth' of AIDS and the projective 'knowledge' of its ideally interpellated spectator, who already 'knows all he needs to know' about homosexuality and AIDS. It is the principal and serious business of this spectacle to ensure that the subject of AIDS is 'correctly' identi- fied and that any possibility of positive sympathetic identification with actual people with AIDS is entirely expunged from the field of vision. AIDS is thus embodied as an exemplary and admonitory drama, relayed between the image of the miraculous authority of clinical medicine and the faces and bodies of individuals who clearly disclose the stigmata of their guilt. The principal target of this sadistically punitive gaze is the body of 'the homosexual'.

The homosexual body

Psychoanalysis understands identification as a process whereby the subject 'assimilates an aspect, property, or attribute of the other and is transformed, wholly or partially, after the model the other provides.' Further, 'it is by means of a series of identifications that the personality is constituted and specified.'[16] But the substantive process of identify- ing operates in two modes: the transitive one of identifying the self in relation to the difference of the other, and the reflexive one of identify- ing the self in a relation of resemblance to the other. The homosexual body is an object that can only enter 'public' visibility in the transi- tive mode, upon the strictly enforced condition that any possibility of identification with it is scrupulously refused. In the register of object- choice, the homosexual body inescapably evidences a sexual diversity that it is its ideological 'function' to restrict. In the register of gender, it exposes the impossibility of the entire enterprise. Feminised in contempt, the homosexual body speaks too much of male 'heterosexual' misogyny. Masculinised, it simply disappears. It is thus constituted as a contradiction *in objecto*. Psychoanalysis will pose this 'problem' in a very different way, since the body with which it deals is 'not some external realm but something that is internal to the psyche. Psychoanalysis does not conceive of perceptions as unmediated registrations of the reality of a pregiven body. Rather, it has a libidinal theory of perception'.[17]

The 'problem' then, is the body itself, radically mute, yet rendered garrulous by projective, desiring fantasies all around it, which, as Leo Bersani reminds us, are 'a frantic defence against the return of dangerous images and sensations to the surface of consciousness'.[18] More precisely, these 'desiring fantasies are by no means turned only towards the past; they are projective reminiscences'.[19] Indeed, the very notion of a 'homosexual body' only exposes the more-or-less desperate ambition to confine mobile desire in the semblance of a stable object, calibrated by its sexual aim, regarded as a 'wrong choice'. The 'homosexual body' would thus evidence a fictive collectivity of perverse sexual performances, denied any psychic reality and pushed out beyond the furthest margins of the social. This, after all, is what the category of 'the homosexual' (which we *cannot* continue to employ) was invented to do in the first place. The social sight lines of sexuality are thus permanently tensed against 'mistakes' that might threaten to undermine the fragile stability of the heterosexual subject of vision. Hence the inestimable convenience of AIDS, reduced to a typology of signs that promises to identify the dreaded object of desire in the final moments of its own apparent self-destruction. AIDS is thus made to rationalise the impossibility of the 'homosexual body', and reminds us only of the dire consequences of a failure to 'forget'. . . . Hence the social *necessity* of the 'homosexual body', disclosed in the composite photography of nineteenth-century penal anthropology and sexology, and contemporary journalism. Hence also the voice of a contemporary English ex-police pathologist in a London teaching hospital, inviting his students, in the familiar pedagogic manner, to identify the physical symptoms of homosexuality, especially the 'typical keratinised funnelshaped rectum of the habitual homosexual'.[20] Other constitutional symptoms of the 'habitual homosexual' include softening of the brain. It is this order of 'knowledge' of the 'homosexual body' that precedes most clinical AIDS commentary and seeps out into the domestic register through the mediating services of medical correspondents, who report back from the clinical front lines on 'our' behalf and ceaselessly refer us to the diagnostic AIDS diptych. In these densely coded *tableaux mourants* the body is subjected to extremes of casual cruelty and violent indifference, like the bodies of aliens, sliced open to the frightened yet fascinated gaze of uncomprehending social pathologists. Here, where the signs of homosexual 'acts' have been entirely collapsed into the signs of death-as-the-deserts-of-depravity, there is still some chance that reflexive identification with the merely human fact of death might interrupt the last rites of psychic censorship, with the human body *in extremis*.

Thus, even and especially in the *clair-obscur* of death itself, the 'homosexual body', which is also that of the 'AIDS victim', must be publicly seen to be humiliated, thrown around in zip-up plastic bags, fumigated, denied burial, lest there be any acknowledgement of the slightest sense of loss. Thus the 'homosexual body' continues to speak after death, not as a *memento mori,* but as its exact reverse, for a life that must at all costs be seen to have been devoid of value, unregretted, unlamented, and—final indignity—effaced into a mere anonymous statistic. The 'homosexual body' is 'disposed of', like so much rubbish, like the trash it was in life. Yet, as always, it is the very excess of the psychic operations informing this terminal 'truth' of AIDS that signifies far beyond its own intentions. And, in these circumstances, ironically, the psychic consequences of the savage social organisation of 'sexuality' in the modern world can only serve ultimately to make instruments to plague us all. For it is precisely the displacement of epidemiology by a moralised etiology of disease, which regards AIDS as an intrinsic property of the fantasised 'homosexual body', that is likely actively to encourage the real spread of HIV by distracting attention away from the well-proven means of blocking its transmission. Such attention would require listening to the voices of the 'guilty' ones, would run the grave risk of acknowledging that HIV is no respecter of persons or even bodies. But the spectacle of AIDS continues to protect us against any such ghastly eventuality, as we settle down before our TV screens to watch and to celebrate the long-prophesied and marvellous sight of the degenerates finally burning themselves out, comfortable and secure in our *gesundes Volksempfinden*—our healthy folk feelings.

The spectacle of AIDS

In all its variant forms the spectacle of AIDS is carefully and elaborately stage-managed as a sensational didactic pageant, furnishing 'us', the 'general public', with further dramatic evidence of what 'we' already 'know' concerning the enormity of the dangers that surround us on all sides and at all times. It provides a purgative ritual in which we see the evildoers punished, while the national family unit—understood as the locus of 'the social'—is cleansed and restored. Yet, as Jacques Donzelot has argued, 'In showing the emergence of "the social" as the concrete space of intelligibility of the family, it is the social that suddenly looms as a strange abstraction'.[21]

Venerealising AIDS, the spectacle reduces 'the social' to the scale of 'the family', from which miniaturised and impoverished perspective, all aspects of consensual sexual diversity are systematically disavowed. We are thus returned to the question of 'sexuality' in the modern world, but with a wholly different point of view from that which sustained earlier twentieth-century campaigns—conceived in terms of a right to privacy—on behalf of 'sexual minorities'. For it is precisely the concept of privacy that is the central term of familialism, now used to challenge the authority of the traditional liberal distinction between 'public' and 'private', which has defined the consensus view of how the spatial relations of 'the social' have been thought for well over a century. That consensus is now up for grabs.[22]

The category of 'homosexuality' has, in any case, constituted a serious 'problem' in relation to laws and social policies drawn up in the terms of a supposedly physical public/private distinction. Legitimated, to some extent, in the technical sphere of the private, it has been all the more problematised in the public domain. AIDS commentary demonstrates this very clearly, insofar as it is invariably addressed to a 'family' that is also 'the nation'. Hence the extraordinary fact that even after 1000 cases of AIDS, the British government has yet to direct a single item of information, advice or support to the constituency most directly affected by the consequences of HIV since the early 1980s—gay men. This is evidently because we are not recognised as a part of the 'social', from which we are paradoxically excluded by virtue of our partially legalised 'private' status. And let us not forget that we are talking here about at least 5 per cent of the overall population of the United Kingdom. The spectacle of AIDS is thus always modified by the fear of being too 'shocking' for its domestic audience, while at the same time it amplifies and magnifies the collective 'wisdom' of familialism. AIDS commentary thus provides a unique perspective on the contemporary government of the home, which is experienced from within as a refuge of 'privacy', and in the defence of which its members agree that it can hardly be sufficiently regulated. In this manner all aspects of 'public' life are gradually annexed and subsumed by the precepts and 'etiquette' of privacy at the very moment that its most eloquent advocates are drawing their curtains against what they perceive as a hostile and dangerous outside world.

Yet, as we have seen, the home itself is also recognised as a site of potential inner corruption, and the prosecution of the 'public' by the 'private' is ideally personified in the fantasy of the 'homosexual body', whose sexual object-choice is displaced into the calibrated signs of AIDS. This body is as repulsive as the task of policing recalcitrant desire requires it to be. The spectacle of AIDS is thus placed in the service of the strongly felt need for constant domestic surveillance and the strict regulation of identity through the intimate mechanisms of sexual guilt, sibling rivalries, parental favouritism, embarrassment, hysterical modesty, house-pride, 'keeping-up-with-the-Joneses', hobbies, diet, clothes, personal hygiene, and the general husbandry of the home. These are the concrete practices that authorise consent to 'political' authority, and it is in relation to them that the entire spectacle of AIDS is unconsciously choreographed, with its studied emphasis on 'dirt', 'depravity', 'licence', and above all 'promiscuity'. Yet the proliferating agencies and voices that offer their 'expertise' on behalf of 'the family' are inevitably as uneven and inept as is the actual maintenance of power in the home itself. 'The family' is thus frequently provided with mutually conflicting and contradictory messages from the very experts to which it has granted authority. Hence, for example, the glaring contemporary British conflict between popular consent for sex education in schools and an imperative against any form of education that is held to 'advocate' homosexuality. 'Public' sex education thus comes to duplicate the 'knowledge' of the 'family', which is duly inscribed in the national curriculum with the full force of law. In a very similar way, the strong lobby in favour of 'AIDS education' in schools, and far beyond, is equally compelled to ignore the actual experience of most people with AIDS, or the communities most vulnerable to HIV infection, lest they also be accused of 'advocating' homosexuality. Here, as in all similar instances, the concept of 'advocacy' speaks from a discourse of sexual 'acts' by which the 'innocent' might become 'corrupted' and turned into 'habitual homosexuals'. Such a concept functions within the powerful anti-Freudian project that aspires to erase all notions of desire from the epistemological field of 'family', that is, 'public', life.

In these circumstances, the spectacle of AIDS operates as a public *masque* in which we witness the corporal punishment of the 'homosexual body', identified as the enigmatic and indecent source of an incomprehensible, voluntary resistance to the unquestionable governance of marriage, parenthood, and property. It is at precisely this point that opposition to the familial sovereignty of AIDS commentary can be posed most effectively. For, as I have argued, the overall spectacle of AIDS places its own audience at direct risk of HIV infection by distracting attention away from the demonstrably effective means of preventing its transmission. At the same time, the tremendous discursive responsibility that is placed upon the notion of 'promiscuity' throughout AIDS commentary renders it especially vulnerable to challenge when it is isolated from the propping imagery of venerealised death. It can easily be demonstrated, for example, that HIV is not a venereal condition, since it is not necessarily or exclusively sexually transmitted. It is not difficult to grasp the fact that if every disease that can or may be sexually transmitted were classified as venereal, the list would include all the most common known medical ailments, as Kaye Wellings has pointed out in relation to the earlier venerealising of herpes in the 1970s.[23] It must also be forcefully pointed out on every available occasion that those posing 'monogamy' as a preferable alternative to prophylactic information are in turn responsible for increasing the spread of HIV by mischievously suggesting that monogamy affords some kind of intrinsic 'moral' defence against a retrovirus. In such ways the entire authority of the spectacle of AIDS could be undermined by the protectionist rhetoric of the spectacle itself. This also permits the wider affirmation of sexual desire and diversity in the presentation of safer sex as an emancipatory and life-saving protectorate for the nation, posed in actively democratic terms that enlarge conceptions of the self beyond the narrowing confines of 'citizenship'. In these respects the challenge of AIDS re-education exemplifies the insight of Ernesto Laclau and Chantal Mouffe that what is being exploded in the postmodern period:

is the idea and the reality itself of a unique space of constitution of the political. What we are witnessing is a politicisation far more radical than any we have known in the past, because it tends to dissolve the distinction between the public and the private, not in terms of the encroachment on the private by a unified public space, but in terms of a proliferation of radically new and different political spaces. We are confronted with the emergence of a *plurality of subjects* whose forms of constitution and diversity it is only possible to think if we relinquish the category of 'subject' as a unified and unifying essence.[24]

By insisting on the psychoanalytic perception of the *psychic reality* of desire, we may avoid the shortcomings of a sexual politics that continues to see 'gay oppression' as a unitary and distinct phenomenon that might easily be rectified and remedied through direct political and legislative interventions, however intrinsically expedient these may be in relation to the only too concrete institutions that currently secure the meaning and practice of 'justice'. The spectacle of AIDS teaches us, however, that it is the structure, epistemology, and 'decorum' of 'sexuality' itself that have inexorably led us to the tragic impasse in which we find ourselves, where seemingly unified 'sexual minorities' are widely and routinely regarded, in their entirety, as disposable constituencies. This point cannot be sufficiently emphasised. For let there be no mistake: the spectacle of AIDS calmly and constantly entertains the possible prospect of the death of all western European and American gay men from AIDS—a total, let us say, of some twenty million lives—without the slightest flicker of concern, regret, or grief. Psychoanalysis may alert us to the psychological processes that can be activated in particular, complex historical circumstances in order to endorse an indifference that casually dehumanises whole categories of persons. To turn back now to the prospect of a politics rooted in the subjectivity of public/private space can only serve to strengthen the powerful emergent forms of a secularised fundamentalism that will not cease to prosecute its own 'projective reminiscences', picked out in the spotlights of its own displaced desires. In the meantime, all those who threaten to expose the brutal, hypocritical, and degrading implications of contemporary 'family values' and 'standards of decency' will undoubtedly continue to be stridently denounced—quite accurately—as 'enemies of the family'.

Increasingly, AIDS is being used to underwrite a widespread ambition to erase the distinction between 'the public' and 'the private', and to establish in their place a monolithic and legally binding category— the 'family'—understood as the central term through which the world and the self are henceforth to be rendered intelligible. Consent to this strategy is sought by tapping into lay perceptions of health, sickness, and disease, unevenly accreted down the centuries, and sharing only the common human fear and disavowal of death. Health education thus emerges as the central site of hegemonic struggle in the coming decades—a struggle that refuses and eludes all known lines of previous party-political allegiance and observance. A new and essentially talismanic model of power is emerging, offering to protect subjectivities carefully nurtured in folklore and superstition, now re-articulated in a discourse of ostensible medical authority. We are witnessing the precipitation of a moralised bio-politics of potentially awesome power—a cunning combination of leechcraft and radiotherapy, eugenics and a master narrative of 'family health'—with social policies that aspire with sober fanaticism to the creation of a modernity in which we will no longer exist. The spectacle of AIDS thus promises a stainless world in which we will only be recalled, in textbooks and carefully edited documentary 'evidence', as signs of plagues and contagions averted—intolerable interruptions of the familial, subjects 'cured' and disinfected of desire, and 'therapeutically' denied the right to life itself.

7. Photography and AIDS

The instant association of AIDS with death—death *from* AIDS*—rather than a consideration of the problem of *living with* AIDS, is part of the dominant agenda for thinking AIDS in contemporary Britain. It is this largely unconscious agenda which is my subject, and the role which photography has played in establishing its authority—the authority of the *morbid* which, as Michel Foucault has pointed out, 'authorises a subtle perception of the way in which life finds in death its most differentiated figure'.[1] The absolute difference of death has by now become closely identified with the effects of HIV infection and the social groups in which it has emerged. AIDS has been widely interpreted as if it were an intrinsic property of these groups, which are seen as actively threatening rather than *vulnerable,* with the outward and visible signs of infection taken as evidence of their supposed inner and secret depravity. The representation of AIDS gives the lie to any oversimplified assumption that the emergence of pathological anatomy and the modern medical sciences of virology and immunology have led to a complete transformation of the concept of disease 'away from the metaphysics of evil, to which it had been relegated for centuries'.[2] The most cursory reading of the history of sexually transmitted diseases demonstrates clearly that the tendency to regard illness as a sign of moral judgment has been displaced rather than replaced at the level of lay perceptions of health by the emergence of modern clinical medicine.[3] In this respect the representation of AIDS is a site of complex struggle between rival and competing estimations of disease and, at a further extreme, of our estimation of the range and meanings of human sexuality. The entire subject of AIDS has been used to shore up and reinforce the ideological fortresses of the Nation and the Family, as if they were under a state of unprecedented siege. In this respect we should

pay particularly close attention these days to the twin rhetorics of defence, which promise to protect the national family unit from both the
powerful projective fantasy of imminent foreign invasion and the equally
powerful introspective fantasy of sexual desire erupting in the bosom
of the home with literally fatal consequences. The family is the central
locus of concern in British AIDS commentary—but not the families of
the more than 90 per cent of people with AIDS, who are gay men or
intravenous (IV) drug users. The family at the heart of AIDS commentary is an ideological unit, as yet supposedly unaffected, but held to be
threatened by the 'leakage' of HIV infection which, like nuclear fallout,
is widely and erroneously perceived to be everywhere about us, a deadly
miasma of contagion and death.

The concept of the family enjoys absolute centrality for modern social
policy makers and their enforcement agents. It is presented as that which
precedes them—their object, that on which they work, invested with
the full ideological weight of Nature. Yet the family is nothing of the
kind, and its apparent stability in the field of public representation only
evidences its primarily *instrumental* role as a rigorously disciplinary
and pedagogical environment in which subjectivities are shaped and
moulded, though not without resistance. As Gayle Rubin observes, a
'domino theory of sexual peril'[4] ensures that anything which can be
represented as a threat to the family can be used to justify punitive legislation and scandalised outcries 'on behalf' of a general public which is
universally represented as entirely and unproblematically heterosexual.

In the 1987 general election campaign, the Conservative Party published a poster which appeared throughout the United Kingdom. It
showed three red books, lined up horizontally, with their titles on display: '*Young, gay & proud*', '*Police: Out of School!*' and '*The playbook for
kids about sex*'. Above them a caption asked, 'Is this Labour's idea of a
comprehensive education?', while beneath them voters were earnestly
exhorted to 'Take the politics out of education', and 'Vote Conservative'. Three strands are densely woven together: in the centre, the notion
of official institutional support for challenges to the authority of the
police, an unacceptable and horrifying threat to the central agency of
law and order, which is simultaneously 'our' most immediate and effective defensive recourse against those who threaten to corrupt and molest
'our' children, who in turn are held rigidly as parental property rather
than as individuals with their own rights. It is axiomatic to this position that 'our' children are entirely nonsexual. This fashionable return
to a pre-Freudian agenda for thinking about childhood is congruent

with the dominant structures of the New Victorianism and its theory of sexuality which continually offers us the spectacle of a heterosexual population threatened from all around by the sinister spectre of perversion, now equated with Labour Party policy, supposedly encouraging and promoting homosexuality.

We find just the same siege mentality at work in the government's AIDS information campaign, with its exclusive targeting of heterosexuals (despite the fact that, at the time of writing, there has been only one definite case in the United Kingdom of AIDS caused by HIV infection contracted sexually between a man and a woman, neither of whom was bisexual, or an IV drug user).[5] We cannot, however, afford to simply dismiss such fears as absurd, since they so evidently speak to and for the vast majority of the population. Behind the election campaign and the AIDS campaigns lies a complex of anxiety which is both social and psychic: social insofar as it is culturally transmitted and expressed, and psychic insofar as it responds to deep levels of sexual repression and guilt. Nor is the mentality of modern familialism easily open to modification, since the central identity of the parent is massively dependent on such fears and is largely stabilised by them. Hence the bizarre yet powerful convergence of popular assumptions about AIDS, regarding it simultaneously as a blessing in disguise and at the same time a threat to the very fabric of society, if not the future of the species itself. We are dealing here with profound beliefs concerning pollution, beliefs which as Mary Douglas explains:

> function to keep some categories of people apart so that others can be together. By preserving the physical categories, pollution beliefs uphold conceptual categories dividing the moral from the immoral and sustain the vision of the good society. Our analytic task is to unwind the causal theories until they reveal who is being kept out and who is being kept in.[6]

The physical and conceptual categories constructed and defended by AIDS commentary are readily apparent from the second paragraph of the Government's leaflet designed for national family consumption, which states: 'AIDS is not just a homosexual disease'. Note the 'just', and its barely concealed note of regret. Seven years into the AIDS epidemic, we hardly need to be ordered not to die of ignorance: it is the nature of the carefully orchestrated and institutionalised 'knowledges' about AIDS that are most immediately threatening. These 'knowledges' constitute a level of general AIDS awareness achieved at the direct cost of accurate risk perception or any recognition of the enormity of human suffering already occasioned in social groups which familial ideology cannot perceive as fully human. Yet familialism is not without its own internal stresses. The grimly pathological nature of much family life, for adults and children alike, is impossible to square with the banal yet dominant cultural family-ideal of maximised gender distinctions and absolute paternal authority, exercised in a domestic space of pure and uncontaminated heterosexuality. According to this picture, it is the child's moral duty to replicate the parent of its own biological sex, before settling down to the given world of labour relations and the renewed task of sexual reproduction. In this Real-Life world of humanoid Action Men and Barbie Doll marriages, it is hardly surprising that we are constantly faced with stories like that of the 'Toy Boy Love Massacre', which reveal the family in a very different light. What is most interesting here is the position of the imaginary spectator which is highly ambiguous. We read of a wife who leaves her husband, an ex-policeman, for a younger 'Toy-Boy' lover. The husband finds out and murders his wife and entire family before killing himself. Quite apart from the implied situation of domestic tension, it is far from clear whether we are intended to identify with the wronged-but-pathological husband, or with the faithless-but-independent wife. The viewing angle on such stories is radically unstable as the dominant cultural fantasy of family life. Such instability is however immediately resolved in relation to AIDS. Thus we are unambiguously asked to sympathise with the vicar who proclaims that 'I'd shoot my son if he had AIDS'. The accompanying photograph sets up the scene of such a crime, with the father pointing a shotgun at his son, above another caption which informs us that 'He would pull trigger on rest of family, too.' Let us consider this scenario. A father, who is also a priest, is saying that he would rather murder his son than acknowledge and accept the fact that the boy is gay and terminally ill. This is not held up as an example of psychotic barbarism, but on the contrary, is offered as an example of Christian moral probity. The familial message is clear: better to kill your own son than accept that he is 'queer' and already dying. This is the domestic register of the morality which speaks of the *contras* in Nicaragua as 'freedom-fighters' and which rushes to denounce 'busybody' social workers stepping in to steal children from their parents—unless it is denouncing the same social workers for their 'irresponsibility' in failing to protect the same children from the same brutalising and murderous families.

For more than five years, groups in the voluntary sector and on the fringes of the National Health Service, in the Family Planning Association, and elsewhere have struggled to achieve some kind of public recognition of the realities of AIDS. As ever, preventative medicine has been struggling against the priorities of clinical practice and the expectations of a 'magic bullet' vaccine.[7] The AIDS agenda established right across the entire media industry, and backed up by massive recent government interventions, has now succeeded in creating widespread AIDS awareness—of a kind. This awareness has been constructed around a triad of terms which are every bit as medically inaccurate as they are socially misleading and politically loaded. To begin with, we are endlessly obliged to imagine 'the AIDS virus', and by courtesy of the transmission electron micrograph we can even see it. In 1985 *The Face* referred to it as 'the spectre of the decade'.[8] In these circumstances it is absolutely crucial to distinguish between HIV infection and the various unpredictable consequences it may have in human subjects, including damage to the central nervous system, AIDS-related conditions (ARCs), total dormancy, and the wide variety of life-threatening conditions which result from damage to the body's immune system, known collectively as AIDS. The collapsing together of HIV infection and AIDS ensures that AIDS takes up both meanings and is itself perceived as a threatening condition to other people, thus creating a totally unjustified fear of people with AIDS themselves. This in turn supports the routine description of people with HIV infection *and* people with AIDS as 'AIDS carriers', with the highly misleading implication that HIV leads automatically and inexorably to AIDS, together with the strong suggestion that both conditions are contagious and transmissible by casual contact, as the ancient connotations of 'the carrier' so forcibly and mischievously imply.

From the earliest days of this epidemic, it has been the original social positions of the groups most devastated by it that have determined the ways in which the whole subject has been understood and treated— though 'treatment' in this case must also include the years of inaction, and underfunding, as much as any actual policy decisions and their consequences. HIV is thus made to appear to dictate social policy with the full authority of its medical and virological nature, and it is endlessly used as a kind of ideological glove-puppet—being made to speak on behalf of bigoted moralists in a ventriloquistic performance of great ideological sophistication and complexity. Thus children themselves are frequently recruited to the cause of making the lives of other children with HIV infections ('AIDS kids') that much more difficult than they need to be. Here at least we can clearly recognise the miserable and impoverished model of the family defended by familial politics—a model which hardly begins to deal with the actual diversity and complexity of human social, sexual, and parenting relations.

The photographic narration of AIDS reinforces the before-and-after conventions of traditional medical photography with the before-and-after conventions of standard photojournalistic practice. An emphasis is all but invariably placed on the question of fatality. This might not be so surprising, given that both HIV and AIDS remain currently incurable and irreversible, were it not for the fact that the vast majority of people with AIDS have a life-expectancy of years and spend most of their time much like everybody else, indistinguishable from the rest of the population. The AIDS agenda requires, however, that AIDS should reveal itself as the stigmata of the doomed and the damned, the concrete visible evidence of the deserts of depravity. Hence the tremendous emphasis on the physical transformation of Rock Hudson's face and body, when the entire story of his fight against AIDS was venomously constructed as the wages of sin and hypocrisy. What is at stake today is an ongoing struggle between the deeply embedded cultural picture of AIDS as retribution, and a model of health which suggests the possibility of individuals and whole social groups taking control of the circumstances and definitions of health and disease. The devastating silence which surrounds the lives of most people with HIV, ARCs, or AIDS suggests that the social constituencies which they are made to represent are officially regarded, in their totality, as disposable. Hence the fetishistic and obsessive concentration on death. Indeed, there is no way in which a person with AIDS can hope to enter the public space of photographic representation save as a sign of mortality, regardless of their own responses to AIDS. The correct site of AIDS thus emerges as the hospital or hospice, which join the prison as the just and proper latitude for the perverse. At the same time people with AIDS with particularly disfiguring symptoms will be privileged above all others insofar as their features can so easily be made to relay the values of all the surrounding commentary. And as usual, the photojournalist is confirmed in his or her role as the 'courageous' and 'intrepid' explorer of secret and forbidden realms—even bearing the torch of humanism! Thus Bob Mahoney in *Looking Death in the Face* describes how, on an assignment to photograph a gay man with AIDS, 'the job became painful, especially as [his] appearance deteriorated. In the end I had to make myself take the pictures.'[9] It is precisely that *compulsive* making of pictures, the sense of AIDS as 'a good story', that photography has so firmly established. I am not aware of a single photojournalistic

AIDS narrative published in the United Kingdom which does not collude in every respect with the overall discursive tendency to criminalise and stigmatise the hapless subjects. In another AIDS story we are told by an editorial voice-over:

> The mild-mannered detective pursuing the culprit in this mystery story is photojournalist Matt Heron. He's a good choice for the case, broadly expert where wide expertise is needed . . . 'I caught the intrigue of this bug,' Matt says. 'I'm devoting my time to uncovering the riddle of this puzzle, going to Central Africa if that's what it takes. Somebody should.'[10]

Needless to say, there is no question of photojournalists lugging their Leicas to London or Washington to explore the scandalous unavailability of drugs for people with AIDS, or to the head offices of the insurance companies which refuse insurance coverage to people with HIV infection, or to the streets of San Francisco and New York where hundreds of homeless people with AIDS sleep out rough every night of the week. What we are typically shown is a face we already know and recognise from AIDS commentary—the face of death, staring out at us with an expression of unbearable intensity and complexity. Whatever such people might be thinking, is silenced by the full weight of an agenda which constructs them unambiguously as morbid and above all *admonitory* signs of the deadly danger of sex outside the confines of the family. The unconscious of such photography is brutally direct: Homosexuality = AIDS = Death. Whether we are shown black Africans or American gays, the person with AIDS is invariably imprisoned within the demeaning category of the 'victim', in which he or she is stripped of all power and control over the actual complex meaning and dignity of an individual's life. In this manner the entire experience of living with AIDS is censored, and the diseased body is transformed into a signifying husk which is only there before our eyes to evidence the 'knowledge' of AIDS commentary which both precedes and exceeds the life of the person in the photograph, whose living being is ruthlessly obliterated. Such images repeatedly reinforce the wider cultural and political victimisation of people with AIDS by sentencing them to the black-and-white testimonial space of the 'AIDS victim'—further validating the entire, monstrous agenda which requires that people with AIDS should always appear as monsters in order to satisfy the sickeningly brutal and thinly veiled revenge fantasies of the upright guardians of 'public' decency.

This, of course, is precisely how particular groups have always been marginalised in the field of photographic practices—caught up in a documentary iconography which effortlessly transforms gay men into 'tragic queers' or 'dangerous perverts', just as blacks emerge as either docile and 'childlike', or else sinister and 'untrustworthy'. Yet at the same time a new and aggressive identity is appearing among people with AIDS, especially in America, where more than 60,000 people are currently living with AIDS and over 300 are dying every month in New York City alone. But as photography transforms people with AIDS into 'AIDS victims', they themselves are actively contesting and resisting the discursive structures which they have been made to embody. Sometimes the collision is dramatic, as in the recent case of the *Guardian*'s framing of the diary of a man who wrote clearly and positively of his rejection of the morbid fatalism surrounding his diagnosis as 'The Diary of a Condemned Man'. It is critically important to recognise that the condemnation here is taking place on the 'other side' of the lived experience of AIDS—among photographers, journalists, subeditors, and politicians. Beneath the text of the diary, a photograph appeared showing a group of men at a demonstration carrying the banner of New York's People with AIDS Alliance. This was clearly intolerable to the picture-editor of the day, who attempted to force the recalcitrant image back in line with his professional agenda by using a caption which read: 'Immunised against embarrassment: American AIDS victims'. Here once more we can identify the unconscious of AIDS commentary at work, struggling to suppress the affirmative identities of groups such as the People with AIDS Alliance and ACT UP in America and Frontliners and Body Positive in Britain, forcing them back in line with the morbid and essentially silent role which is so obviously required and expected of them. However, the 'embarrassment' here comes from within the AIDS agenda, faced with the truly terrifying spectacle of people with AIDS who calmly and confidently reject the entire pernicious ideological framework by which they have been hitherto contained. The 'AIDS victim' is the final discursive product of the AIDS agenda. Crushed, submissive, mute, he or she accepts and justifies the 'punishment' of AIDS for the unforgivable capital offence of daring to live beyond the narrow and sadistic intelligibility of familial consciousness. By contrast, the person with AIDS affirms and confirms the actual diversity and richness of human affectional and sexual experience. At this moment in time a great and historical struggle is taking place around the meaning of AIDS. Photography is one of the many cultural means by which it is being waged, challenging and interrupting the degrading spectacle of official AIDS photography. There should be no doubt in anyone's mind that the outcome of this struggle will ultimately decide who controls the most basic definitions of what it means to be a human subject—black or white, male or female, adult or child—in the modern world.

It is therefore imperative that we accept and celebrate the social, racial, and sexual diversity of our species, since it is at the level of the species that AIDS commentary offers its most extreme and apocalyptic vision. This involves devising cultural means to reinforce and encourage those behavioural changes which are the only effective means for minimising the transmission of HIV. Unfortunately, but revealingly, the dominant AIDS agenda continues to imply that it is sex *as such* which is dangerous, rather than particular forms of unprotected sexual behaviour, especially fucking. It should go without saying that it is impossible to successfully persuade people to explore the multiple erotic possibilities of safer sex from a perspective which is radically anti-erotic. We have to establish safer sex as an enlargement of our lives, rather than a restriction. This is especially difficult among heterosexual men, whose identities seem so frequently to be confined by the most limited notions of 'real' sex as unrestricted penetrative intercourse. The world does not divide up neatly between the chaste and the promiscuous, any more than it can be fully and humanely understood in terms of the Righteous and Damned. The last thing we need at this of all times is an increase in the censorship of sexual materials which can help to promote the cause of safer sex. When sex is regarded as intrinsically dirty and degrading, it will undoubtedly become dirty and degrading, and those who continue to call for ever-increasing censorship of explicit sexual materials must ultimately shoulder a large part of the responsibility for the increase in HIV infection among those who use sex as a weapon because they have never been allowed or encouraged to explore and experiment with their sexuality in any other terms. In this respect lesbians and gay men continue to provide a more mature, and flexible, and above all honest model for social and sexual relationships than is currently sanctioned anywhere else in British culture. Which in turn is precisely why AIDS has come to seem a blessing in disguise to those who are most profoundly threatened by the promise of guilt-free consensual sexuality, since its emergence among gay men can, ironically, be used against us on the grounds that it is our sexuality *per se* which causes AIDS. This argument can prosper only among those who hold to the primitive belief that the social group in which a virus emerges is in effect its cause, a belief which is entirely in keeping with the overall tendency of familialism to think of the modern world in terms of almost medieval superstition and grotesquely over-simplified dogmatism. Viruses are not choosy about whose blood they infect.

It is these positions which guarantee the continual harassment and mistreatment of people with HIV and AIDS, causing them untold suffering in relation to housing, employment, and medical treatment. The systematic persecution of people with AIDS and the tenacity of an agenda which remains silent on the subject of their ordinary day-to-day lived experience will undoubtedly come to be regarded at some later date as one of the most glaring indictments of late twentieth-century British culture. In the meantime, however, we have to work, especially at the level of representation, to transform an agenda which so belittles and impoverishes us all. We have to shift the terms of the entire AIDS debate now, before it is too late. For the sake of the thousands who have already died, and their families, and friends, we have to ensure that a whole new agenda for thinking AIDS is established, so that the morbid chorus which speaks in such gloating ways of 'AIDS victims' and 'AIDS carriers' will be fully and publicly exposed to the same contempt and humiliation which they reserve for those whose voices they have so far so effectively silenced. We will know that day has arrived only when a text which talks of people 'dying of AIDS' is automatically corrected to 'people living with AIDS'.

Conclusion

The changing imagery of AIDS is largely determined by the social history of the epidemic, which responds slowly and unevenly to new information concerning the biochemistry and natural history of HIV that has emerged in recent years.[11] For example, it is currently estimated by the Centers for Disease Control that the average time between infection and diagnosable AIDS symptoms is approximately eight years, though it should always be emphasised that such statistics are never predictive for individuals.[12] Moreover, this delay may be subject to upward revision.[13] At the same time a number of factors have effectively contributed to a significant increase in the average life-expectancy of people with AIDS in both Britain and the United States. First, it is clear that good standards of patient care, and the practice of patient-centred medicine, play an important role in improving the quality and length of life of people with AIDS. Second, the emergence of new treatment drugs has played a significantly positive role, though as Dr Mathilde Krim,

the founding chair of the American Foundation for AIDS Research (Am-
FAR) pointed out early in 1988: 'Drug development has been very slow.
We have tens of thousands of people sick . . . and only 2,900 of them are
in government clinical trials.'[14] Third, the Report of the US Presidential
Commission on AIDS and the emergence of effective activist organisations such as ACT UP have drawn attention to the gross inadequacies of
the US government's and the pharmaceutical industry's responses to the
epidemic, as well as signalled the outrage of the most severely affected
social constituencies.

In sum, it is vital to understand that HIV was widely transmitted for
at least a decade before its existence was even suspected, and that the
profile of AIDS today closely reflects the transmission of the virus some
ten years ago. Yet such relatively simple and intrinsically uncontroversial
information is not widely known, or its significance appreciated. In the
United States it would at least seem that a certain liberal consensus is
now generally supportive of people with HIV or AIDS. It remains doubtful, however whether popular medical or political understandings have
significantly improved. In this context we should consider the active
role played by frequent and widespread representations that construct
and relay the supposed 'meaning' of AIDS. In January 1988, the *New
York Times Magazine* could give over its main story to the subject, but
only as an entirely personalised and privatised account.[15] We are thus
shown an image of free-lance journalist George Whitmore, who has HIV,
relaxing with his cat: 'I'm one of the lucky ones. I haven't even been
hospitalised yet.' Then Whitmore is seen again in another photograph,
staring rather glumly at a lab full of high-tech equipment in the New
York Medical Centre, together with a research assistant who acts as a
Virgil-like guide to the complex underworld of biomedical information,
while also asserting biomedical authority within the text. Both photographs emphasise Whitmore as an individual patient, facing a medical
reality which is threatening and mysterious, and over which he exercises
little or no control himself.

It is the cumulative effect of such 'human interest' stories that remains so problematic, for they almost invariably abstract the experience
of living with AIDS away from the determining context of the major institutions of health-care provision and the state. By being repeatedly in-
dividualised, AIDS is subtly and efficiently de-politicised. For example,
you would never suspect the existence of huge national support groups
and other organisations created largely by and for people with HIV and
AIDS, or the vast network of information and treatment drugs that they
have developed for themselves.

The photographic iconography of AIDS in countless newspaper and magazine articles in the United Kingdom and the United States still massively conforms to what I have described elsewhere as 'the AIDS diptych', which narrates AIDS according to two sets of images: one focusing on colour-stained electron-microscope derived images of HIV, usually misdescribed as the 'AIDS virus', and other signs of biomedical technology and authority; the other relentlessly constructing people with AIDS as 'AIDS victims', physically debilitated and preferably disfigured.[16] Such images not only mystify the actual complex history and reality of the epidemic, they also serve to naturalise some government and medical policies at the expense of others. We are thus invited to imagine a world of supposedly disinterested medical research, with patients' best interests always in the foreground. Yet in reality, research is generally dictated by the profit motive, rather than people's medical needs. This was brilliantly exposed by the Gran Fury collective in a parody of *The New York Times* entitled *The New York Crimes,* produced by ACT UP for a demonstration against the intransigent neglect of AIDS by New York's City Hall. Across a full-page image of a scientific petri-dish, with an anonymous lab technician's hand clad in a rubber glove and holding out a pipette, we read a quote attributed to a spokesman from a leading pharmaceutical company: 'One million [people with AIDS] isn't a market that's exciting. Sure it's growing, but it's not asthma.' At the bottom of the page, we read the simple message: 'This Is to Enrage You'. The juxtaposition of words and image provokes us to think about how 'science' may indeed be photographed, not simply as a field of incomprehensible yet heroic research, but as a site of complex conflicting values, beliefs, and methods. This is precisely the history that most AIDS photojournalism suppresses.

Much of the uncertainty and confusion surrounding most aspects of AIDS may also be attributed to the development of 'official', and often state-funded, AIDS information materials. For example, the New York State and New York City departments of health have for several years distributed leaflets and posters that show a fairly wide cross-section of the population under a banner statement: 'AIDS does not discriminate'. Such an approach is to some extent understandable, given the dominant journalistic construction of AIDS as intrinsically connected to gay male sex or the sharing of intravenous drug equipment. Yet by showing a mixed group of women and men, albeit of different racial origins, we are left with a new set of mystifications. For it is clear that HIV has had an overwhelmingly disproportionate effect in population groups that were already profoundly marginalised long before the epidemic began—

particularly African Americans and the Hispanic community. Of course AIDS itself does not discriminate, but nonetheless discrimination in relation to the availability of adequate health care provision and health education remains a major factor in determining one's risk of HIV infection. This is especially true of societies such as the United States, which so conspicuously lacks the provision of socialised medicine: a lack that goes much of the way to explain the seriousness and extent of the national epidemic.

Having refused for years to heed the advice of AIDS service organisations in the voluntary sector, the British government's Health Education Authority (HEA) recently launched a new campaign of photo-based ads that seek to establish the distinction between HIV and AIDS. Yet the way in which the HEA has sought to clarify this important point still conforms to the larger ideological agenda of most public AIDS commentary in the west. Throughout the British press, for example, we were shown an image of a stereotypically glamorous young woman, with a caption underneath that reads: 'If This Woman Had the Virus Which Leads to AIDS, in a Few Years She Could Look Like the Person Over the Page'. Turning the page, we find exactly the same photograph, but this time with the terse caption: 'Worrying, Isn't It'. The implied meaning is clear: we are meant to be worried by the fact that a beautiful (and sexually available) woman might have HIV, 'we' being heterosexual men. A woman with HIV would certainly not find it 'worrying' that she looks perfectly well.

It is almost impossible to imagine any other group of people living with a manageable yet chronic disease who could be presented as a public problem for the simple reason that they look, and to all extents and purposes are, well and healthy. Moreover, such images demonstrate the long-term consequences of the confusion of HIV and AIDS, and the tendency to think of people with chronic disease in terms of infectious illness. Thus people with HIV are made to embody the powerful and misleading notion of 'AIDS carriers'. Well or ill, they are reduced to the status of *deterrents,* used to frighten people about sex, in a manner which taps into deep-seated misogynistic anxieties concerning female sexuality, and guilt about sexual pleasure. Thus people with HIV are tacitly understood to be in some way 'guilty' for having been infected, while HIV is also understood as a reflection of excessive or immoral sexual behaviour. In this way the fantasy that HIV affects only certain types of people (prostitutes, the 'promiscuous', the 'unfaithful', and so on) is protected. Supposedly 'ordinary' women and men are thereby reassured that there is nothing for them to worry about. But HIV is not necessarily associated with particular types of people or any sexual acts except unprotected intercourse, and risk comes as one writer puts it, not from how you label yourself but from what you *do*.[17]

Many of the problems of the photography that I've discussed derive from ways in which the various institutions that generate photographs— from photojournalism to 'art' photography—have traditionally represented lives and social groups that are usually culturally visible only as 'deviants' or 'exotic'. Thus the widespread notion that intravenous drug users constitute a recognisable type obscures the fact that many people may inject drugs at some time or other. Yet photography rarely attempts to explore the wide latitude of intravenous drug use, or of sexual practices, and instead seeks refuge in easily identified stereotypes—especially when it is employed by other institutions, including the press and the state, that have a major investment in just such stereotypes. As a result we rarely gain any real sense of the scale or complexity of the epidemic, for this would involve a visually immediate acknowledgement of the actual diversity of drug use and sexuality in everyday life, a diversity which is evidently very threatening to many institutions, especially those that have a major investment in policing and defining our perceptions of ourselves and the world we live in. Thus we also see little or nothing of the scale of community-based support and activism for people with HIV and AIDS, for such images would likewise threaten to interrupt the pious sentimentality with which this epidemic is quietly and tastefully celebrated. Instead we see 'AIDS victims', isolated, often hospitalised, frequently near death, in the face of which they are shown to be meek and—most dishonest of all—accepting. It is in this context that we might usefully recall the words of Michael Callen, who has lived with AIDS for seven years. As he points out, this type of single-minded emphasis on fatality 'denies the reality of—but perhaps more important, the possibility of—our survival'.[18]

In any case, photography's conventional eye has long fixed the look of disaster in the likeness of passive, suffering 'victims', in both news and documentary images. Heroic or pathetic, the 'victim' invariably waits, dependent on the faint chance of relief or remedy, understood to be beyond his or her personal control. Hence the 'victim' is constructed as a universal category, constituted in images which are accepted because we recognise that we are all ultimately subject to the same common order of mortality. Yet as James Baldwin argues, this acknowledgement should be the source of our dignity as a species, rather than a pretext for oversimplification, since the awareness 'that isolation and death are certain and universal clarifies our responsibility'.[19] The photographic construction of the 'AIDS victim' on the contrary depicts AIDS as always *someone else's* problem, rather than a *collective* social issue. Thus the most familiar range of photographic images of people with AIDS functions to protect and defend audiences from recognising that AIDS might ever be a reality for themselves. Nor is this specific to the signification of AIDS. For example, the image of a Sudanese child dying of starvation may be used to represent the failure of the rain season, or to embody the intractability of a 'Marxist regime', but almost never to signify the direct social consequences of western capitalist financial and political policies.[20] Moreover, the chronically sick have generally tended to be presented as emblems of disease rather than as people who are often as much in control of most aspects of their lives as anybody else.[21]

Nonetheless there is growing awareness in both Britain and the United States of the yawning gulf between the political and psychic realities of this epidemic and the impoverished and punitive imagery through which its public face is habitually registered. It is not surprising that this awareness has been keenest among those most deeply involved in the complex realities of AIDS, understood as a biomedical, political, and cultural phenomenon. In the United States both Jan Zita Grover and Douglas Crimp have written eloquently of the emergent cultural response to AIDS among progressive artists and photographers, while others including Kristen Engberg have—like Grover—curated major exhibitions.[22] In Britain, a number of photographers are also working to establish an understanding of the wider network of social, economic and political factors that play such a major role in determining the situation of people living with HIV and AIDS. For HIV-related disease is never 'just an illness', as Susan Sontag has claimed.[23] On the contrary, throughout the west it has engaged the most vicious forces of racism, misogyny, classism, and homophobia, in ways that cannot be adequately explained by recourse to the history of medicine alone, as many commentators are now attempting to do.[24] At any given moment, the epidemic should also always be thought of as a still-life that is every bit as rich and complex as that of any seventeenth-century Dutch artist: a still-life that contains many bottles of drugs, together with the multinational pharmaceutical industry that generates and markets them, and the government agencies that regulate (and frequently inhibit) their availability. The imagery of AIDS includes keys to properties illegally reclaimed by fearful and bigoted landlords; job contracts terminated by prejudiced employers;

interminable application forms for every aspect of welfare, social security, and sickness benefits; rejected health insurance and life insurance claims; travel-passes for the disabled; and the collective cultural, political, and personal achievements of thousands of groups and organisations around the world working on behalf of the rights and needs of people with HIV and its many consequences. Not least, the AIDS tableau should finally include some suggestion of the constant avalanche of photographs that continue to do so much to undermine the confidence and dignity of people attempting to live their lives with all the humour and courage that they can collectively muster. Writing as a woman who has used photography to explore her own situation as someone living with cancer, British photographer Jo Spence insists that:

> not only do we need to use photography to try to make visible what is not being talked about by those in power . . . but the other side of the coin . . . that only by using photography to ask new questions can we then begin to understand the systematic denial of the reality and fantasies of groups and individuals who have plenty to say, who have been silenced, or who are still fighting to speak.[25]

In all of this it is still important to avoid the conclusion that photography has simply 'misrepresented' AIDS, with the implication that at the end of the day there is indeed a clear, unitary visual 'truth' of the epidemic that might be directly accessible to the camera. Photographers are particularly well positioned to interrupt the constant flow of images that conflate HIV and AIDS and to challenge the crude and cruel version of the epidemic that continues to regard AIDS as a moral verdict rather than a medical diagnosis. For if we accept that photography participates in the practice of representation that forges our identities, we should be as sensitive to its potential to produce subjects as we are to its undoubted capacity to define objects.

8. 'AIDS' or 'HIV Disease'?

Most readers of *Capital Gay* will be familiar with the history of how the Acquired Immune Deficiency Syndrome was first identified in the United States in 1981.[1] Doctors in New York and Los Angeles had independently reported significant clusters of cases of two previously very rare medical conditions—pneumocystis carinii pneumonia (PCP), and a form of cancer known as Kaposi's sarcoma (KS). The only connection between these, and a number of other rare diseases being reported amongst otherwise healthy young gay men, was their known association with damage to the body's immunological defences. Because these clusters were first identified among gay men, they were at first collectively described as Gay Related Immune Deficiency (GRID). It was eventually recognised (and not without considerable resistance on the part of some doctors and epidemiologists) that the underlying cause of these clusters of rare diseases was not specific to gay men, especially after it was discovered that the unknown agent responsible for them could be transmitted via blood transfusions. Thus, in 1982, the Centers for Disease Control (CDC) in Atlanta, Georgia officially classified the condition as Acquired Immune Deficiency Syndrome, by which name it is still widely described.

The Human Immunodeficiency Virus (HIV), which is responsible for AIDS, was not isolated until 1983, and not made public until the following year. In all of this it is important to remember that doctors, and members of the gay community were working backwards in a detective manner, in order to establish the agent responsible for AIDS, and to understand its possible modes of transmission in order to protect people. Thus it was that Michael Callen and Richard Berkowitz wrote their ground-breaking pamphlet 'How to have sex in an epidemic' with a preface by Dr Joseph Sonnabend, in 1983, on the assumption that some sexually transmitted factor was responsible for many if not all cases of AIDS. That was the originating moment of what we all now know as safer sex. Nonetheless, even now in 1988 the distinction between HIV and AIDS is still far from universally understood, and AIDS is widely regarded as if it were a single disease, rather than a syndrome, which refers to a huge range of conditions which may emerge in the wake of HIV infection, and damage to the body's immunological defences.

Hence the need to repeat that AIDS is not a single condition, and that different people diagnosed with AIDS will not, therefore, necessarily share medical or clinical experience. AIDS can be experienced in a wide variety of sequences and combinations of what are known as 'opportunistic' conditions—conditions which have taken the 'opportunity' (horrible word) of damage caused by HIV. It should also be stressed that most of the conditions which may lead to an AIDS diagnosis are present in all of us, but are held in check by our immune systems. It is this set of relatively straightforward facts which is difficult to communicate to many people because of the way in which AIDS was first identified and classified back in 1982. Many of the most basic misunderstandings about AIDS stem from a failure by journalists and others to appreciate the sheer diversity of medical experience, and the complexity of issues raised by a syndrome. To describe AIDS as if it were a single disease is an easy option, but it obscures almost all the real issues faced by individuals with AIDS, and has led to any number of misleading assumptions and ill-informed beliefs about almost every aspect of the epidemic. For example, many people still talk about 'catching AIDS', and the belief that there is an 'AIDS test' remains unfortunately widespread.

There are thus strong reasons why we should consider following the example of doctors who have by-passed the notion of AIDS, just as AIDS by-passed the earlier classification of GRID. They talk of HIV infection, referring to the specific and limited modes of transmission of the virus, and HIV disease, referring to the disease of the immune system itself, and referring to the wide spectrum of subsequent medical conditions which may arise in the wake of HIV infection. There is another compelling reason why we should consider this as a significant advance. As knowledge concerning the effects of HIV grew in the 1980s, it became clear that a large number of people with HIV were becoming seriously ill, though they did not have illnesses which are officially classified as AIDS. The revision and enlargement of the diagnostic category of AIDS by the CDC in August 1987 has not really improved the situation of all those people who still find themselves diagnosed as people with AIDS

Related Complex (ARC), sometimes known as AIDS Related Conditions. A diagnosis of ARC is in some ways even more difficult for many individuals to live with than a diagnosis of either HIV infection or AIDS. ARC is widely seen as an 'in-between' condition, halfway between HIV and AIDS. This only encourages the use of absurd terms like 'full-blown AIDS' to refer to people with symptoms of the syndrome, and implies that people with ARC have 'half' or 'semi-blown' AIDS!

It is clear that nobody set out to deliberately construct this Chinese Box of medical categories, with all the confusion and misunderstanding which they tend to reinforce. The easiest and most logical way forward would surely be to gradually abandon the categories of ARC and AIDS altogether, and to encourage the adoption of the simpler—and more accurate—distinction, between HIV infection and HIV disease. In this way large numbers of people would be spared the totally unnecessary stress involved in an ARC diagnosis, which is a cruel and sadistic category with which nobody should in future be obliged to identify their experience of HIV disease. This would also have the advantage of undermining much of the demonising mythology surrounding the present classification of AIDS. It would also make the task of HIV education far easier, and by making the epidemic more comprehensible to more people, might help in the crucial task of preventing further infections, and improving the general quality of life of everyone affected by the consequences of HIV infection and HIV disease.

9. 'The Day After Hiroshima': Reflections on official British and Swedish AIDS education materials and government policies

Whilst it is important to understand the global impact of AIDS, as it was described at the World Health Organisation's Summit Conference in London in January 1988, I would like to emphasise that it is equally important to realise that each country affected by HIV has its own distinct epidemic, shaped according to its own national culture, access to health-care provision, health education strategies, and so on. In this respect we must recognise that the Swedish AIDS epidemic is quite distinct from that in Norway, or the Netherlands, or Britain. Furthermore, the epidemic is lived differently in Stockholm for example than in Vasteros or Malmo. We should always remember that an epidemic is a complex social and bio-ecological phenomenon. At the same time we should try to relate HIV and AIDS to the wider local framework of disease and health-care provision in any given society.

It may be instructive to begin by comparing the situation in Britain to that in Sweden. In Britain we have approximately ten times as many cases of AIDS as there are in Sweden. However, since our overall population is seven times larger, the rate of cases per 100,000 is not so very different. Yet the social context of the British epidemic could hardly be more unlike that in Scandinavia. For example, antenatal care has stagnated in many regions for more than thirty years.[1] The Royal College of Physicians recently reported that more than 2000 premature infants die unnecessarily each year in England and Wales due to cuts in hospital equipment, and staff shortages.[2] In the West Midlands, 93 per cent of hospital buildings are officially described as being in poor repair. Fire standards are not met in 33 Scottish wards for elderly and physically handicapped people.[3] Cancer treatment which was routine for women in their sixties ten years ago is no longer available. In October 1988 a government Minister of Health, Mrs Edwina Currie, was widely reported when she gave a speech recommending old people to start knitting warm clothing in order to avoid hypothermia in the coming winter!

At the same time, the social constituency most directly affected by HIV and AIDS has been subjected to the most punitive homophobic legislation seen anywhere in Europe since Germany's notorious Paragraph 175, in 1935. In the field of AIDS education, the government has recently announced plans to dis-fund the country's largest and oldest AIDS service organisation, the Terrence Higgins Trust, which in any case only receives a mere £100,000 from the State in order to finance all its health-education materials, buddying services, telephone hotlines, and so on. The Department of Health has also censored the government's own Health Education Authority's AIDS education materials, produced for school teachers, and a book for professional health educators, on the grounds that these do not sufficiently follow the government's 'moral agenda' for dealing with AIDS. Sadly, such measures are only likely to *increase* the transmission of HIV in Britain, by denying people access to information which alone can save lives. It would seem that the strong national current of homophobia, which has wrecked and sometimes destroyed lesbian and gay lives in Britain for centuries, will ironically now lead to the deaths of heterosexuals themselves.

I therefore hope that I make myself clear when I say that I am only too well aware of the tremendous challenge facing everyone in the task of HIV education in these difficult times. Like others in Britain and around the world, I proceed from a sense of great respect for the values and achievements of social democracy in Sweden, especially since I come from a country with a grossly unrepresentative political system, in which the very notion of a genuinely democratic party politics has all but broken down in the course of the last decade. A country where direct government censorship of the mass media has become a commonplace, where whole levels of local government have simply been abolished if they disagreed with government policies, and where increasingly authoritarian attitudes are very widespread. As Hanif Kureishi pointed out recently, our little 'Prague Spring' of the 1960s is long gone, and England (if not the UK as a whole), is nowadays an 'intolerant, racist, homophobic narrow-minded authoritarian rat-hole, run by vicious suburban-minded materialistic philistines, who think democracy is constituted by selling off . . . council houses and shares'.[4]

I would remind you that we are dealing with a seemingly new virus, which emerged in the West amongst gay men and injecting drug users at some time in the early 1970s, when its existence was, of course, entirely unknown and unsuspected. According to the Centers for Disease Control in Atlanta, Georgia (USA), the average length of time between infection by HIV and an AIDS diagnosis, is eight years in otherwise healthy people. This means that AIDS statistics today reflect transmission events which took place eight years ago in many cases. Thus, whilst cases of AIDS amongst young people are still comparatively rare, we should note the significance of the time-delay factor. Many were clearly infected as teenagers. The future of AIDS will only be determined by the success or failure of our primary prevention strategies today. In this context I would only repeat the statement by Dr Allan Brandt that 'there will be no simple answer to this health crisis'. As he argues, no health promotion campaign based on fear has ever been effective, and no single intervention—not even a vaccine—'will adequately address the complexities of the AIDS epidemic'.[5]

The difference of the Swedish response from that in Norway, or Denmark, or even Britain, could hardly be more striking. The Swedish government's AIDS Delegation has invested most of its funds (and its faith) in HIV testing, as if this were intrinsically the most effective means to prevent the transmission of HIV. This seems to me to be a delusion, and a delusion which is potentially extremely dangerous in the long-run—both for the Swedish people, and for other countries which might be tempted to follow the Swedish example. Do not misunderstand: I am arguing neither for nor against HIV testing *per se,* I am however insisting that we should consider the nature, purposes, and consequences of HIV testing very seriously, and certainly more so than appears to have been the case in Sweden.

There are at least two strong arguments on behalf of the HIV antibody test. First, epidemiologists need to assay the incidence and prevalence of HIV in order to direct appropriate resources to those groups which are most in need, whoever and wherever they may be. Second, the test is important in order to guarantee access to treatment for individuals in need, whoever and wherever they may be. But the HIV test is not, in itself, whether results are positive or negative, a guarantee of any kind concerning subsequent behaviourial change, as several independent surveys in Europe and the USA have demonstrated. It is the quality of the accompanying counselling which may help save lives, and this is rarely discussed in Sweden. If you have adequate counselling, you may not need the test. Swedish AIDS education advertisements repeatedly emphasise people's fears and anxieties but with the extraordinary assumption that a negative HIV test result will automatically resolve and alleviate them.

On the contrary, testing sadly tends only to reinforce people's fears, as is widely demonstrated by the international phenomenon of compulsive repeat-testing amongst the 'worried well'. Nor, I believe, should we encourage complacency amongst those who have had the good fortune to discover that they are seronegative. A negative test result may frequently lead to an entirely false sense of security, and the resumption of very unsafe sex indeed.

Whilst Swedish AIDS publicity stresses that HIV testing is voluntary, it is in fact widely regarded as a routine matter of standard medical practice. Laws which require individuals to have the test, if they have had sex with someone known to be seropositive hardly help matters, especially since they do not recognise any distinction between safe, and *potentially* unsafe, sex. Such legislation can only serve to undermine confidence in the wisdom and sense of concern of the Swedish government, especially on the part of those most immediately and directly affected by the epidemic. Nor does the overall policy take any account of the straightforward statistical problems of sensitivity and specificity (true positives and false negatives) involved in the large-scale testing of population groups in which HIV remains very rare. This problem has been admirably summarised by the World Health Organisation.[6]

There is also a fundamental contradiction between Swedish attitudes towards HIV testing, and attitudes to safer sex. Young Swedes are strongly recommended to take the test if they are worried about AIDS, or if they are starting a new relationship. Yet a negative test result is only likely to undermine the need for safer sex, especially in population groups with little or no direct experience of AIDS. Testing should never be regarded as an obligation. If testing is regarded as obligatory, it can hardly be described as voluntary. This brings me to what I regard as the central delusion about HIV testing, namely, the fantasy that in spite of HIV, life can go on very much as before. The notion that one can identify everyone with HIV, and then forget all about AIDS, strikes me as offensive and dangerous. As one American doctor stated recently 'It is like the day after Hiroshima—the world has changed and will never be the same again'.[7] The powerful idea that everyone with HIV can be identified can only damage the prospects of effective safer sex education, which is the only proven means to prevent transmission. You cannot test HIV out of existence.

In recent years I have observed the international emergence of two basic approaches to AIDS education—which I have described elsewhere as the Terrorist Model and the Missionary Model.[8] The former regards

HIV rather like an illegal immigrant, or a hijacker (or perhaps as a Russian submarine in this case, slipping invisibly into Stockholm harbour). The solution is invariably understood as a barrier or a net, in the form of prophylactics or HIV testing or a combination of both. The latter regards HIV as a species of heathen—a degenerate or a pervert, who must be converted to the moral virtues of Christian marriage, to celibacy or monogamy. What is extraordinary and specific to the Swedish AIDS response is its vigorous simultaneous deployment of both these models, and the differing strategies they invoke. Yet if I may paraphrase the American doctor whom I quoted earlier, it is clear that there has never been a society anywhere on earth in which the patterns of sexual behaviour were exclusively restricted to monogamy or celibacy—and it is, to say the least, highly unlikely that either Britain or Sweden in the 1990s will become the first.

Young people everywhere need and deserve a model of AIDS education, which faces the complex reality of actually existing social and sexual relations which can draw on the forces within youth culture which can make safer sex both *sexy* and *fashionable*—allowing young people to experiment, as experiment they must, but without putting themselves or one another at risk. Cindy Patton has pointed out, risk comes from what you do, not how you label yourself.[9] As I have written elsewhere 'If sex were not pleasurable, people would not be at risk, and we cannot help people if we deny all pleasure in sex.'[10] We should all remember the character in the Woody Allen film who, when informed that sex without love is 'an empty experience', replied that 'as empty experiences go, it's one of the best'. Such sentiments may of course offend some people, but we have to decide whether we think that the sensibilities of a small, if vocal, minority, are more important than other people's lives.

Sadly, the subject of sexual behaviour is once again surrounded by a thick fog of moralising, ruthless sentimentality, and plain hypocrisy. There are few people in this world who have only ever had one sexual relationship. Yet their exceptional experience is held up to the rest of us as if it were an intrinsic good, and a model for everyone else to emulate. We know that marriages and other relationships can go wrong. In such circumstances we all have to start again sooner or later, looking for a sexual partner or partners. We also know that many 'successful' marriages are more-or-less sexless, and survive because one or both partners has sex elsewhere. This is the context in which we have to plan safer sex information. As an American journalist points out 'the idea that people need powerful external controls to say 'no' is characteristic of this and every other era of sexual conservatism. In this regard the political right wing has played a powerful role in influencing the limits of acceptable public discourse'.[11] The political right may have set this agenda, but it is certainly not their monopoly, as debates in both Britain and Sweden demonstrate. We should recall that only sixty years ago it was more permissable to contract a sexually transmitted disease in private than it was to talk about it in public. If these are the 'Victorian values' which Mrs Thatcher, and many others who would not describe themselves as conservative, wish to reimpose on us, then the prospects for effective AIDS education look decidedly bleak.

Yet this is evidently not the way in which the Swedish government wishes to proceed. On the contrary, it provides Noah's Ark, Sweden's leading AIDS service organisation, with six times more money than the British government gives to the Terrence Higgins Trust. Noah's Ark also receives a further £1,000,000 to £1,500,000 from the Red Cross, and additional funding from other sources. The Swedish government has also given a quasi-legal status to lesbian and gay relationships and has recently financed what is widely regarded as the finest lesbian and gay social centre in Europe. Such measures remain of course entirely unthinkable in Britain. Yet whereas Sweden has tended to follow the general social democratic principle of decentralisation in other areas of social policy, consulting with individual social groups on matters which affect them—in relation to AIDS all this has been reversed. The Swedish government appears to have completely forgotten its honourable former principle that the state should not attempt to do what other social organisations can do better. This is especially noticeable in relation to policy decisions concerning injecting drug users and their sexual partners. Swedish drug information and social policy was entirely de-centralised in recent years, until the emergence of HIV, which is clearly understood to require central government intervention on a national scale. It is as if nothing had really been learned from hard-won previous experience. This situation is strikingly different to that across the border in Norway, where politicians initially approached the national Council for Gay Health, and other gay organisations, to invite them to draw up the country's AIDS education programme, including the excellent materials for all Norwegian school pupils.

One need only compare the AIDS education pamphlets produced for Norwegian schools to those produced for Swedish schools to recognise the enormity of the difference between the two national responses. The cultural relations between Norway and Sweden are rather like those between Scotland and England, but I cannot believe that the two countries are so very different that Norway has visible, articulate lesbian and gay teenagers, whilst Sweden apparently has none. The absence of visible gay teenagers who, after all, are the group of young people most at risk from HIV, from such materials in Sweden, closely resembles the similar amnesia affecting the British government, which demanded the withdrawal of AIDS education materials for schools for the explicit reason that they dared to acknowledge the existence of lesbian and gay teenagers. However, in relation to AIDS education such a refusal to acknowledge the reality of sexual diversity is not merely moralistic—it is potentially dangerous. Indeed, it is difficult to avoid the conclusion that a society which prefers to pretend that gay teenagers don't exist would not miss them were they all to disappear. It is important to realise the full significance of the fact that many people consciously or unconsciously consider AIDS to be an extremely convenient phenomenon, ridding the world of regrettable and unwanted minorities.

Fortunately I am sure that British and Swedish youth are not so stupid as their parents in such matters. Most young people know perfectly well that their aunt Mary is a lesbian, or that Roger and Peter who run the local garage are gay, or that Michael or Helen or Thomas in their school class are gay or lesbian. Few young people think of gay teenagers as if they were aliens from outer space, and if they do, it is a sad reflection on the power of bigotry and ignorance at home over genuine education at school and from life. AIDS education materials which fail to adequately address the real difficulties facing gay teenagers today will quite rightly be dismissed in their entirety as inadequate and untrustworthy by most young people. If AIDS educators omit gay youth from their considerations, they run the very serious risk of undermining their message amongst the rest of the population, as well as leaving young gay people feeling more isolated and vulnerable than ever. AIDS education would be much improved if adults were obliged to watch safer sex videos and to read leaflets written for them by their children, who generally have a much more sophisticated understanding of risk factors.

By telling teenagers to stick with one sexual partner, and to take an HIV test if they are worried, Swedish AIDS education fails to recognise that neither of these options provides a realistic solution to the issue of HIV. Besides, both messages are in conflict with the urgent task of establishing safer sex as a central and indispensable element of youth culture. We have to produce AIDS information which emphasises the pleasures of safer sex rather than the fear of death. On the whole young people are very good at helping one another through difficult times. We will certainly not help them to help one another if we continue to pretend that HIV testing and the number of one's sexual partners are the central issues in AIDS education. People will not take to safer sex if it is continually presented as an *injunction,* and regarded as essentially negative. Nor should we imply that safer sex is boring and mechanical—something like putting on a diving-costume in order to have sex. Unfortunately a large number of people who have rushed in to talk about the need for safer sex, and to make videos and write pamphlets are working to a pre-AIDS agenda, and are actually far more concerned in stopping what they see as 'promiscuity', than in stopping AIDS. Perhaps many adults take refuge in the fantasy of perpetual testing because they are in fact afraid of safer sex themselves, and the possibly threatening implications of increased eroticism, and a challenge to traditional gender roles?

I fear that if Sweden continues with its current policies, the only result will be a generation of severely sexually disturbed young people, and a large number of AIDS cases, which might have been avoided. Besides, do we really want to encourage people to settle down for life with their first sexual partner primarily out of fear of HIV? It is difficult to imagine a more sure-fire recipe for marital misery, violence, and (presumably unsafe) extra-marital infidelity. No one chooses to enter a relationship which will go wrong, any more than anyone chooses to get sick. If AIDS education materials continue to pump out the ridiculous message that everyone can and should settle down for life with the first person they fall in love with, or have sex with (and these are frequently not the same person) we are turning our backs on everything that we have learned about human sexuality and relationships in the twentieth century. Is this the great 'morality' which we wish to communicate? If so, it reflects very badly indeed on our ethical standards. In any case, as we all know deep down if we are honest with ourselves, neither a wedding ring nor a vow of fidelity is or ever will be an effective prophylactic against this, or any other virus.

This is why we urgently need to develop a community model of safer sex education, which will give adults and young people alike a new sense of collective achievement and self-esteem both of which derive from the sure and certain knowledge that we have faced a difficult and unprecedented situation and not pretended that there is a single, simple answer to all our problems. At the moment a certain 'common sense' prevails in Sweden, a common sense which has led to the closing of saunas, the mass screening of pregnant women, and the making routine of HIV testing for everyone. But there is never only one common sense. For example, we need only consider the new legislation on infectious diseases in Sweden, which suggests that a person with HIV is actually contagious, and a threat to society. The vital distinction between contagious disease and infections with specific and limited modes of transmission is thus denied and increasingly punitive measures are put into effect. Yet the Danes have recently abolished their old infectious disease legislation. We might equally contrast Swedish attitudes towards prostitutes at this time to the situation in The Netherlands, where prostitution was legalised in 1987, and a number of seropositive prostitutes were given licences to work on the sensible grounds that someone who has contracted HIV is likely to prove a particularly good safer sex educator. And in any case, prostitutes tend to be highly conscious of the risk of sexually transmitted diseases, and all over Europe have organised HIV education for themselves. If prostitutes are stigmatised, they are put at greater risk because they are denied access to the information which can save lives. We should also note that most prostitutes are more at risk from shared needles, or sexual contact with injecting drug users, than from any other source. It is *they* who are vulnerable. The Danish and Dutch governments are not stupid, and they recognise that we cannot legislate HIV out of existence. The great danger now in Sweden is that punitive social policies and legislation will drive HIV underground, and people at greatest risk of HIV infection will not feel free to take the test, and will thus be denied treatment which might prolong their lives.[12]

Whilst we know that everyone who has unprotected sex, or who shares needles is potentially at risk of HIV infection, it is not the case that we are all equally at risk. The inability to recognise that HIV was widely transmitted amongst gay men and drug users in the West for many years, long before its existence was recognised, has led the Swedish authorities to direct far more attention to those least at risk than to those who are in fact most vulnerable. We all know that HIV is not intrinsically a 'gay plague' as the British press still loves to describe it; but a response which fails to acknowledge that injecting drug users and gay men are most at risk has surely missed the point? The fear of an anti-gay 'backlash' is often used in Britain and in Sweden to justify existing policies. But this is surely extremely cynical. Is it better for governments to make life even more difficult for the communities already devastated by HIV, than to guarantee to protect their basic human rights and to lead the fight against prejudice?

So, as Cindy Patton has argued, we must all learn to think of ourselves as safer sex teachers. Such an approach gives people confidence to exercise real choices in their lives, and allows us not to be constantly terrorised by this wretched virus. We need accurate, non-judgemental information, which explains the modes of transmission of HIV. We need to treat people as adults, and to recognise that we can all calculate the risk of HIV infection in our lives, be it great or small. We also need to establish the opportunity to talk about our feelings, including our fears, in order to change attitudes, rather than smothering or denying our emotions with the pretence of a simple technological solution.[13]

Sweden, like Britain, urgently needs to re-think all aspects of national AIDS education. This does not mean that governments should start hiring new commercial advertising agencies, for this would only repeat the most basic errors in previous campaigns. If we reject those with the most experience of AIDS education, in favour of supposedly 'professional' advertising companies, we will only end up with the familiar type of over-generalised messages aimed at a vague and oversimplified 'general public', with which nobody can easily identify.

Instead of trying to frighten people into not having sex, we should be trying to encourage people to have safer sex. When bigots claim that this is 'encouraging promiscuity' we need to be able to point out very clearly that the human race has not needed government AIDS education on television in the past in order to enjoy sex.

By far the most effective safer sex education takes place in small face-to-face group sessions, where people can ask the questions they want answered, and share their experiences and feelings. This will be expensive, but will undoubtedly prove cost-effective in the long run as new cases of HIV infection are avoided. It cannot be sufficiently stressed that the success of safer sex education today will only be reflected in the AIDS statistics at the end of the century. In the meantime we can begin to evaluate our work in a number of ways. These include a full understanding of the distinction between HIV and AIDS, and an equally full understanding of the HIV antibody test. We will also know that our education projects are really working when people feel sufficiently confident to reject advice and information which is more concerned with stopping sex than stopping AIDS. People must be actively encouraged to make their own assessments of AIDS education campaigns, and to distrust those which contain factual inaccuracies, or conflicting messages. Safer sex campaigns must be taken out of the hands of advertising agencies and politicians and doctors who have no experience whatsoever in the field of health promotion, and must be produced in full consultation with community groups and representatives. We should demand accurate information and adequate resources as our collective right. Above all we need to avoid the types of advertising which are vague and unclear, for example the Swedish message to holiday-makers returning home, which asks them if they have 'exchanged experiences on holiday'? It would be much better to point out to visitors travelling overseas that they can play a role in the international struggle against HIV, and encourage them to have a really good—safe—time!

In conclusion, I can only repeat that the Swedish obsession with testing can only serve to promote an attitude of 'sex as usual' amongst those who test negative. The widespread, routine use of HIV testing in populations at low risk of infection is sadly only likely to make Swedish society increasingly hysterical and neurotic about all aspects of sex, and this will help nobody, least of all those with HIV or AIDS, who are most in need of support. Perhaps we can make some good from the tragedy of AIDS by using safer sex education to enlarge rather than still-further decrease the possibilities for human relationships. Some people unfortunately persist in blaming AIDS on the supposed weakness of what they think of as 'traditional' morality. On the contrary, I think we should emphasise that it is precisely the narrow and cruel standards of an inflexible moralism which threatens to make AIDS into a still greater tragedy— by making it so difficult for many people to talk openly and honestly about sex by blanketing all aspects of human sexuality in a dense cloud of ignorance and guilt. Rather than surrendering to a small minority of ignorant bigots, who wish to exploit AIDS to their own purposes, and turn the clock of history back one hundred years, we must be vigilant to resist and overcome sexual guilt in our work as AIDS educators, rather than reinforcing it. For let there be no mistake, it is ignorance and guilt and prejudice and fear which are the biggest threats to AIDS education, and the best allies HIV can possibly have.

10. Cross-Over: A film by
Staffan Hildebrand

In the glossy publicity materials which accompany Swedish filmmaker Staffan Hildebrand's latest film, *Cross-Over,* we can read how, in the course of filming, he took the hand of a man dying from AIDS. He recalls thinking 'that I definitely, once and for all, will be contaminated and die'. Hildebrand's fears are not of course unreal, or uncommon, and they subtly inform every aspect of his film—from the 'experts' he selects to speak, the words that he retains on his soundtrack, the locations in which he films, and the overall message that his film conveys. Given the authority of television in the modern world, and the vital need to produce effective AIDS education materials, we should consider *Cross-Over* very seriously indeed—especially in relation to its intended audience, young people.

Cross-Over belongs to a familiar genre of documentary filmmaking which I have described elsewhere as 'AIDS-safari journalism'.[1] We are whisked around the world at great speed to a wide variety of exotic locations, from Manilla to The Bronx. Yet the picture we see everywhere is effectively the same, since such films proceed from the profoundly misleading assumption that we can and should think of AIDS as a uniform, global phenomenon, rather than as a series of quite distinct epidemics, affecting different societies and cultures in very different ways. It is therefore hardly surprising if *Cross-Over* seems to be little more than a public-relations exercise on behalf of the Swedish government's AIDS Delegation view of the subject. This is particularly regrettable, since the official Swedish response (with its emphasis on personal anxiety and fear) to HIV and AIDS is so dramatically unlike that of any other Scandinavian country.[2]

If Hildebrand had made a film which had addressed his own fears in public we might at least have had an opportunity to think seriously

about how we might discuss, analyse, and dispel some of the irrational feeling—and policies—which are provoked by AIDS. Instead, we
have yet another film which oversimplifies almost every aspect of the
epidemic, and tends only to reinforce ill-informed public anxieties, by
making the epidemic seem even more terrifying for many viewers than it
already is. Instead of thinking seriously about what we might learn from
the experience of other countries, Cross-Over offers us the picture of a
global epidemic without any significant variations. Nor does it manage
to include anything positive or productive in the form of health education. Above all, Cross-Over fails to establish the relevance of any of
its material to the situation facing contemporary Swedish teenagers—
who are supposed to be its primary audience. Hildebrand appears to
have learned nothing from the wide experience of the RSFL, or the 1986
and 1988 international AIDS conferences held in Stockholm and rather
than facing a difficult situation, his film takes refuge in lazy, sentimental
stereotypes. Like other Safari hunters before him, he has brought home
the film equivalent of a worn-out zebra-skin rug, a few bales of silk,
and lots and lots of glamorous, misleading images which tell us next to
nothing about the societies which they supposedly represent.

At the beginning of the film Martin Sheen's husky American voice
informs us that 'Something has happened. What is it? How does it affect
us? . . . Can we protect the young generation? . . . Can we stop drugs?
Only the future will tell.' This litany of questions is evidently not addressed to young people themselves, but speaks over the tops of their
heads to other adults. There is also already a lot of confusion around. For
example, what does it mean to ask 'Can we stop drugs?' Which drugs
are we supposed to be concerned about? It is obvious that AIDS education has been hijacked in the opening moments of the programme by
a blanket anti-drugs agenda, which is an unhelpful distraction. Justice
Michael Kirby from Sydney, Australia, makes the point that AIDS is 'a
challenge to humanity', but Hildebrand clearly fails to understand that
its challenge is experienced in an enormous variety of different ways, according to differing circumstances. Instead of providing viewers with a
real opportunity to understand the circumstances which determine the
differences between AIDS in Sweden for example, and AIDS in Swazi-
land, a single set of images is abstracted from a multitude of international
sources, and is offered as the single, indisputable 'truth' of AIDS.

Thus AIDS is almost invariably presented in Cross-Over in the context
of hospital treatment. Yet in the west the majority of people with AIDS
spend less than 20 per cent of their lives in hospital after their initial

diagnosis. AIDS is lived within the community, yet *Cross-Over* failed to show us any sign of how most people with AIDS live their ordinary day-to-day lives. This is obviously a clear reflection on the beliefs and values of Staffan Hildebrand and his team. It is also highly misleading and irresponsible in a film aimed at people who are unlikely to have any direct experience of the epidemic. It is therefore most regrettable that the first man with AIDS shown in the film is not even given a name, let alone a nationality. He simply exists in the anonymous world of those dying in hospital, according to the film's ideological requirements. A black woman with AIDS, also in hospital, comments, 'I don't understand. If they only understood pain. . . .' But there is precious little evidence of any real understanding of AIDS in *Cross-Over,* except on the terms of its own narrow preconceptions.

The film then cuts to an American man with AIDS, once more (of course) in a hospital bed. He tells viewers: 'Stay away from drugs, promiscuity. Follow what you feel inside and you'll be alright. You can't fail if you follow what you feel is natural.' It should however be pointed out immediately that the man is talking dangerous nonsense. Which drugs are we supposed to stay away from? What does he mean by 'promiscuity'? If you split up with a lover and start a new relationship, is it alright not to have safer sex because of what you 'feel inside'? Is it okay not to use a condom because 'what you feel is natural'? The speaker was evidently chosen because what he says reflects the film's main agenda. This agenda is at least as muddled and contradictory as the speaker's comments, which can unfortunately only serve to further confuse viewers rather than to educate them. As a health education tool it is therefore not only useless, it is counterproductive. You would never guess from *Cross-Over* that all round the world hundreds of thousands of people have been actively engaged in developing effective HIV prevention strategies for many years. Nor does the film provide even the remotest suggestion of the scale of organisation and response in the communities which have been most devastated by AIDS (especially amongst gay men), throughout Europe, the USA, and far beyond. Hildebrand refuses to acknowledge the existence of any position which does not faithfully echo his own entirely negative and fatalistic perspective. He is presumably aware that if he actually interviewed someone with genuine experience from any of the leading AIDS service organisations, such as the RSFL in Sweden, or the Terrence Higgins Trust in London, or the PWA Coalition in New York, his own ignorance and confusion would be only too clearly exposed. Such glaring omissions from a film which claims to offer a global overview of the AIDS pandemic are inexcusable. They also guarantee that his film can only possibly be taken seriously by those with very little direct experience of the international situation, or those who have a prior interest in restricting public perceptions of AIDS.

In The Bronx district of New York City we were informed, to the sound of Doom music familiar from a thousand science fiction and horror films, that every sixteenth person is infected. Indeed, one could write a review of *Cross-Over* which simply analyses the use of music in establishing just this kind of analogy. A black taxi-driver explains that local youths don't want to go to school, and that they take drugs. This, I suppose, is intended to be deeply shocking. But what is shocking is that the film makes no attempt to establish why young people in New York feel so deeply alienated. A policeman states that 13, 14 and 15 year olds carry guns. But so what? What does this tell us about HIV or AIDS? The film describes drug addiction, prostitution, homelessness and poverty as 'the perfect environment for the virus to thrive'. Whilst this is obviously true, in the context of large cities like New York which lack adequate social services, it hardly explains the situation in Scandinavian cities. Indeed, the strong implication that AIDS is a syndrome which we should associate with extremes of social deprivation offers the inescapable message to its audience that HIV poses little or no threat to young, white, Swedes. On a personal note, I was particularly irritated to see a few moments of a demonstration by ACT UP (AIDS Coalition To Unleash Power). One would certainly never imagine from *Cross-Over* that ACT UP has done more work putting pressure on the Reagan administration to release much needed treatment drugs to people with AIDS in the USA, and to publicise their plight, than any other organisation. ACT UP is a sophisticated and articulate coalition of doctors, nurses, civil rights lawyers, and concerned people; its political analysis of AIDS is, in my experience, much the most important and incisive that can be found in the United States. If Hildebrand had spent just one-tenth of his budget, and spent two weeks with ACT UP, his viewers might have learned something positive and valuable about human courage in the face of great adversity (mostly deriving from murderous government inaction) in the USA and elsewhere. He would not, however, have found any voices to mirror the shallow position represented in *Cross-Over,* so ACT UP becomes conveniently reduced to a little demonstration. It was ACT UP that paved the way for the 11 October 1987 march on Washington, the largest civil rights protest in the history of the United States, with well over half a million people participating. Such a picture of organisation and articulate challenge to government policies hardly fits in with Hildebrand's picture of pathetic 'victims' surrounded on all sides by beaming doctors, eager to help.

Europe is presented in *Cross-Over* by familiar clichés and stereotypes: 'Time for a shot of the Eiffel Tower boys!' According to the voice-over, 'Europe had earlier warning than the United States and Central Africa'. This again is preposterous nonsense, and completely misleading. We are told that there is a 'generation gap', but it is far from clear whom it affects, since most of the young people we see seem highly confident and well informed, even if the film's editing emphasises a continually negative line: 'You can't trust anyone', and so on. This is of course profoundly unhelpful, and only like to undermine young people's confidence that there is anything they can do to avoid HIV infection, or to support one another. One boy spoke of the need to change morality and encourage love and 'deep relations'. But love has never exactly lacked advocates in 'official' culture, and it is far from clear how young people are supposed to establish these 'deep relations'. Does Hildebrand seriously propose that all young people should settle down for life with the first person to whom they feel sexually attracted? This seems to be one of the prevailing messages of *Cross-Over,* and it is of course both absurd and potentially dangerous. Dr Didier Jayle spoke eloquently on the need for clear information, and against trying to frighten people into behavioural change. He seemed to have wandered in from another film altogether. Or perhaps the filmmakers simply failed to understand what he was saying. One real opportunity was lost when a young man who said that he would not use a condom was simply dismissed. But if we take AIDS seriously, we have to take those who don't share our beliefs seriously as well. If the film had stayed with this young man, and explored his attitudes, something useful might have been gained. Instead, the chance to consider resistance to safer sex was simply thrown away.

Throughout the film we are constantly presented with situations which are treated in this same deeply superficial manner. On the one hand we are told that AIDS is a terrible global catastrophe, but as soon as a concrete issue emerges the film dashes off in the opposite direction as fast as possible. Thus British and American tourists in South-East Asia describe their fears of contracting sexually transmitted diseases from prostitutes, while the situation of those most at risk—the prostitutes themselves—is ignored. A young man in Manilla is found to puppet the *Cross-Over* line that the only solutions to AIDS are condoms or monogamy. But what does this mean? Are condoms available in The

Philippines, and how much do they cost? Is monogamy a feasible option in that society? What is the position of women? What of gay men? All the really important questions are neatly brushed away under the carpet. Thus in Brazil we see the so-called 'princes of the night', young male prostitutes. Yet nobody asks them if they have received useful safer sex education. Nobody talks about the situation of gay teenagers, or thinks to ask how these boys got involved in prostitution. It is simply assumed that they are the innocent 'victims' of older men. We learn from one doctor that Brazilian men do not identify themselves automatically as bisexual or homosexual. But why should they? Brazil is not Stockholm, and it is profoundly racist to imagine that the comparatively modern categories of sexual identity which apply in white, western societies are equally applicable in other parts of the world. The scene where a doctor tells one teenage boy, 'You are infected. Are you afraid of dying?' was one of the most distasteful and insensitive things I have ever seen on television. At such moments one becomes fully aware of the real consequences of the film's relentlessly sentimental obsession with death. It is all very well to interview Dr Jonathan Mann from the World Health Organisation, and to quote his words concerning possible treatments in the future. But what of treatments which exist today, and are unavailable to people with HIV and AIDS right now? This is not simply a problem of exotic faraway places. Why is aerosolised pentamidine, the major prophylactic drug against pneumocystis carinii pneumonia (the leading cause of death among people with AIDS), not available in Stockholm, when anyone in America who is fortunate enough to have medical insurance can obtain it on prescription? This is not a question to detain or concern Staffan Hildebrand.

These problems were most extreme in the section of *Cross-Over* which dealt with a place which was curiously described as 'Central Africa'. This is not a country in my atlas. Does the situation in Malmo represent the position of 'Northern Europe'? *Cross-Over* effortlessly depicts the inhabitants of this mythical land as more or less sex-crazed: 'I must have a girl-friend wherever I go to look after me', reports one black lorry driver, and we see seemingly endless shots of black women dancers in bars, and so on. But is this really so very different to European attitudes and behaviour? I think not. Dr Samuel Okware solemnly denies that homosexuality is seen in Africa. Well, it may not be seen, but it certainly exists, even if (as in Brazil) few central or eastern African societies have adopted western sexual categories, and the social identities which they encourage. In any case, black men having sex exclusively with one another are presumably at much less risk of HIV infection in those parts of the world where transmission is predominantly through heterosexual intercourse.

The film takes its name from the situation in Sydney, Australia, 'where an estimated 55,000 people in this city alone are infected'. We are also told that there is 'a growing international gay community' and much prostitution and injecting drug addiction. Sydney is thus a 'cross-over point', according to the film, with the strong implication that gay men are somehow the cause of HIV and AIDS. Rather than showing gay men as the most threatened, they are depicted as threatening. This, of course, speaks volumes about Hildebrand's underlying attitudes. We do at least see one female counsellor working with young male prostitutes in a highly supportive way, asking them 'How's work tonight?' At least one felt that some youths have access to good safer sex information. This non-moralistic line is immediately forgotten however as soon as the filmmakers themselves get involved with the boys 'on the game'. One of these boys, aged 15, explains how he ran away from home, but the interviewer never stops to ask him *why* he left.

The majority of young male prostitutes in the First World get involved in the sex industry for the simple reason that their families have thrown them out onto the street for the 'crime' of being gay. *Cross-Over* chooses to ignore the central role of homophobia in putting such young people at risk, and presents them as innocent heterosexuals, driven into prostitution by vague forces which are never named. As is often the case in *Cross-Over,* this particular young man seems much more sensitive and intelligent and well-informed about AIDS than his interviewer. After all this whizzing around the world, the crew must have been pretty jet-lagged, but even this does not excuse or explain the way in which AIDS is presented as an intrinsic problem of homelessness and prostitution, whilst these problems are never analysed as structural social phenomena, with concrete causes. Nor does it excuse the accumulating implication that HIV is not in fact a problem for the well-off, or those who have never been involved in the sex industry.

Similar problems afflict the film's depiction of AIDS in San Francisco, where, we learn, 98 per cent of AIDS cases are amongst gay men. This is certainly true of downtown San Francisco, but if one takes the subway a few stations out to the suburb of Oakland for example, one finds that gay men constitute only a minority of cases. It is precisely this tendency to over-simplify and to over-generalise which is so infuriating about *Cross-Over.* The film tells us that in San Francisco 'anger, desperation and suicide have begun to be replaced by a new mood of optimism. . . . The city is slowly winning the war on fear.' It is certainly not winning the long-running war against ill-informed filmmakers, who think only in terms of hospitalisation and death, and never stop to film community organisations which have struggled for many years against the effects of dreadful films like *Cross-Over*, with their endless parade of doctors and scientists, and their indifference to the role of safer sex educators and health promotion. There is nothing in *Cross-Over* about long-term survivors, nothing about San Francisco organisations such as Project Inform or Stop AIDS which have provided the only effective community-based challenge to the type of fatalistic garbage churned out by well-meaning but deeply ignorant liberals such as Staffan Hildebrand. Nor have they only provided education, for without such groups many thousands of people with HIV and AIDS would not have had access to the treatment drugs on which the quality of their lives depends.

Like the Swedish AIDS Delegation, the makers of *Cross-Over* seem to have learned little or nothing from those who have most experience in the field of AIDS prevention. The history of health education demonstrates only too clearly that you cannot frighten people into behavioural change.[3] A vast amount of money has been wasted in the making of *Cross-Over*, which will only serve to reinforce ignorance and prejudice. It is a very sad reflection on Swedish AIDS policy that such a film should appear, eight years into the epidemic. It is even more regrettable that this film is likely to be shown to young people in schools who have little access to more reliable and helpful information, such as the exemplary 1988 Danish film *The One I Love*, which does more on its small budget in just five minutes than the whole dreary and depressing length of *Cross-Over*.

11. Politics, People and the AIDS Epidemic: And The Band Played On

The very length of Randy Shilts's account of the first six years of the AIDS epidemic in the US suggests something of the scale and complexity of the issues he tackles. It is an epic of a book, impossible to ignore, and it will cast a shadow across all subsequent interpretations. It is also, by turns, heartbreaking and infuriating, shrewd and naive, extremely uneven and wildly inconsistent. All the more reason, then, to scrutinise it as closely as Shilts considers his leading characters, who he lines up from the first page like the cast of a disaster movie.

In fact, *And The Band Played On* is two books, condensed somewhat uneasily into one. In the first, Shilts tells the scandalous story of the indifference of the American government and institutions to a tragedy, the enormity of which has still not been fully recognised. Evidence comes from the Dean of the University of California at San Francisco, who observed in 1985 that 'at least with AIDS a lot of undesirable people will be eliminated'. Then there was the blood-supply industry which refused to acknowledge the grim consequences of viral transmission.

Shilts relays the words of a health-care worker who says of federal policies that 'we are seeing people take any opportunity within the law to avoid providing care.' He writes of the bath-house owner who, in 1984, told a group of doctors in San Francisco: 'We make money at our end when they come to the baths. You make money from them on the other end.'

In the second book within this book, Shilts charts the responses of American gay men to AIDS, a story which he weaves around the lives of numerous key figures—doctors, activists, and so on. Shilts's approach seems clearly based on the principle implied in his early quote from Emerson that 'all history resolves itself quite easily into the biography of a few stout and earnest persons'. Sadly, everything he reveals elsewhere about the political and medical research institutions of the US strongly suggests otherwise.

With the blinding clarity of hindsight, Shilts divides the world neatly into heroes and villains. To him, heroes are those who demanded that gay men should give up sex altogether, while anyone who questioned this prescription is branded a villain (and generally dies a horrible death within a few chapters). Shilts's historical individualism is matched by his complete dependence on the notion of 'leadership', again either noble or wicked. The complex history of AIDS thus emerges like a medieval legend, a tale of good and evil leaders locked together in mortal combat.

Huge community organisations such as Gay Men's Health Crisis or the People With AIDS Coalition suddenly emerge inexplicably from nowhere. But Shilts leaves them in the background because he is evidently not interested in issues of community health care or education. Indeed, he explicitly damns the very strategies of choice that are based on knowledge of the mode of transmission of HIV, strategies which have proved so immensely successful. Anything that throws doubt on his model of leadership, he tritely and insultingly dismisses as 'AIDSpeak'.

Straddling the two narratives is the now notorious *grand guignol,* figure of Patient Zero, who Shilts offers as the male Typhoid Mary of HIV, and onto whom he appears to have projected all his own unresolved anger, sorrow and pain. Patient Zero embodies the familiar mass-media stereotype of the vengeful 'AIDS carrier'. While it is obvious that not all gay men initially behaved well or even sensibly in response to AIDS, Shilts's attempt to locate a single named individual as source and cause of AIDS offers no more than a bizarre inversion of the wider tendency to blame all gay men collectively.

Thus we find Patient Zero thinking to himself as he shares one day in 1982: 'Who had done this to him? Certainly someone had. They had passed him the virus that meant he was going to die.' This, we should recall, was a year before Luc Montagnier isolated HIV in Paris, and two years before the public announcement!

In any case, Shilts cites repeatedly the early evidence concerning an incubation period of five-and-a-half years, which means that the men who developed AIDS soon after having sex with Patient Zero were mostly already infected.

Sadly, such glaring epidemiological inconsistencies abound, and are compounded by Shilts's casual aetiology, which repeatedly and unquestioningly returns us to a primitive 'dark continent' of Africa, which of course fits in with his general tendency towards the gothic, if not the frankly racist (as spelled out more clearly in an interview in *Village Voice*).

Both Larry Kramer and Michael Callen, who have played major roles in AIDS education in the community, are chipped down in order to fit in with Shilts's model of the heroic leader.

Such a treatment explains much of the immediate and profoundly contradictory impact of *And The Band Played On*. It also sadly explains much about its tremendous international success.

1989 ————

12. Missionary Positions:
AIDS, 'Africa', and race

The discursive regularities of Western AIDS commentary are nowhere more apparent than in the construction of 'African AIDS'.[1] In *Newsweek* in 1986 a French doctor was quoted as saying: 'It's difficult using these words, but (in Africa) we risk an apocalypse.'[2] A year later the *Guardian* described a 'leading doctor' in Uganda who 'believes that next year will be apocalyptic'.[3] Again in 1986, *Newsweek* informed its readers that in Kinshasa, 'Some joke that the French acronym for AIDS, SIDA (*Syndrome d'Immune-Deficitaire Acquis*), stands for *Syndrome Imaginaire pour Decourager les Amoureux*.[4] In the same year *The Times* reported that the citizens of Kinshasa joke that 'the French acronym for the illness actually stood for *Syndrome Imaginaire pour Decourager les Amoureux*'.[5] And as recently as July 1988, Alex Shoumatoff flew all the way back from Zaire to reveal in *Vanity Fair* that 'there is a joke in Kinshasa that SIDA stands for *Syndrome Imaginaire pour Decourager les Amoureux*'.[6]

Such repetitions already suggest something of the *mise en discourse* of 'African AIDS', and its potential for fomenting displacements. In a three-part series of reports entitled *Africa's New Agony,* Prentice Thomson set the familiar stage: 'young men suddenly grown old, haggard mothers with sickly children clinging to their backs. . . . For the foreseeable future, they will be confronted by a hideous, unimaginable disaster.'[7] A doctor in Burundi states that: 'Telling people that they could die from a sexually transmitted disease is unlikely to have much impact. They think it's just the church preaching at them. But if we tell women that they may give birth to infected children who will die because of parental promiscuity, there may be a chance of changing their behaviour.' The situation in 'Africa' is offered as a premonitory image of 'our' future in Europe and the United States, as planes fly out carrying away 'the seeds of infection, to be planted on foreign soil'.

In the third article, headlined 'Nightmare of a raddled city', Kinshasa is the central focus, with its 'unenviable name of the AIDS capital of Africa', where 'Even today, donor blood is not comprehensively screened for the AIDS virus. Tragic but predictable then, that 31 per cent of children with AIDS in a city hospital had a history of blood transfusions. Tragic, too, that a fatal flaw in the maternal instincts of most African women leads them to choose injections rather than pills for sick babies.' According to the article, many men, if not most, have numerous liaisons with different women, including prostitutes, who have been clearly identified in Kinshasa and elsewhere as reservoirs of AIDS infection. . . . 'Promiscuity and lack of medical resources have made Kinshasa the AIDS capital of the world.' The sudden leap from being 'AIDS capital of Africa' to 'AIDS capital of the world' is strongly indicative of the anxieties which inform and motivate such commentary, which need to be unpicked in some detail.

It is evident that Prentice's narrative and iconography operate within a long discursive tradition which finds perhaps its most complete description in Joseph Conrad's *Heart of Darkness*.[8] The former's 'young men suddenly grown old' are indistinguishable from the latter's dying man who 'seemed young—almost a boy—but you know with them it's hard to tell'.[9] The image of 'hideous, unimaginable disaster' also speaks directly of an Africa constituted in inscrutability, a 'treacherous' domain of 'lurking death' and 'hidden evil'. Its people are so hopelessly sunk in depravity and licentiousness that education is impossible, unthinkable. These 'people' can only be frightened into measures which supposedly will save their lives. Yet these measures amount to only one thing— monogamy, understood as the only effective prophylactic against HIV infection. Two points immediately stand out. First, if 'Africa' is as saturated with HIV as is suggested, monogamy as such is unlikely to provide any protection against transmission. The text is telling us that these 'people' can and must die, but they should at least have the 'decency' to do so within the moral conventions of Christian marriage. Second, the text concedes that these 'people' are only too well aware of the missionary imperative: 'They think it's just the church preaching at them.' What we actually learn here is that the population of Burundi operates a highly sophisticated decoding of Western 'information', understanding its motives only too clearly. Any seeming concern for the lives of the populations described is entirely secondary to the larger ideological imperatives of Western AIDS commentary, as it redraws the epidemic in the likeness of older colonial beliefs and values, targeted at the assumed (white) reader. I use the term 'AIDS commentary' to refer to the complex discursive field in which AIDS is used to signify the interests of many different institutions, from government to the Press: commentary that may be characterised by 'its repetitions, its slippages, its omissions, its emphases, its 'no-go' areas, its narrative patterns, and so on'.[10]

Rather than acknowledge the actual diversity and complexity of human sexuality, this commentary exhorts us all to reduce the numbers of our sexual partners, rather than address the potentially embarrassing question of sexual behaviour. Such commentary is far more interested in stopping promiscuity than it is in stopping the transmission of HIV. Committed in advance to the hypothesis that HIV originated somewhere in Central or Eastern Africa, such journalism wreaks its own sadistic 'revenge'. Hence the otherwise frankly extraordinary picture of 'a fatal flaw in the maternal instincts of African women', who somehow are supposed to have understood the modes of transmission of HIV long before the research teams at the CDC and the Pasteur Institute in Paris. The maternal fecundity of this imaginary 'Africa' becomes the target for particular hatred. Thus any woman whose sexuality cannot immediately be classified within the terms of Christian monogamy becomes a 'prostitute' and, as such, deserves to die. Moreover, she is the author of her own destruction, rather than someone who has herself been infected by a man. 'Africa' emerges, as in Conrad, in 'a wild and gorgeous apparition of a woman'. A woman, moreover, whose fascination speaks too much of Western sexuality, and its ever-attendant poles of disgust and attraction, contempt and desire.

A year later Peter Murtagh wrote a similar three-part series entitled 'AIDS in Africa' for the *Guardian*. Each section begins with the image of a woman—a prostitute, a woman with AIDS, and a nurse. The opening lines prepare us for the familiar genre of AIDS-safari reportage: 'The best time to observe the Nairobi hooker is at dusk when the tropical sun dips beneath the Rift Valley and silhouettes the thorn trees against the African skyline.'[11] According to Murtagh, East African truck drivers 'like nothing better than to round off a day's work by visiting a prostitute'. Prostitutes, truck drivers and their respective families are all carefully distinguished from 'the general population'. Writing of British soldiers stationed in Kenya, he describes how 'The futility of trying to keep the soldiers and women apart was evident last week by the numbers of men from the 2nd Battalion of the Parachute Regiment in the bars and discos of Nairobi.' This certainly gives the lie to his report in the same newspaper a month later, where he claimed that 'prostitutes, who are regarded as the main potential AIDS carriers likely to have contact with soldiers, follow the troops to wherever they take their leave'.[12] One cannot avoid asking who is following whom.

In his second article, 'Death is simply a fact of life', Murtagh introduces Josephine Nnagingo, who 'lives in a mud and wattle farmhouse in the middle of her family's field of banana trees not far from Kyotera, a few miles from the shores of Lake Victoria in southern Uganda'. She is dying from AIDS, and 'the wasting of her shrunken body has made her head appear outsized, and her dress is now too big for her. Her arms and legs are desperately thin, and she moves only with pain.' In some districts, 'deaths in the houses have prompted survivors to flee in the belief that the buildings themselves are in some way responsible for the illness'. Recourse to witchdoctors, herbal remedies and talismans are all detailed, together with the warning that because hospitals are overwhelmed, and patients prefer to live at home in their villages, 'figures for the numbers of AIDS deaths may not be accurate'.

His series ended with a final article entitled 'Sickening of a continent', in which one doctor concludes that 'if we do not beat AIDS it will be the end of a continent'. This sits ironically beside a description of a Catholic nurse, Sister Miriam, who 'cannot bring herself to advocate the use of condoms'. Church teaching is one man, one woman, and no sex before marriage. " 'I'm not going to go against theology," she said.' Another nurse can identify people with HIV 'by the way they look. They have a kind of listlessness.' Yet we already know these scenes, from a host of sources which, like Conrad, depict the spectacle of black Africans 'dying slowly . . . nothing but black shadows of disease and starvation. The black bones reclined at full length and slowly the eyelids rose and the sunken eyes looked up at me, enormous and vacant.'[13] It is as if HIV were a disease of 'Africanness', the viral embodiment of a long legacy of colonial imagery which naturalises the devastating economic and social effects of colonialism in the likeness of starvation-bodies reduced to 'bundles of acute angles'.[14] Hence the significance of a recent advertising campaign on behalf of the British charity, the National Campaign for the Prevention of Cruelty to Children (NSPCC), which shows the emaciated body of a small child with the accompanying caption: 'Four years old. Seriously underweight for her age. Scavenging for food where she can find it. And she's English.' For 'English' read 'white'. Whilst such adverts evidently derive from very different institutional sources, they nonetheless draw upon presumed long-standing 'knowledge' concerning the supposedly correct relations between England and 'Africa', between whites and blacks. This 'knowledge' is constituted in the complex discursive legacy of British colonial history, sedimented over the course of many centuries, and centrally involved in the formation of British national cultural identities, as much in their acceptance as their contestation. Hence the need to understand that the language of metaphor that informs so much African AIDS commentary carries a very specific ideological cargo, and nowhere more so than in talk of the 'heart of Africa'.

Alex Shoumatoff's lengthy *Vanity Fair* article 'In search of the source of AIDS' begins with a piece of typical scene-setting:

> The heart of Africa is stricken. The 'AIDS belt' is spreading, and the disease that has already claimed the lives of thousands of men, women, and children will claim millions more. *Vanity Fair* sent Alex Shoumatoff on a journey of exploration along the equator, where he met the fatalistic bar-girls of Kinshasa, the exhausted doctors of war-shattered Uganda, the folk-healers of Guinea-Bissau, and the plague-ridden smugglers of Lake Victoria. Is this a nightmare vision of our own future?

And set against a photograph of a vast expanse of water we read the caption: 'Lake Victoria, deep in the heart of darkest Africa, is on some level, perhaps only mythical, the font of AIDS.'

'How curious it would be,' thinks Shoumatoff idly to himself, 'if the source of the Nile and the source of AIDS prove to be one and the same, that huge teeming lake in the dangerous heart of darkest Africa.' He asks about the number of local cases, but 'having been through this several times before in the Third World, I know it is futile to expect reliable figures'. The Ugandans he talks to think that HIV is transmitted 'mainly by sex but sometimes by witchcraft against debt welshers'. They are thus set up as authentic 'natives'—unreliable, superstitious, in a word, primitive. Arriving in Bissau he notes: 'There were no whores on the premises, as there usually are in African hostelries.' There is a striking parallel here to the earlier observation by an American doctor describing the situation in Kigali in Rwanda where 'The small number of prostitutes who are inconspicuously present on the streets are believed to be a prime source of spreading AIDS.'[15] The figure of the prostitute is necessary, as presence or absence. The local Director of Public Health informs Shoumatoff that:

> the patients and their families were not being told what they had. Most of the public did not know that nasty little microbes were

on the loose, threatening to kill them. They still believed that gas, the spirits, were the cause of sickness and death. In some ways [he] observed, the viruses had a lot in common with the iras: they were invisible, their existence has to be taken on faith, and one was powerless against them.

Quite apart from Shoumatoff's evident inability to distinguish between microbes and viruses, we should immediately note the infantalising tone. In the logic of racism, it stands to reason that one talks to childlike black Africans about 'nasty little microbes' rather than modes of transmission. Yet countless surveys demonstrate that irrational beliefs concerning the (non-existent) threat of miasmatic contagion from HIV are at least as prevalent in the West as any Ugandan faith in iras. It is particularly unpleasant to find people's lay beliefs held up for mockery in a context in which they have evidently been systematically denied access to any other sources of information—they 'were not being told what they had'. The complete failure to recognise this double standard is hardly surprising from a writer who casually wonders if the local 'weaseloid carnivores' had been tested for retroviruses. Shoumatoff also casually accepts the notion of a Simian origin for HIV, six months after the definitive rejection of the theory by the same Harvard scientists who first proposed it in 1985.[16] Such a cavalier attitude towards virological evidence is entirely in keeping with the belief that the current crisis of public health and health-care provision may be attributed to the 'withdrawal' (as he curiously puts it) of Belgian colonial authority in 1960 rather than to the long-term effects of colonialism itself. This is rather like attributing the current economic crisis in Vietnam to the 'withdrawal' of American troops rather than to the Vietnam wars and the subsequent punitive denial of Western funding.

However, as we have seen, Shoumatoff 'knows' his Africa, just as he 'knows' that 'the Western gays who participated in *la ronde* of bar sex and promiscuity were in fact suffering from an infectious-disease burden very similar to Africans'. Once the notion of 'promiscuity' has been medicalised in this way, a royal road of analogy is opened up between the different groups first affected by HIV. Already regarding black Africans and gay men as effectively interchangeable, a convenient 'intestinal-parasite co-factor theory' can be invoked, claiming that 'Africans, Haitians, and many Western homosexual men are riddled with amoebas'. Thus Africa becomes a 'deviant' continent, just as Western gay men are effectively Africanised. Returning to Masaka, in Uganda, our intrepid hero finds that 'the only place still open is a bar, where we wash down chapatis with Bell beer. It is the most degenerate scene, the closest thing to Sodom I have ever seen. Guys completely bombed, with girls on their laps, etc. Obviously nobody cares about getting AIDS.' Everything here hangs upon the unelaborated 'etc.', for if getting drunk with a girl on one's knee is Sodom, then Sodom is an extensive province indeed. According to *Newsweek* in 1986 it undoubtedly extends well into Tanzania, where the town of Kashenye in the Kagera region 'was like Sodom and Gomorrah' with 'wild parties, orgies'.[17]

Equatorial Africa is so primitive ('unreliable') that 'most tribes don't even seem to have a word for homosexual', although 'homosexuality is very taboo'. This observation is strikingly similar to that of an anthropologist from Berkeley who recently commented in the *Guardian* that in Brazil 'a great many men who engage in same-sex interactions simply don't identify themselves as homosexuals or bisexuals'.[18] It is clear that the relatively recent emergence of the classificatory system of western sexuality is by now as completely taken for granted and de-historicised as Linnaean taxonomy.

Shoumatoff concludes his article with a familiar valedictory slipstream of *de rigeur* anxieties. 'I thought of how HIV must have become airborne—airplane-borne—moving from continent to continent: tens of thousands of revellers flying down to Rio for Carnival, for instance. I imagined this archetypal communicable disease travelling along the mutually manipulative interface of the First and Third Worlds in countless copulations', through the Far East and on into 'the Arab world, where the predilection for buggery will provide a brisk amplification system'. He also ponders mightily on 'the unprecedented merging and mixing and growing together of the world's population in the last four decades', and it struck him that:

> for a microcosm of the melting-pot process, one had to look no further than this completely booked and waitlisted Rome-New York jumbo 747. Among the four hundred passengers winging their way to the great land whose politically admirable but epidemiologically lamentable motto is *E Pluribus Unum* were Indians and Arabs, Venezuelans, Poles, Africans, Israelis, Italians, Turks and Bulgarians, not to mention Americans of assorted hues and stripe—a rich cross-section of the human cornucopia—statistically three people aboard ought to be carrying the virus.

All of this might seem a good case for international HIV screening, if one is not aware of the World Health Organisation's detailed statistical analysis of the problems of sensitivity and specificity (accuracy in identifying true HIV positives and true negatives) which are inseparable from large-scale HIV testing.[19] As the WHO consultation points out, 'HIV screening programmes for international travellers would, at best and at great cost, retard only briefly the dissemination of HIV both globally and with respect to any particular country.' Besides, the imagery of 'airborne' HIV only serves to draw attention sooner or later to profound unacknowledged fears concerning the (non-existent) miasmatic transmission of the virus, which are rationalised and displaced across the field of international travel. This in turn seems to be closely connected to an equally deep-seated fear of racial miscegenation. How else should we account for the patently absurd fantasy that international travel is a function of jet propulsion? The 'forgetting' that is going on here concerns a far simpler mode of transport in a far earlier period—the galleys and galleons of the international slave trade, which carried another 'cross-section of the human cornucopia' across from Africa to the Americas. It is the power of disease to effect such displacements and 'forgettings' to which we should now turn our attention.

AIDS in 'Africa' versus 'African AIDS'

The rising rates of HIV infection and AIDS in Central and Eastern Africa have been widely recognised since the early 1980s, with the highest cumulative numbers of cases in descending order from Uganda, Tanzania, Kenya, the Congo, Burundi, Rwanda, Zambia, and Malawi, to Zaire. It is important to recognise that every country affected by HIV has its own epidemic, shaped by a multitude of variable local factors, amongst which the circumstances of the population groups affected first by the virus are the most important. In this respect the notion of 'African AIDS' already obscures the specific characteristics of the different AIDS epidemics in these countries, constructing them in the spurious unity of an 'Africa' which is immediately denied any of the cultural, social, economic and ethnic diversity which is taken for granted in Europe and North or South America.

As a cultural and psychic construction, 'African AIDS' exhibits at least five consistent aspects. First, it speaks of a peculiar and special affinity between a virus and a continent. Second, it reads the modes of transmission of HIV as signs of a generalised and homogenous African 'primitiveness', whether sexual or medical. Third, it singles out the alleged 'mis-reporting' of African HIV and AIDS statistics as further evidence of 'backwardness' and 'unreliability'. Fourth, it equates black Africans and western gay men as wilful 'perverts' who are equally threatening to 'family values'. Fifth, it regards 'Africa' as the source of HIV infection in the sense of origin and of cause. Whilst none of these aspects are individually specific to the issue of AIDS, their collective configuration is, I believe, unprecedented. The construction of 'African AIDS' tells us much about the west, and its major strategies of self-knowledge, rooted in systems of difference and otherness. But even more importantly, it serves to justify and validate the continued, genocidal indifference to the long-term consequences of HIV infection in any population group other than white, western heterosexuals. It is here that we can map out the complex relations between racial and sexual boundaries which legitimate and make possible the casual contemplation of the virtual extinction of all black Africans and all gay men.[20]

1 The infectious continent

Patrick Brantlinger has acutely observed how:

racism often functions as a displaced or surrogate class system, growing more extreme as the domestic class alignments it reflects are threatened or eroded. As a rationalization for the domination of 'inferior' peoples, imperialist discourse is inevitably racist; it treats race and class terminology as covertly interchangeable or at least analogous. Both a hierarchy of classes and a hierarchy of races exist; both are the results of evolution or of the laws of nature; both are simpler than but similar to species; and both are developing but are also, at any given moment, fixed, inevitable, not subject to political manipulation.[21]

'African AIDS' emerges with a similar effect of inevitability, condensing the distinct issues of a virus with clearly established modes of transmission, and a syndrome of many distinct opportunistic conditions which may appear in the wake of HIV's progressive weakening of the body's immunological defences. Hence the relentless misclassification of 'African AIDS' as a disease, a seemingly 'natural' result of sexual 'treachery' which is also aspective of the 'treachery' of Africa itself. The symptoms of this 'African AIDS disease' are also immediately identifiable as evidence of some innate 'African-ness'—lassitude, extreme weight-loss, huge staring eyes—the only too familiar signs of famine, but in this instance supposedly caused by excessive (sexual) appetite. The identification 'African' thus slides directly into the diagnosis, 'AIDS'. An entire continent may be infected because its peoples and its physical geography are held as one. 'African AIDS' thus legitimates and 'proves' the fantasy of intrinsic correspondences between environment, character, and physical health—constructing 'Africa' as an undifferentiated domain of rot, slime, filth, decay, disease, and naked 'animal' blackness. This infernal and unhygienic territory is the perfect imaginary swamp in which a new virus might 'percolate', as Shoumatoff so revealingly speculates—a virus which eventually kills by transforming all its 'victims' into 'Africans', and which threatens to 'Africanise' the entire world.

2 AIDS and 'the primitive'

Writing of Africa, *Newsweek* recently reported that 'Today, in the zones of highest infestation, AIDS pervades everyday life.'[22] It is highly unlikely that the same journalist would ever describe London or New York as 'infested' with AIDS. The heads of the poor may be infested with lice, and a rotting corpse may be infested with maggots. Thus First World cities are merely 'affected' by AIDS, though black or Hispanic or gay communities within them may be 'devastated'. The rhetoric of infestation is reserved for a continent which is always known in advance to be polluted and pestilential. The images of liquidity and putrefaction which are so indispensable to 'African AIDS' commentary speak of a coital condensation in which Africa, understood as the font of human life, is confused with Africa the supposed 'font of AIDS'.[23] This maternal Africa is subject to the phantasmatic projections of her Western 'sons', locked in the double difference of race and gender—white and male, repulsed and desiring. The flow of Africa is the flow of the mother's body, the atavistic source of life and death.

The evolutionary model of the social sciences which was established in the second half of the nineteenth century grounded a narrowly restrictive picture of 'higher' human nature in a series of contrasts with 'the primitive'. To leave Africa is to be purified, to return to 'the light', which is also repression. 'African AIDS' must therefore always be presented as *sui generis,* a completely different disease from AIDS in the First World. Indeed, most commentators have preferred almost any explanation of the 1:1 AIDS ratio of man to woman in most African countries, rather than that of heterosexual transmission. These 'explanations', including cannibalism, bestiality, ritual scarification, violent sex and so on, bear a striking similarity to the 'weird customs' catalogued by Rider Haggard and his contemporaries. As long ago as 1985 Dr Angus

Dalgleish reported on behalf of an extensive field survey conducted by researchers from the London Institute of Cancer Research, that 'We investigated and ruled out all other factors in the disease's spread—except heterosexual activity.'[24] Yet the cultural logic remains: 'primitive' Africa generates 'African AIDS'—'civilised' Europeans and Americans (white, heterosexual) are safe.

3 Fun with figures

'Primitive' Africa is also inscribed in the field of epidemiology. The 'under-reporting' of HIV and AIDS statistics from African nations has long been a familiar trope in 'African AIDS' commentary, generally attributed either to 'poor facilities' or the mendacity of individual governments. Yet it should be recognised that by their nature, such figures can never be precise, and further, that their relative accuracy is no more characteristic of Zaire or Uganda than of Texas or the United Kingdom.

For example, there are strong social and economic disincentives to HIV antibody testing in Britain, where ignorance and prejudice abound against those known to be infected. Nor is there any legislation (or hope of legislation) to protect the most fundamental rights to employment or housing or insurance for infected individuals or members of the social constituencies in which HIV was widely transmitted before its existence was known or even suspected. We should also recognise that most people at high potential risk of infection have long since taken measures to minimise any chance of viral transmission. Hence the dramatic fall in new infections among gay men in Britain and elsewhere in recent years. In such circumstances the only reason for testing would be to obtain drug treatments, in the form of anti-virals, immune-stimulants, or prophylaxes against individual opportunistic conditions. Sadly, financial cuts in the National Health Service have frequently made these unobtainable in Britain.

UK doctors also frequently fail to diagnose AIDS, since they mistakenly assume that it is only to be found in the inner cities, or because their acceptance of sexual stereotypes means that they simply don't realise that their patients are at risk. In both circumstances the larger cultural climate surrounding the epidemic affects HIV and AIDS statistics by reinforcing highly misleading notions about 'the promiscuous' or 'gay men' or 'injecting drug-users', as if these were all instantly identifiable. The widespread shaming of people with AIDS in the First World, together with their families, lovers and friends has also led many doctors to attribute deaths to individual opportunistic conditions, rather than naming the syndrome on death certificates, in order to 'spare' the bereaved. This is entirely understandable, and moreover may be clinically correct. But it does not serve to clarify the epidemiological profile of the British AIDS epidemic. A recent report that 'doctors should no longer assume the elderly do not get AIDS' only further reinforces the ignorance and naivety among many doctors concerning the actual complexity of sexual and drug-using behaviour, across all social barriers of class, race, age and gender.[25] In such circumstances the repeated emphasis on the 'under-reporting' or 'mis-reporting' of 'African AIDS' statistics only serves to reinforce prevailing notions of African 'primitiveness', whilst masking the brutal forces which constantly skew European and American figures concerning the incidence and prevalence of both HIV and AIDS.

'Primitive' Africa also emerges in relation to countless anecdotes concerning 'dirty' hospitals, 'out-of-date' medical equipment, the sharing of syringes, and so on. What is at stake here, however, is not the fact of poverty or the effects of post-colonial disruption throughout central Africa, but the implication that 'African AIDS' can be explained away as a by-product of 'African medicine', with the assumption that Western medicine is invariably 'better' and more 'advanced'. Everything in this distinction depends upon the value we place on the look of high technology. Whilst experimental drug trials take place widely in the United States, they are restricted to those who can either afford them, or who are fortunate enough to be insured. The fundamental injustice of American private medicine is thus erased by the image of gleaming chromium. This is particularly regrettable since it also obscures the fact that health insurance is unavailable to those categorised as members of 'high-risk groups'. In this manner, demographic factors such as gender, marital status, and even postal localities have been substituted for actual risk factors, which include the possible sharing of needles, and the question of whether individuals are having safer sex or not. In the meantime, fears that the US public health system may collapse under the strain of the epidemic will continue to reflect the originating mythology of 'African AIDS', rather than the prior structural inadequacies of American health-care provision.

4 Monstrous passions

In 1897 the missionary Joseph Johnston noted that he had been 'increasingly struck with the rapidity with which such members of the white race as are not of the best class, can throw over the restraints of civilization and develop into savages of unbridled lust and abominable cruelty'.[26] Another missionary 'believed that merely witnessing heathen customs could be dangerous: "Can a man touch pitch and not be defiled?' "[27] The narrator in Conrad's *Heart of Darkness* struggles to explain: 'You can't understand. How could you?—with solid pavements under your feet, surrounded by kind neighbours ready to cheer you or to fall on you . . . how can you imagine what particular region of the first ages of a man's untrammelled feet may take him into by the way of solitude?'[28] In all these texts, and countless like them, we may identify 'the heavy, mute spell of the wilderness', drawing white men 'to its pitiless breast by the awakening of forgotten and brutal instincts, by the memory of gratified and monstrous passions'.[29]

These passions, too monstrous to name, are outwardly sanctioned in the projective image of Africa as the 'wild and gorgeous apparition of a woman'.[30] As early as 1758 Linnaeus had contrasted the 'caprice' of Africans to the 'customs' of Europeans.[31] Lacking 'restraint', like Conrad's Mr Kurtz, or merely deprived of neighbourly 'customs', the white man is uniquely vulnerable to the temptation to 'go native'. Yet this temptation is always ambiguous, since it is at once a return to nature, and the unnatural. Moreover, the 'monstrous passions' which Africa awakes have evidently already been 'gratified'. A series of complex analogies thus become possible in colonial discourse. For the childlike 'primitive' is immediately identified as a sexual adult and as a sexually active child. There is also a close parallel between the anthropological attention to African sexuality, illustrated in the lantern-light of eugenic theory, and the equally spectacular inventory of 'the perversions', so painstakingly catalogued by the early sexologists. Blacks and 'perverts' alike were held to share the characteristics of unbridled sexual rapacity and low cunning. They might also however be led to at least the semblance of normality— the former as a result of missionary zeal, and the latter by 'therapeutic' initiatives.

In spite of the widespread acceptance of more pluralistic models of both human societies and sexuality in the twentieth century, the national-popular of the West remains strongly influenced by the notion of a single, linear model of human cultural evolution, and an equally over-simplified picture of normative psycho-sexual 'development'. At many levels of popular culture, including folklore, children's fiction, cinema, the Press, and gossip and jokes, blacks and gay men remain curiously linked—the two great indispensable Others in the operations of postmodern governmentality.[32] Given the widespread revival of evangelical Christian and 'pro-family' currents in contemporary Anglo-American political culture, we may fairly detect significant parallels between the hystericised anxieties concerning the 'threat' of white colonialists 'going native', and modern fears about the possibility of 'innocent' heterosexuals 'going gay'. At a time when homosexuality in Western societies is once more regarded as a critical 'problem', AIDS has been widely used to reinforce the boundaries of object-choice. Hence the widespread tendency of Western governments to emphasise the 'threat' of HIV 'leaking' from the social constituencies affected most severely by AIDS into the newly designated 'heterosexual community'.[33] The recent emergence of this extraordinary category is only comprehensible as an expression of the cultural paranoia which still regards HIV as an innately black or gay condition, the scourge of 'perverts', against which only 'the family' can prevail.

Ronald Hyams has argued that 'the willingness of Victorian Britons to endure the deprivations involved in working overseas probably depended quite crucially on the easy availability of a range of sexual consolations'.[34] It is only too easy to identify the psychic structures of denial and defence which register transgression on such a scale—the 'horror' of 'going native', which is in turn closely paralleled in our times by excessive responses to the intrinsically unremarkable fact of sexual diversity. Just as the figure of 'the prostitute' is habitually regarded as a source rather than a victim of disease, so we may trace out the patterns of displacements which offer us a carnal Africa as the 'source' of AIDS, transported home to the bosom of the white Western family via the 'monstrous passions' of 'perverts' and 'the promiscuous'. Anything which threatens this fantasy must be ruthlessly denied. Anything which suggests the actual complexity and diversity of human sexuality must be censored. Hence the discursive necessity for a non-Western point of origin for AIDS, and the requirement that 'perverts' be held reponsible as culpable intermediaries.

5 Fons et origen

Infectious disease has long provided the fundamental epistemological model for Western medicine, with its familiar narrative of identification/diagnosis, treatment, and cure. Indeed, it is precisely this model that historians have already used to 'explain' the history of AIDS, which is frequently compared to the earlier histories of syphilis and cholera in such a way that the specific dimensions of racism, misogyny, and homophobia are entirely erased from consideration.[35] With the gradual recognition that environmental change has improved life expectancy and public health more effectively than medical interventions, this model has been faced with something of a crisis. This has been reinforced by the parallel recognition that the major threats to late twentieth-century Western health have not been infectious diseases. In this respect HIV has proved something of a godsend, being widely used to reinstate the authority of a particular medical model of treatment, together with its attendant doctor/patient relations, calculations of risk, and so on.

This in turn has tended to deflect attention away from questions of preventive medicine to the possibility of developing a vaccine. It is of course important to recognise that if virologists were able to prove that HIV 'mutated from an ancestor virus that caused little harm in humans, or is derived from a closely related virus in animals, then a theoretical chance exists that the ancestor virus might be used to develop a vaccine to protect humans'.[36] This is not however how 'African AIDS' commentary has dealt with the question of the possible origins of HIV. By the late 1980s 'many researchers are agreed that the evidence for AIDS originating in Africa is weak'.[37] Robert Biggar of the US National Cancer Institute has pointed out that there is no conclusive evidence that HIV 'originated in Africa, since the epidemic seemed to start at approximately the same time as in America and Europe'.[38] However, as Cindy Patton explains: 'The unconscious belief that a strange new virus could not have arisen from the germ-free West led researchers on a fantastic voyage in search of the origin of HIV in Haiti and then in Africa'.[39]

Sander Gilman has also argued that 'We need to locate the origin of a disease, since its source, always distant from ourselves in the fantasy land of our fears, gives us assurance that we are not at fault, that we have been invaded from without, that we have been polluted by some external agent.'[40] Whilst it is possible to disarticulate the tangled web of racism and homophobia which work to resist or obscure acnowledgement of the intrinsically unremarkable modes of transmission of HIV, we should certainly not conclude that AIDS is not a real and terrible epidemic throughout Central and Eastern Africa. The analysis of the social and psychic construction of 'African AIDS' has unfortunately led some commentators to deny the actual scale of AIDS in Africa.[41] At present it seems unlikely that the origins of HIV will ever be precisely established. Yet even if they were, we should not make the absurd mistake of blaming the people of that cultural and geographical locality for its emergence. Indeed, we should constantly be on our guard against any such attempts to blame those affected first by an infectious disease, as if the source of a virus were somehow its *cause*.

Conclusion

The construction of 'African AIDS' tells us little or nothing of AIDS in Africa, but a very great deal about the changing organisation of sexual and racial boundaries in the West, where AIDS has been widely harnessed to the interests of a new hygienic politics of intense moral purity. This new politics aspires to realign national-popular identities, replacing the vulnerable barriers of class identities which can no longer be easily policed with strongly pathologised distinctions between sexual 'normality' and 'perversion'. As Europe draws together in the likeness of a federation, and the Soviet Union is increasingly accepted as a legitimate nation-state, Africa has been effectively demonised in a post-colonial discourse of perpetual catastrophe and unnatural disasters. This undifferentiated apocalyptic Africa has proved an ideal site in which to find and 'see' disease. 'African AIDS' thus condenses ancient fears concerning contagious disease, together with vengeful fantasies concerning 'excessive' sexuality, understood in essentially pre-modern terms as both the source and the cause of AIDS.

Besides the callous insult which such commentary adds to the tragic injuries of HIV-related disease and human suffering, this reconstitution of 'African AIDS' sadly only serves to increase the likelihood of HIV transmission in the West by deflecting perceptions of risk away from the domestic sphere of white heterosexuals. The racism and homophobia which Western culture has visited on racial and sexual minorities for millennia now threaten to turn back on heterosexuals themselves, in their seeming refusal and inability to acknowledge the realities of HIV infection and disease.[42] It would appear that we are witnessing a fundamental reorganisation of Western racism, as the constitutive colonial analogy between race and class is dissolved, and African blackness is reconceptualised as an analogue of the sexually perverse. The relations which emerge between First and Third World blacks is one of the many instabilities which this new alignment opens up. The role of black gay men in this emergent configuration may well prove to be of decisive importance, for they occupy a space of maximum contradiction, since the majority of black and Hispanic American men with AIDS are gay, whilst in Africa black men who only have sex with one another should be regarded as a low-risk population group for HIV.

The recent insistence by the Primate of Kenya, the Most Rev Manesses Kuria, that AIDS 'is a disease from the sin of homosexuality' suggests a regrettable reaction to the implications of 'African AIDS' commentary. This ironically only further serves the interests of Western principles of governmentality. Imposing the restrictive categories of Western sexuality on a global scale threatens to obliterate cultural alternatives which, equally, provide secure social and individual identities.[43] The picture of 'African AIDS' is also largely responsible for the climate of increasing hostility and violence to Western lesbians and gay men, of which the notorious 'Helms Amendment' and Section 28 of the British 1988 Local Government Act are the most extreme examples.[44] Cindy Patton has described the 'Queer paradigm', according to the logic of which 'AIDS has such power as a supposedly "gay disease" that anyone who gets it becomes "queer" by association.'[45] Yet 'African AIDS' is a two-way street, presenting black Africans and gay men as mutual surrogates, whilst steadfastly refusing ever to consider AIDS from the actual lived positions of either group. As 'official' state racism directed against the black populations of the First World is slowly delegitimised, AIDS is evidently being used to validate the drawing of new lines of power and popular consent which require the fabrication of new Others, to bolster 'healthy' familial identities. The British government already feels sufficiently confident in these strategies to legislate binding distinctions between supposedly 'pretended' and 'real' families. How Western gay men and Africans can respond to this crisis in both their cultural representation and their objective circumstances remains to be seen. But we should all note as a matter of considerable urgency that when supposedly 'democratic' governments feel free to criminalise the so-called 'promotion' of homosexuality, they are equally at liberty to prosecute the 'promotion' of anything which might be construed as inimical to 'public health' or 'family values', or 'tradition', which may be rewritten daily. In such circumstances it is salutary to recall how Joseph Conrad reversed the terms and values of an earlier moment in the history of racism when, at the beginning of *Heart of Darkness* he invited his readers to imagine the Romans arriving in Britain two thousand years ago, at 'the very end of the world, a sea the colour of lead, a sky the colour of smoke . . . and going up this river with stores, or orders, or what you like. Sand-banks, marshes, forests, savages—precious little to eat fit for a civilized man, nothing but Thames water to drink. . . . They must have been dying like flies here.'[46] All the evidence suggests that people with AIDS in Africa are treated with all the care and support that their communities can provide. There can be few more starkly telling contrasts in the modern world than between the way in which black African societies treat their sick and dying, and the spectacle of the tens of thousands of Americans with AIDS, few of whom can afford such drug treatments as are available—many of whom are homeless and living out on the streets of New York, Los Angeles, and every major city in the United States. In Britain, changes in the Social Security Act (1986) have reduced the income of people living with AIDS by up to two-thirds, whilst treatment drugs are frequently unavailable, and standards of personal care are highly uneven. In all of this it seems that people with HIV and AIDS are entirely dependent on the limited resources of private charity, rather than the fundamental estimation of needs and rights to adequate health care provision that obtain elsewhere in the National Health Service.[47] Who in this picture are the 'primitives'? Who the 'barbarians'?

Missionary positions: AIDS, 'Africa', and race

This article is dedicated to Paula A. Treichler, whose work on HIV/ AIDS provides continual inspiration. Her article, 'AIDS and HIV infection in the Third World: a first world chronicle' in Phil Mariani and Barbara Kruger (eds), *Remaking History,* New York, DIA Foundation, 1989, appeared too late for me to refer to it in this article. I strongly recommend it to anyone interested in the complex tragic subject of 'African AIDS'.

13. Young People and AIDS

The conviction in May of four men for the murder of 14-year-old Jason Swift was widely reported in the British daily press. 'Vilest Of The Vile' bellowed the *Sun,* while the *Independent* was somewhat more restrained: 'Four found guilty of killing boy in homosexual orgy'.[1] The nature of the crime was, of course, deeply repugnant, yet the press reaction entirely missed the story's underlying significance. The *Independent* described how Jason 'worked as a rent boy after leaving home to escape being bullied by his family because of his effeminacy'. The *Sun* concurred: 'Jason, a timid, effeminate child', ran away from home 'because of bullying'. Nonetheless, most papers felt confident to quote the boy's family as a moral authority, as if the family's behaviour had been entirely beyond reproach. An 'effeminate' and 'timid' boy . . . we all know what that means. . . .

In the course of the trial the prosecution described 'a world most decent people would never dream existed'. By this he evidently referred to the world of men who have sex with rent boys, rather than the world of families from which a 13-year-old feels he has no choice but to run away. This is the sickening hypocrisy that surrounded the public commentary on Jason's all too short life.

His story demonstrates only too clearly that the supposedly 'decent' world of the family, and that of child abuse and child prostitution are intimately related. Moreover, the trial reports reveal a frightening inability to imagine the situation from Jason's point of view, from the position of a gay teenager growing up in a hostile and aggressively homophobic society.

According to the government's own Office of Population Censuses and Surveys, 37 per cent of marriages in 1987 will end in divorce, and 41 per cent of marriages will be between teenagers.[2] Furthermore, a survey by the Imperial Cancer Research Fund shows that 9 per cent of men now under 20 had sexual intercourse before the age of 15, and 67 per cent before the age of 18. These statistics are double the figures reported by men now in their 40s concerning their sexual behaviour as teenagers. The survey also found that less than 2 per cent had had homosexual intercourse.[3]

Unfortunately it is not easy to obtain statistics which provide an accurate picture of the age profile of people with HIV and AIDS in Britain, but we know that in the United States only 1 per cent of people with AIDS are in the 13–19 age group. However, a recent article points out the danger of imagining that HIV only affects adults. For example, in the state of Minnesota, 25 of a total of 1045 people with HIV are teenagers. It is also highly significant that 40 per cent of people with HIV in the region are aged between 20 and 29. Of these, the vast majority are gay.

The Minnesota Department of Health has given its largest grant for HIV/AIDS education among young people, and especially gay teenagers, who can lack self esteem and are often isolated. When we talk about the 'vulnerability' of gay teenagers we should be clear that we refer to their vulnerability to the effects of homophobia at home and at school. As Leo Treadway, an American AIDS educator, points out: 'we have to recognise that you can't simply talk about AIDS without talking about sexuality and the existence of lesbian and gay teenagers'.[4]

In Britain we need to recognise the inevitable consequences of our bizarre and cruel national refusal to support effective AIDS education amongst the young. People like Mary Whitehouse and Victoria Gillick are not just quaint eccentrics, they are dangerous, and their claims to speak on behalf of 'traditional moral values' should be closely scrutinised in relation to the rates of unwanted pregnancies, and now HIV, amongst teenagers. As one writer on the subject of teenage motherhood, concludes: 'If there is a single most common reason for teenage pregnancy, it is the inability of children to talk to their parents, and vice versa'.[5] Hence the vital role of sex education in schools, however inadequate it may sometimes be. And whilst AIDS statistics remain low among teenagers the figures of people with AIDS in their twenties makes it clear that many were infected in their teens.

Effective HIV/AIDS education for young people has to recognise that home is the last place where useful sex education is likely to take place for most teenagers. It must also acknowledge that not all teenagers have homes in the first place. For example, every year some 8000 young people leave state care with no protection, and no families to turn to, whilst no one has the faintest idea how many teenagers leave home because of parental violence, incest or their family's homophobia. However, we do know that 80 per cent of care-leavers in the UK are unemployed, whilst 40 per cent of the homeless are care-leavers.[6] Of these, no fewer than one in six are likely to have been sexually abused whilst 'in care'.[7]

This appalling situation has been made even worse by the recent changes in Social Security regulations which reduced benefits for school leavers in 1988, removing any provision for board and lodgings, on the misguided and callous assumption that all teenagers have families to house them until the age of 25.

These cuts are matched by a similar clampdown on family benefits. Junior Health Minister David Mellor's recent demand that the Health Education Authority should work 'fully within government policies', and abandon health education modelled on community development, suggests a terrifying inability even to begin to appreciate the complexity of the task facing HIV/AIDS educators in Britain.

Competition among Tory ministers to out-Thatcher one another in front of the Prime Minister is likely to create even more difficulties for the young, and especially the homeless, and can only ultimately contribute to the increased transmission of HIV amongst teenagers, who it seems are the latest victims on the High Altar of political careerism and the worship of Family Values.

If rent boys such as Jason Swift are to be regarded as victims, then we must be clear that they are victims of the long-term casually accepted and politically legitimated evil of homophobia throughout British society, an evil that may be found in all classes and population groups, and which seems perfectly prepared to deny any kind of responsibility for the health and safety of gay teenagers whose very existence it evidently prefers to forget. AIDS service organisations must not collude with this neglect, or be intimidated by charges of 'promoting' homosexuality. They must do all they can to help and support the same young people so many of us once were.

14. Community Responsibilities

The American critic Douglas Crimp has recently pointed out that most individual and social attitudes towards AIDS depend on whether the epidemic is regarded simply as a natural, accidental catastrophe, or whether it is seen as the result of gross political neglect: 'an epidemic that was allowed to happen'. For some, perhaps the majority, AIDS is understood as a problem that only affects a minority within a minority. For others, it is a crisis that should be recognised in everyone's lives, especially those of all gay men.

Given the generally abysmal track record of British medical journalism since the beginning of the epidemic, few of us have much understanding of the complex ways in which medical research and social policy have been dictated by financial and political factors, rather than the needs of people living with HIV disease. Most social aspects of HIV have also been consistently badly reported outside the gay press; and since it is unlikely that most men who have sex with other men actually read gay newspapers or magazines, this means that ignorance and misunderstanding are also widespread in the gay community.

For those like myself, who have witnessed the virtual decimation of an entire generation of gay men in the United States, including many dear friends and loved ones, the experience of direct loss has been the major motivating factor in our personal involvement. Most gay men in Britain are still statistically unlikely to have knowingly had much direct experience of HIV disease, especially outside London. The consistently low rates of new cases of HIV infection among gay men since 1984 show that it has not been direct personal experience but the growth of non-government AIDS service organisations all round the country that has determined the success of the safer sex revolution in our lives. These have resulted from the real strengths of British gay culture but most of all our everyday lives and friendships.

Yet we constantly hear that straight society has nothing to learn from us, that our lives are 'exceptional', that we only took up safer sex when we actually saw our friends dying in front of our eyes. Such an interpretation is not only deeply ignorant and insulting, it is also profoundly tragic, for it strongly suggests that homophobia will continue to prevent many heterosexuals from even trying to learn from our collective example. In these regrettable circumstances I believe that we have a continued responsibility to try to make other people listen to us, so that they will not have to go through the terrible losses with which many British gay men from all walks of life are now sadly familiar. Nonetheless, it is to one another that our most important responsibilities continue to lie, for the simple reason that no one else really gives a damn.

First, we should remember that there is no natural or inevitable unity among gay men, and that there are many reasons why some people find safer sex difficult, especially if they are isolated and cut off from other people, either geographically, or because of their social oppression. The current HIV antibody status of everyone who has had sex in the past fifteen years, and in particular in the long years before HIV was even known to exist, is a matter of sheer coincidence. I had a lot of sex in New York in the early 1980s and I am here writing this column. A close friend with whom I often stayed is now dying. It is as simple as that. And for New York one might as well read London or Glasgow. This is why HIV disease remains an issue for all gay men, regardless of our known or perceived HIV antibody status. Those of us who chance to be seronegative have an absolute and unconditional responsibility for the welfare of seropositive gay men. Would they have written us off if we had happened to get infected? This is the question we should all ask ourselves.

It is also vital that debate concerning possible treatment options reaches as many people as possible. When questions of possible treatment options are literally matters of life or death, we must learn to respect decisions which differ from our own. This is especially important in relation to the situation of people living with AIDS, since the Medical Research Council has so entirely abdicated its responsibility to conduct clinical trials for possible new treatments for opportunistic conditions such as MAI, CMV, and a host of others. It is hardly surprising if people living with HIV disease or AIDS frequently turn to complementary medicine. Non-biomedical treatments should be subject to the highest standards of scrutiny, but such evaluations are often unimportant to people who have chosen to reject what they regard as the limitations of western science. It should always be remembered that the

painful and often difficult decisions that occur at all levels of orthodox treatment—for example, the decision facing an individual offered a
place on a placebo-based randomised clinical trial—are no less seriously
undertaken than decisions to explore other avenues of possible benefit.
As the author of *The Natural History of Quackery* has observed: 'Quite
a lot of "quacking" today emanates from unexpected sources, which include medical journalism and our royal colleges. Perhaps a kindly motto
would be: "Never bust a quack unless you have something better to offer
the patient".'[1]

It is crucial that discussion of preventative medicine, health education, biomedical research, and complementary medicine take place in
the public domain. We should furthermore insist as a non-negotiable
condition: that people with HIV and their advocates are consulted at all
stages of health promotion, treatment and research. There has been far
too little debate concerning the scandalous lack of research on new anti-
HIV and anti-AIDS drugs in the UK, or the ethics of research protocols.
Those of us who continue to draw attention to these issues do so because
we are convinced that knowledge is a weapon for all of us in the fight
against AIDS. As the New York activist Mark Harrington wrote earlier
this year: 'AIDS advocates are not doctors. We are learning as we go, and
we will make some mistakes along the way. Nothing that is written or
said about AIDS should ever be accepted uncritically. Scepticism, constant questioning and relentless challenging of established authorities
are our only way to find out what works'.[2]

15. Safer Sex as Community Practice

Throughout the 1970s and 1980s many lesbians and gay men have been deeply involved in sustained and sometimes difficult debates concerning questions of sexual identity, representation and cultural politics.[1] In retrospect it almost seems as if we had been limbering up in advance to face the immensely complex and challenging problems raised by HIV disease, and the international 'pro-family' politics of the past decade. There can be little doubt that these debates over theory have substantially improved our understanding of much of the political and cultural hysteria that surrounds us, and have helped us plan effective strategic interventions on behalf of people living with HIV disease, and their various communities.

The formal title of the panel of the Fifth International Conference on AIDS in Montreal at which I gave a version of this chapter in mid-1989— 'Eroticism, Safer Sex and Behaviour Change'—involves three distinct terms, two of which are fundamental, and one of which, the third, is frequently highly misleading. Day after day at major conferences on AIDS, and in literally hundreds of published articles, we have witnessed the ways in which the institutions of behavioural psychology and quantitative social science have recoded their latent racism, misogyny and homophobia across the fields of epidemiology and health education— into which they have lately trespassed in search of sweeter funding pastures. Hence at Montreal we were invited to consider issues such as: 'Smoking as a Risk Factor for Heterosexual Transmission of HIV-1 in Haitian Women', and 'Hypermasculinity as a Predictor of Sexual Risk Behaviours in a Cohort of Gay Men', and the claim that: 'Childhood Gender Nonconformity Predicts HIV-1 Seropositivity in Homosexual Men'. It would appear from this that regardless of whether a gay teenager tries on his mother's shoes or his father's tweed jacket, he is equally doomed.

Frankly, one might as well consider ownership of the 'Judy Garland at Carnegie Hall' double album as a predictor of HIV seropositivity, or indeed the possession of a pair of Levi 501 jeans. When considering the gay communities in which HIV was widely transmitted for at least a decade before its existence was even suspected, any aspect of our cultural lives might be selected as significant indicators or 'risk factors' by researchers who, by doing so, reveal only the depths of their ignorance of the diversity of gay culture. It is hardly surprising that many safer sex educators are infuriated by such inane 'research' at a time when resources for effective health promotion are so hard to come by, and when so many lives are potentially at stake.

Of the hundreds of research projects presented at the Fifth International Conference on AIDS, only three considered the role of health care providers from the perspective of clients. AIDS has evidently provided many social scientists with a hitherto unparalleled 'opportunity' to survey the behaviour of gay men. This amounts to nothing less than a grand recapitulation of just the type of deviance theory that originally constituted the modern 'homosexual' as an object of surveillance and 'knowledge'. It is therefore high time that we evaluate the methods and values of this disease-inflected scrutiny of our lives as exhaustively as its curious investigations of ourselves. This is especially important because behaviourism so critically lacks any theory of desire, for which it substitutes a mechanical and simplistic notion of 'sex', taken as an *a priori* reality that blinds researchers to the multiple, uneven, shifting relations of desire to sexual behaviour and identities, both in the lives of individuals and desiring collectivities.[2]

Effective safer sex education requires a sensitive awareness of the finely nuanced variations of sexuality, understood as an extremely complex site of overlapping and frequently conflicting sexual desires, behaviour and identities in which irreducible and unconscious forces find expression in a multitude of specific concrete historical and cultural circumstances. Eroticism—that is, the pleasures of the body—is rooted in desire and desiring fantasy, while it is invariably articulated through practices that are intimately connected to contingent cultural forms and institutions. Located thus, eroticism cannot simply be switched on or off, or subjected to arbitrary redirection. Indeed, one of the profoundest insights offered by psychoanalysis is the recognition that we should have little faith in any attempt finally to demarcate between what is, or is not, sexual—between what may or may not be desired, and experienced, as sexual pleasure. The main problem with casual notions of 'behaviour change' is their inability to approach this primary domain of sexual fantasy, on which the substitutions and displacements that constitute safer sex must be established and libidinised. For what does it mean to say that we 'know' that HIV exists, in the face of pleasures that precisely threaten to destabilise and dissolve the conscious knowing self? Indeed, sexual gratification requires the abandonment of the very levels of self-conscious awareness that behaviourism attempts to redress. While it may be easy to have safer sex on an initial encounter, how do we sustain it over time, how do we translate the shallow notion of 'behaviour modification' into actual erotic practices, consistent with the great complexity and diversity of individual and collective sexual fantasies?

As gay men, we were initially vulnerable to an increased rate of the transmission of HIV because we tend both to fuck and get fucked. This is the only 'mystery' of gay sex. At the same time, our generally marginalised position has encouraged a certain frankness and articulateness about sexual behaviour which should properly be considered as exemplary. It is one of the larger ironies of our times that HIV has coincided with an especially fierce conflict between rival definitions of sexual morality in the West, most evident in the increasing gulf between heterosexual expectations of marriage and the reality of sexual relationships. Indeed, marriage has perhaps never been more culturally idealised than in the period of no-fault divorce laws. In all of this we may observe that a fundamental conflict is being waged between a widespread and radical demand for an enlargement of culturally legitimate estimations of human sexual relations, and the institutions and discourses of a largely secularised, yet nonetheless potent, Christian cultural tradition. Lesbians and gay men are inevitably positioned at the very heart of this conflict, since on the one hand we represent the possibility of a more open model of sexual relationships cemented in an ethics of mutual consent, and on the other we constitute the very embodiment of all that is perceived to be most threatening to supposedly 'traditional' values, many of which are of comparatively recent origin. This is the context in which we should emphasise Crimp's[3] forceful argument that gay men's promiscuity 'should be seen instead as a positive model of how sexual pleasure might be pursued by and granted to everyone if those pleasures were not confined within the narrow limits of institionalised sexuality.' In all such formulations it remains important to emphasise that 'gay men' do not represent a simple homogeneous social category, and that our sexuality contains the same diversity—both qualitatively and quantitatively—as that of any other population group defined by sexual object-choice.

The origins of safer sex

It is instructive to remember that gay men invented safer sex, long before the identification of HIV or the widespread availability of HIV antibody testing in the West. Callen's groundbreaking *How to Have Sex in an Epidemic* offered both a theory and a practice of risk reduction that has stood the test of time remarkably well, and represents an approach to safer sex education that continues to contrast strongly with the vast majority of UK and US government-funded initiatives, that might collectively be regarded under the heading: 'How to Give up Sex in an Epidemic'.[4] Meanwhile, both British and American government officials continue to claim that their interventions were responsible for the dramatic fall in new cases of HIV infection among gay men, in spite of the overwhelming epidemiological evidence that this took place on both sides of the Atlantic long before either government began their belated respective campaigns.[5] As Evans and others observe: 'The part played by the information campaign funded by the government in bringing about modifications in homosexual lifestyle seems to have been small. The most substantial changes had occurred before the campaign started.'[6]

Since the earliest years of the epidemic, safer sex education among gay men has been most successful when rooted in the recognition that HIV is a community issue, requiring a community-based response. The motivation behind the non-government safer sex campaigns that led to the original fall in the incidence of HIV was the recognition that safer sex should be established as a practice for all gay men, regardless of known or perceived HIV antibody status. Such an approach contrasts strikingly with 'official' messages, generally targeted at isolated individuals who are assumed to be uninfected. Such 'official' campaigns seem to regard safer sex as if its adoption were akin to a personal decision to change one's brand of toothpaste, or perhaps to become a vegetarian. For example, in England the Health Education Authority's (HEA) first venture into the field of AIDS education for gay men early in 1989 simply exhorted us to 'Choose Safer Sex', as if this had not been a central aspect of gay culture for years. Moreover, advertisements as part of this campaign only appeared in the gay press, and thus never reached men having sex with men who have little or no gay identity.

Sustaining safer sex

The real issue facing safer sex educators working with gay men is how to sustain safer sex over time, especially since there is some evidence that social and other factors may combine to undermine its importance.[7] The terrible scale of personal grief and loss must play a central role in this context for many individuals, especially those who do not have ready access to community-based support and counselling facilities. As Ben Schatz, Director of the American public interest law firm *National Gay Rights Advocates,* has pointed out, we sometimes speak of the gay community's achievement in cutting down new cases of HIV infection to 'only' 2 or 3 per cent per annum, whereas we should be horrified by the potential loss of life that such statistics continue to imply.[8]

It is painfully clear that in relation to the need for effective health education, gay men are still not officially regarded as a part of the 'general public' by the state or large sections of the press, in spite of the fact that in Europe, Australia and North America we have been far more terribly affected by HIV than any other section of the population. This places a tremendous weight of responsibility on non-government AIDS service organisations which are largely founded and financed by gay men. We thus face the curious paradox of a situation in which the government in Britain can praise the work of organisations such as the Terrence Higgins Trust and the gay community as a whole, which in all other circumstances is not even acknowledged to exist, save as a general 'threat' to the rest of the supposedly heterosexual population. Yet to obtain minimum funding, such non-government organisations have frequently found it convenient to turn their backs on the long-term volunteers who contributed so much to their early success. This 'degaying' process, as Cindy Patton has described it, does not automatically resolve the immediate problems of internal management and funding which it is ostensibly designed to address.[9] Furthermore, the human resources of AIDS volunteers are limited in relation to the long-term stress of such work, and 'burn-out' is an increasingly serious factor across the entire field of HIV/AIDS-related volunteer work. In these grim circumstances, we must ask ourselves what exactly the state is for. Certainly official government-funded AIDS 'information' campaigns throughout the West have consistently preferred the promotion of ideological and frankly moralistic nostrums to effective health promotion.

Unfortunately, Britain's ludicrous indecency and obscenity laws means that it is more or less impossible to develop the kinds of frank and sexually explicit safer sex materials that abound in countries such as Denmark or the Netherlands. This situation is complicated by the fact that the 'de-gaying' of nongovernment AIDS service organisations, and the power of conservative doctors within them, has guaranteed a widespread timidity in this vital area: one which is frequently reinforced by the fear of losing such relatively small sums of public money as have so far been made available, but upon which such organisations are largely dependent. There is thus all the more reason to think about the ways in which safer sex is discussed, publicised and developed, especially since international evidence now demonstrates that effective safer sex education is invariably rooted in the development of collective community values. As I have written elsewhere, community development is effective AIDS education, insofar as worldwide evidence strongly suggests that gay pride has played a major factor in preventing HIV transmission by establishing safer sex not just as a set of techniques, but as a fundamental aspect of gay cultural practices'.[10]

Strategies for safer sex education

In the early years of the epidemic it was recognised that a sexually transmitted agent (or agents) was probably responsible for AIDS. Thus, before the isolation of HIV, gay men in the USA developed guidelines to help minimise the possible risk of infecting one another. Understandably, such guidelines initially listed almost every conceivable sexual practice in relation to possible risk factors. Hence the emergence of the familiar categories of 'high', 'medium' and 'low' risk sexual activities, which formed the model for subsequent materials after the isolation of HIV in 1983 and its public announcement the following year. Such lists have subsequently been expanded and modified in the light of changing epidemiological information, and new knowledge of the natural history of HIV and its modes of transmission. Yet the problem remains that this approach tends to regard safer sex simply as a series of techniques, rather than as a way of life, or as a question of collective cultural practice.

Hence the growing tendency to approach safer sex education in terms of three overlapping objectives. The first of these is to provide the most basic general information concerning which sexual practices are most potentially likely to facilitate HIV transmission. The second is to present this information in the context of specific, easily recognised situations, addressed to groups of gay men, and men who have sex with other men but who do not have a positive gay identity. Third, safer sex education aims to provide a level of general, collective cultural empowerment, encouraging us to be able to identify one another's needs, and to think of ourselves as a community united in response to the epidemic. Hence the significance of Patton's emphasis on the need to eroticise the process of

negotiation that must always precede Safer Sex.[11] As D'Eramo argued in
a leading US gay porn magazine:

> The idea that gay men have no option for sexual expression left
> is a common appraisal, but it simply is not true. Safer sex itself
> cannot motivate us unless we eroticise it and make it more than a
> mere technique. Safer sex, as a motivator, without self-esteem—a
> mix of self-love and caring (gay pride included)—is very limited
> at best, and, at worst, doomed to failure. The crux is what you do
> and why. And what you do is your choice. Abstinence doesn't work
> because when people abstain, they don't learn about safer sex . . .
> and when they get horny enough, they'll go out and break every
> rule in the book.[12]

Individual and community empowerment is thus fundamental to effective safer sex education for gay men and lesbians, especially in countries
such as Britain that so conspicuously lack strong political traditions
founded in notions of civil rights. Furthermore, it is important to combat anti-gay prejudice in all forms of safer sex education targeted at
heterosexuals, in the light of the possibility 'that anti-gay attitudes stand
between media information and public knowledge and public opinion'.[13]
American research conducted in San Francisco demonstrates that in
the reporting of AIDS, the main determinants of media coverage were
initially based on prior attitudes to gay men, which again raises the
possibility 'that anti-gay attitudes constrain the ability of the media to
effectively communicate information about risk factors and how the disease is transmitted'.[14] The same researchers also discovered that: 'as we
expected, education was a significant predictor of knowledge about HIV
transmission, but it accounted for considerably less variance . . . than
attitudes towards gay rights'.[15] There is thus strong evidence to support
the hypothesis that anti-gay, and also probably racist, attitudes tend
to encourage the denial of heterosexual transmission among prejudiced
individuals, and there is clearly an urgent need for cross-sectional studies
of correlations between accurate HIV/AIDS knowledge, safer sex behaviour among heterosexuals and racist and anti-gay prejudice. It would
also be extremely useful to devise research protocols to assess the role of
homophobic and racist attitudes within and between different national
media institutions, comparing television and the press, for example, in
relation to levels of inaccuracy and conflicting information concerning
all aspects of HIV/AIDS. This is especially important since most people
gain such information as they may possess from such primary cultural
sources.[16]

If, as seems highly likely, the routine provision of ambiguous, misleading and conflicting messages throughout the media puts viewers and readers at increased risk of HIV transmission, it is important to devise counter-strategies that might protect them. For example, effective safer sex education should actively encourage everyone to disregard in its entirety any HIV/AIDS education materials or information that continues to speak of the 'AIDS virus' or 'the AIDS test', and thus demonstrates its own inability (or refusal) to distinguish between HIV and AIDS. Other direct indicators of unreliability would include all references to so-called 'AIDS carriers', and a refusal to comply with the demands of the Denver Principles and the international principles established in the 1988 World Health Organisation resolution concerning the avoidance of discrimination in relation to HIV-infected people and people with AIDS.[17] This in turn would constitute an immediate and easily achievable form of individual and collective empowerment that is the prerequisite for adopting and sustaining safer sex over time. Such an approach encourages people to read critically, and to make their own assessments of health education materials and all other sources of supposed 'information'. It recognises that safer sex education should aim to provide not only generalised short-term information but also longer-term focused campaigns and strategies to counteract unjustified fears and anxieties that may derive from cultural sources, including politics and religious fundamentalism, which seek to legitimise prejudice. It also refuses any suggestion that sex is simply an autonomous 'behaviour', like driving, or fixing one's hair. It must continually be asserted that one does not take up, or stick with safer sex in the same way that one might choose a new car, or consider changing one's favourite brand of hair gel.

It is particularly regrettable that many governments have entrusted their national HIV/AIDS education campaigns to commercial advertising agencies, and have turned their backs on the accumulated findings of decades of research in health education and health promotion. As the distinguished medical historian Allan Brandt points out: 'The limited effectiveness of education which merely encourages fear is well-documented.'[18] Yet this is totally ignored by many governments throughout the world. For example, in Britain the HEA has been subject to heavy state presure in relation to all aspects of HIV/AIDS education.

The HEA's most recent campaigns have all shared a common byline: 'AIDS. You're as Safe as You Want to Be'. This significantly places all responsibility for HIV transmission on the isolated individual, and clearly colludes with many other such advertisements, in the implication that people with HIV or AIDS constitute a threat that only the individual can avoid. Yet such campaigns never attempt to provide practical safer sex advice, beyond conflicting messages such as: 'Having fewer partners is only one way to reduce the risk. Safer sex also means using a condom, or alternatively, having sex that avoids penetration.' Encouraging people to talk about sex is at least as important as condom use, and this is especially important for population groups like many British heterosexuals, that may be characterised as hysterically modest and all but pathologically inhibited in their ability to discuss sex. One medium that might almost have been designed to meet the needs of safer sex education, domestic video, is unfortunately subject to far stricter legal controls than in any other European country except for the Republic of Ireland. Most British HIV/AIDS videos have therefore tended to be extraordinarily dreary, with little or no attention being paid to sexual desire or practice.

Homophobia, 'lifestyles' and 'addiction'

The underlying puritanism that determines so much British legal moralism may also be widely found in national safer sex materials, which often seem to be affected by a refusal or inability to acknowledge the diversity of sexual behaviour, even among lesbians and gay men. While it is clear that safer sex aims to minimise the transmission of HIV by preventing semen getting into the rectum or the vagina, this does not mean that effective sex education works by telling people not to fuck. It is certainly not helpful to pretend, for example, that many lesbians do not enjoy both anal and vaginal penetration, or that 'non-penetrative sex' is some kind of ideal goal independent of safer sex, as some feminists strongly imply. Indeed, it should be noted that safer sex education has provided an opportunity for sexual puritans of all persuasions to rush into print and workshops, whether from the perspective of revolutionary feminism or from other forms of evangelical culture. Such strongly directive approaches are only likely to encourage resistance, which can prove very dangerous. We should be very cautious of ostensible safer sex advisers and 'experts' who seem more interested in promoting their particular moral beliefs than in trying to understand and respect the full range of their clients' consensual sexual needs and pleasures.

This is especially important when many of the lesbians and gay men who developed the early models of effective safer sex education are either leaving non-government organisations as the result of burn-out, or because they feel they can no longer work within increasingly bureaucratic structures that are often more concerned with 'not rocking the boat' than meeting the needs of those constituencies most at risk from HIV. It is crucial that lesbians and gay men do not collude with such processes in desperately underfunded non-government organisations, which are often directed by boards and board members who have little or no understanding of the basic issues of safer sex education. For we have an absolute responsibility to our various lesbian and gay communities, in all their diversity, and especially to those whom no one else is prepared to support—gay teenagers, racial minorities, the elderly and the disabled. It is worth pointing out that 15 per cent of people with AIDS diagnosed in Nice are over sixty.[19] While it is frequently, and correctly, pointed out that HIV has had a disproportionate impact on the black and Hispanic population of the United States, this same structure of argument is never employed in Britain to describe the impact of HIV on gay men. This is presumably because gay men are not regarded as proportionally comparable to heterosexuals in the first place. The sheer scale and efficiency of British homophobia often seem all but overwhelming, and insuperable. For example, the leading London weekly magazine, *Time Out,* recently compiled a long list of subjects that are supposedly 'In' and 'Out' for the summer of 1989. Thus sex, we learned, is 'In', together with comics, the singer Madonna, and Batman. Food and political comedy are 'Out'. So, apparently, is AIDS: 'Do you want to be bored to death?' asked *Time Out.*

Such attitudes do not lack more sophisticated exponents. For example, the same team of epidemiologists that reported the fall in new cases of HIV infection among gay men in the UK write of the epidemic from which their statistics derive in a manner that reveals an extraordinary ignorance about human sexuality. Hence their bizarre and insulting hypothesis that 'the profound consequences of HIV infection might have been expected to suppress the expression of a homosexual lifestyle in younger men'.[20] It is precisely such expectations that reveal much about the attitudes of professional social scientists and others involved in AIDS research. What might the readers of the *British Medical Journal,* where their report was published, have made of the claim that 'the profound consequences of HIV infection might have been expected to suppress the expression of a heterosexual lifestyle in younger men'? It is the stark double standard applied to gay men in relation to heterosexuals that is so alarming.

The key term in these and allied debates is that of 'lifestyle', which is frequently used throughout the AIDS literature to refer to gay men in such a way that it protects the unstated but underlying assumption of a 'natural' heterosexuality, from which homosexuality is regarded as a voluntary aberration. This provides an ostensibly 'scientific' legitimation for any amount of scapegoating and victim-blaming.

It is this notion of 'lifestyle' that also unites the discourses of epidemiology and 'official' HIV/AIDS 'education' materials. Ann Karpf has described the emergence of what she terms the 'look-after-yourself' model of health education in the late 1970s. From such a perspective 'illness is the result of harmful individual habits or a "lifestyle" undertaken voluntarily—eating the wrong foods, drinking too much, smoking, lack of exercise, and stress'.[21] The 'look-after-yourself' approach to health education was intended to combat an overly medical view of health, for which it simply substitutes a highly voluntaristic picture of individuals 'taking charge' of their lives, and rejecting previous 'unhealthy' and 'irresponsible' lifestyles. As such, it has been widely instituted in many health education campaigns, although, as Karpf points out, it assumes that individuals possess 'unqualified powers to shape their lives, with their future well-being their priority'. This also involves a virtual suppression of any consideration of the many powerful contingent circumstances that may inform decision-making. It is also a particularly inadequate approach in relation to questions of sexual behaviour, which comes to be seen as a simple arena of conscious choices, rather than as a complex arena of intense commercial and cultural pressures that compete to arouse and satisfy the workings of sexual fantasy. Finally, there is the added problem of creeping moralism that may inform distinctions between supposedly 'healthy' and 'unhealthy' sex, in a rhetoric that can easily slide into frank homophobia. It is especially important to reject spurious and highly misleading analogies between sexual behaviour and chemical addictions. These compound the double error of regarding smoking or alcoholism or narcotic drug use as purely personal, individual phenomena, while suggesting that any form of sexual activity outside the context of a full social and emotional relationship should also be regarded as shameful and damaging.[22] Such an approach is entirely incompatible with the aims and methods of effective safer sex education.

From the individual to the collective

The HIV epidemic also coincides historically with a quite separate crisis in the overall management and 'political economy' of sex and sexuality in the modern world. For example, state-directed HIV/AIDS 'education' campaigns have afforded an ideal opportunity for many governments to develop new strategies in their constant struggle to win popular consent to their larger political objectives in relation to population management and social policy. Not surprisingly, such strategies have stimulated widespread resistance, and it seems that levels of HIV/AIDS-related ignorance, prejudice and denial are highest in those countries such as Britain that have been bombarded with explicitly moralistic and directive kinds of AIDS 'education'. Hence the increased difficulties experienced by non-government AIDS service organisations that are obliged to face and deal with the direct consequences of campaigns which Patton has brilliantly characterised as: 'Too much, too late'.[25] These consequences include a steady escalation of the 'worried well' needing attention, and the drying up of funding for a 'problem' which it is erroneously believed has been resolved via government posters and television advertising.

This is why it is so vitally important to continue to emphasise that safer sex education should be concerned with developing individual and collective self-esteem in relation to erotic practice. For most official HIV/AIDS 'education' has only tended to reinforce negative perceptions of safer sex as a system of imposed constraints, that are only able to be complied with reluctantly, from motives of guilt and fear. It is unlikely that significant numbers of people will be able to sustain safer sex over time from such a perspective. Nor can mechanical behaviourist analyses explain the failure of such campaigns, save in terms of individual 'noncompliance' or so-called 'sexual addiction'. In the meantime, the delusion that HIV is only a risk from extraordinary sources that are external to the lives of decent, ordinary folk is casually reinforced.

It does not require a close psychoanalytic reading of government sponsored HIV/AIDS 'health education' materials to demonstrate their profound dread of an active, autonomous female sexuality, as exemplified in the 'Worrying Isn't it' campaign. Such fear on the part of many heterosexual men is evidently displaced and projected onto gay men, who are literally required to be 'feminised' in much public AIDS commentary. For effective HIV/AIDS education inevitably draws attention to the simple but clearly controversial fact that when everything is considered, all forms of consensual human sexual behaviour amount to much of a muchness. This is seemingly very disturbing to sexual identities that are massively stabilised by exaggerated notions of gender specificity, and the imagined 'otherness' of such supposedly unified categories as 'women' or 'homosexuals'. In this manner, possibly painful divisions in the self may be conveniently projected onto 'other people', and expressed as contempt. This process seems to be far more common among heterosexuals than lesbians or gay men. Indeed, the widespread phobic dread of AIDS that manifests itself daily in tabloid journalism and in the helpless compulsive HIV antibody testing of the 'worried well' is not unconnected to the fantasied perception that HIV infection implies a direct, if mediated, physical relationship with the bodies of gay men or people of colour. Dread of HIV infection thus speaks an excessive fear of transgressing profound social and psychic boundaries that evidently stabilise many aspects of heterosexual identity. That heterosexual identity may often require to be bolstered by the forces of unconscious homophobia and racism is a conjecture that deserves further enquiry. It may well be easier for some people to think of HIV in terms of miasmatic contagion, than to confront the actual modes of transmission that cannot be admitted to consciousness, for whatever reasons.

Notions of HIV antibody testing or quarantine as effective measures for the primary prevention of HIV transmission are in this context only the most transparent re-inscription of those boundaries and categories forged by repression, that are experienced by many as indispensable to their most basic (if vulnerable) sense of self. Thus the struggle to achieve a psychic goal of masculinity or femininity may be rationalised and articulated in the readily available language of disease control. We should also recall that the available categories and identities of modern Western sexuality were originally constituted in a heavily medicalised discourse of sickness and health. Much of the imagery of AIDS was thus ready and waiting, and is by no means specific to the epidemic. When entire societies succumb to the excessive symptoms of sexual repression and anxiety, the consequences can be grim indeed—as the history of HIV/AIDS-related legislation in such countries as Britain, Cuba, Sweden and the USA demonstrates with alarming clarity.[24]

While such theoretical speculation may seem overly abstract to some, it is precisely because we face such a grim reality that we need to exercise all the intellectual adroitness of which we are capable. For Europeans like myself, who have helplessly watched the virtual decimation of an entire generation of fellow gay men, including many dear and much loved friends in cities throughout the United States, it is of the greatest importance to try to understand the continued denial of adequate funding and support for basic health care provision, health education, housing, anti-discrimination legislation and clinical trials of possible drugs for use in the treatment of HIV disease. It is our ethical and political responsibility to try our best, in the midst of a crisis that is frequently all but physically and emotionally overwhelming, to learn such lessons in order to be able to anticipate and counteract such tendencies in Europe, where the provision of socialised medicine and more enlightened social welfare policies have not prevented widespread discrimination against people living with HIV and AIDS, as well as their communities. As increasing numbers of gay men opt for the HIV antibody test as a means of access to good patient management, we can learn from the unexpected consequences of changing attitudes towards testing in the USA. For example, Helquist has recently pointed out that 'organisations, like individuals, may also encounter conflicts. . . . Some AIDS activist groups have found that their seropositive members give top priority to AIDS treatment issues, while seronegative members want to emphasise prevention and policy concerns.'[25]

In the present circumstances, we should emphasise that questions concerning safer sex education and treatment issues are not alternatives, but are strictly complementary, and of equal significance. Effective health education depends on the recognition that safer sex is an ongoing necessity for all gay men, regardless of our known or perceived HIV antibody status. At the same time, the need for ethically acceptable clinical trials for potential treatment drugs is equally an issue for everyone in the various communities affected by HIV disease. For nobody can know for sure if and when they might need them. And as Nick Partridge from the Terrence Higgins Trust has argued, there must be no question of our being any less supportive of people who may contract HIV in the future than we are of people living with HIV today.[26] In the meantime we need to sustain the development of the erotics of safer sex in the context of a morality that is founded on respect for diversity and choice, and which accords with Foucault's rejection of any form of morality that seeks to be acceptable to everyone: 'in the sense that everyone would have to submit to it'—an aim that he identifies as 'catastrophic'.[27] It is precisely that aim which underpins so much official government-sponsored HIV/ AIDS 'education' around the world, a project that aspires to tether sexual identity ever more restrictively to the twin poles of 'the family' and the nation-state.

The erotics of safer sex remain the only effective means by which we can challenge and resist the literally deadly consequences of a stunting moralism that refuses to accept that all our consensual sexual needs are equally valid. This project is necessarily provisional, and closely contingent upon changing circumstances and available resources, including those of creative imagination. Safer sex constitutes both an erotics and an ethics; it has established a set of collective cultural practices that combine the affirmation of sexual desire in all its forms with an active, practical commitment to mutual care and responsibility. As the state and its many attendant institutions continue to look on, indifferent to our plight, we have enlarged our concept of gay identity that was forged in the tradition of gay pride, insisting that gay identity should also now mean safer sex. It is from this perspective that we now evaluate the dominant political and sexual rationalities of our times with a mixture of astonishment and horror. We are astonished by the relentless strategies of naked biomedical policing that now passes for HIV/AIDS 'education' in so many parts of the world. We are horrified by the refusal of the state to accept its responsibilities to the complex population whose allegiance it claims.

As the epidemic worsens, we can only reasonably expect the gulf between these two models of HIV/AIDS prevention, and their respective research methods and priorities, to widen. The situation in Britain is very uneven. On the one hand, it is clear that younger people have a far more open-minded and generally sophisticated approach to questions of sex and sexuality than their parents and grandparents. On the other, it is equally apparent that older traditions—of moralism, of education, of party politics, of sexual and class identities—continue to dominate the field of cultural practice and cultural reproduction. Non-government AIDS service organisations are praised in public by government ministers, yet prevented from undertaking fully effective safer sex education in a period of ever-increasing state censorship. The government has also set its face against all forms of health education rooted in the hated concept of community development, while a leading spokesman for the Medical Research Council, which supervises HIV/AIDS-related biochemical research, has publicly stated that he believes that treatment research raises a 'moral dilemma' since it might 'prolong the lives of people who would be infectious in the community'.[28] The gulf between such 'pure science' researchers and the day-to-day lived experience of directly involved doctors and nurses faithfully duplicates the gulf between the rival models of health education that this chapter has considered. We cannot expect an easy or immediate resolution of these divisions, since HIV/AIDS education inevitably involves issues that are heavily loaded in political and ideological terms, from 'the family', national identity and gay rights to the complex realities of prostitution and injecting drug use in contemporary Britain. The attempted sexual counter-revolution that is such a central plank of British government policy means that effective HIV/AIDS education will continue to take place under the closest scrutiny of politicians and scandal-mongering journalists. The struggle between rival models of safer sex education meanwhile involves fundamental matters of life and death, and in the coming years it is likely to prove, for many, a fight to the death.

1990 ———

16. Re-gaying AIDS

Suddenly and entirely unexpectedly, it has become possible in 1990 to think of Europe as a cultural and social entity
that stretches from Ireland to Greece, and from Sicily to Prague,
Warsaw, Budapest, and even Leningrad. The emergence of confident lesbian and gay movements in central Europe also raises the necessity of
addressing HIV/AIDS education in these countries, whose experience
and needs are in some ways different, and in others similar, to our own.

In February the First European Conference on HIV and Homosexuality took place in Copenhagen, with almost 200 delegates from 19
European countries, including Poland, Hungary and Czechoslovakia.
The title of the conference—'Re-Gaying AIDS'—encouraged discussion
of the importance of a positive gay identity in the struggles against HIV
infection and its consequences. As long ago as 1986, Cindy Patton described the dangers of ignoring the role of gay pride and gay community
values in effective HIV/AIDS work, and of looking only at: 'the actions
and concerns of the professionals who have taken up AIDS as an issue'.
As she argued with passion, our successes:

> are derived from gay activists, not from the professionals who came
> late and reluctantly to the health crisis. If we embrace a revised
> history in which professionals imagine that they conjured safe sex
> out of formulas and studies, we will come even more dependent on
> the medical establishment that is so callous towards women's and
> gay health concerns!

We know from our own British experience that nationalist movements
and political parties are rarely sensitive to sexual politics, and this becomes more difficult still when such nationalist movements are xeno-
phobic, as in many parts of Russia, or deeply traditional in religion and

moral outlook, as in Poland. Whilst we are familiar with the role of the Far Right in preventing HIV/AIDS education in Britain, Benny Henriksson from Sweden gave a paper that usefully analysed anti-gay prejudice on the Left, and the failure of social-democratic or welfare-state policies to respond adequately to the needs of gay men in the epidemic. He stressed that policies emphasising formal social control, and rejecting safer sex, are as common on the Left as they are on the Right, since welfarism involves a culture of purity that is incompatible with a gay culture of pleasure.

Hans Moerkerk, the Director of the Health Education Centre in Amsterdam, expanded this theme in his analysis of the different types of government response to AIDS throughout Europe. For example, he contrasted the frankly political responses in Britain, West Germany and Sweden, to the exclusive bio-medical emphasis in Belgium, Spain, France and the emergent central European democracies. Both approaches are steeped in anti-gay prejudice, and contrast, argued Moerkerk, with the more pragmatic approach in countries such as Holland, Denmark and Switzerland, where: 'the emphasis has not been on prohibition or on other coercive forms of control but on planning, evaluation, pragmatism and consensus'.

The most impressive paper came from the Norwegian sociologist Annick Prieur, discussing the reasons for continued unsafe sex among some gay men. She concluded that:

> When we started this research, some of us were surprised that gay men still had unsafe sex. Why can't they change their sex life, it must be more important to survive than to keep on having sex in the same way as before? . . . We were distanced from gay men's sex life and we didn't know what it meant to have your entire sex life labelled as something dangerous. It was easy for us to conceive of only negative reasons for having unsafe sex. . . . If this were true, unsafe sex would be caused by a lack of self control, by drinking, drugs or just plain madness. This is a view that stems from a simple rational choice model. If people don't behave 'rationally' that must be because they have lost their reason. But the world is not that simple; unsafe sex is also a rational behaviour—but a wider understanding of rationality is needed: including longing and love as motives for action.

Many, many millions of pounds have been squandered on academic research projects around the world that do not begin to approach such a sensitive and practical understanding of the issues facing HIV/AIDS educators in the gay community.

It seemed clear that a more direct networking is necessary between different gay organisations and non-government AIDS service organisations in Europe, especially in relation to knowledge about treatment drugs, clinical trials, and standards of general patient management. For just as I believe that everyone who knows or thinks that they are HIV antibody-negative has an absolute responsibility to support people with HIV, so the gay communities of Europe have an overall responsibility to and for one another. This was admirably shown in relation to Section 28, with demonstrations in Amsterdam and elsewhere. We can and must be equally well-organised in relation to HIV. Moreover, these issues are not going to go away, and there remains much work to be done, not least in forcing lesbian and gay groups which have ignored AIDS to recognise that for the foreseeable future HIV is the major issue for all gay people. This is especially important in countries with statistically small epidemics, where gay men are particularly vulnerable to prejudice, and the denial of treatment drugs available elsewhere. The blueprint for an extended, democratic federal Europe is being drawn up, and it is up to all of us to make sure that lesbians and gay men are not written out of the picture yet again.

17. Practices of Freedom: 'Citizenship' and the politics of identity in the age of AIDS

One of the main characteristics of Thatcherism has been the confidence with which the government speaks and legislates in the name of 'traditional' moral values, in areas which previous postwar administrations have regarded as highly sensitive and complex. Of these, the question of sexuality and 'the family' has been especially important: much of the government's popularity has resided in its successful presentation of 'the family' as uniquely threatened and vulnerable, and therefore in need of stringent defensive measures, mainly from lesbians and gay men who have consistently been presented as one of the gravest threats to this fantasy of uniform 'family life'. In Mrs Thatcher's personal rhetoric, 'family' and 'nation' have long been presented as mutually interchangeable terms in such a way that imagined challenges to the former can also be presented as deeply dangerous for the latter.

Yet AIDS confronts the government with a complex reality that cannot easily be disposed of in such over-simplified terms. We are not dealing with a single epidemic, but with a series of unfolding and overlapping epidemics within and between different population groups, determined by the modes of transmission of HIV in the decade or more before its existence was realised. The result has been a significant tension between conflicting imperatives. On the one hand ministers such as David Mellor congratulate organisations such as the Terrence Higgins Trust in the voluntary sector, whilst on the other, hard-line back-benchers continue to make political capital out of the crudest forms of prejudice, aided and abetted by the ever-dependable services of large sections of the British press. One consequence of this tension has been a bizarre compromise between the government's official moral ideology and the need for effective health education, which seriously suggests that recommending monogamy or celibacy is the best 'solution' to the issue of HIV infection. It is as if the actual complexity and diversity of human sexuality is as much of a problem for the government as the epidemic.

Direct censorship of health education projects produced by the government's own Health Education Authority provides shocking evidence of Thatcherism's unwavering reliance on moral homilies, which are policed at entirely unaccountable levels of executive government. An overriding commitment to a politically expedient vision of 'family values' is being sustained indefinitely, at the direct expense of effective health education strategies. This can only serve to guarantee the increased transmission of HIV, especially among heterosexuals who have been comfortably cocooned in the potentially deadly delusion that they are not really at risk since the beginning of the epidemic. Given the average of ten years between HIV infection and diagnosable symptoms of AIDS, the government's direct legacy of preventable AIDS cases will not be fully apparent until the late 1990s.

The opposition parties have all but failed to challenge the validity of the picture of British social life depicted by Thatcherite fundamentalism, or to question the government's long-term failure to acknowledge the actual complexity of the population that it claims to represent. Political parties in opposition to Thatcherism seem uniformly unable to grasp the political dimensions of the HIV epidemic. The Left has only been able to register AIDS against the criteria of pre-existing policies and priorities. In practice, this has guaranteed an almost total silence on the entire subject. It would not be correct to conclude that the Labour NEC has simply buckled under the pressure of external anti-gay prejudice, real as this is. On the contrary, it has been fully prepared to exploit that prejudice to its own imagined electoral advantage. AIDS may be privately described as a 'disaster' or even a 'tragedy', but it is never publicly identified as an epidemic which in almost every respect has been, and continues to be *allowed to happen*.[1]

Since the early years of the epidemic, lesbians and gay men have been at the forefront of attempts to produce effective health education materials, for all sections of the population. Unfortunately this work has been hampered both by lack of funds, and archaic indecency and obscenity legislation. The Thatcherite model of business sponsorship for private charities has proved a failure, even for the government's own National AIDS Trust (NAT) which has failed to raise funds from the city or other commercial sources. We now face a situation in which the consequences of a decade of inadequate medical reporting in the British press has led to widespread boredom with the whole subject, reinforced by the government attempts to perpetrate its values on the epidemic through its own 'official' advertising campaigns, which are based on a heady brew of sexual puritanism and scare-mongering.

This is exemplified by the typically individualistic approach of the work of the Health Education Authority (HEA), whose advertisements share a common by-line 'AIDS: You're as safe as you want to be'. The situation is further complicated by the fact that the HEA itself has long been under attack from the radical Right, which wishes to present AIDS as a form of direct retribution against those who wantonly fail to live lives of exclusively monogamous heterosexuality. The prevalence of this retributive view is most tragically apparent in the widespread acceptance of the belief that the success of safer sex campaigns amongst gay men may safely be disregarded by the rest of the population because of our 'exceptional' status. The exceptionalist argument holds that gay men constitute 'a community' which adopted safer sex only when we saw our friends dying around us. This is untrue and dangerously misleading, since until very recently indeed it was statistically most unlikely that most gay men had any direct experience of either HIV infection or AIDS in their immediate friendship circles. Yet safer sex was indeed taken up by most gay men in Britain in the mid-1980s, as official epidemiology makes perfectly plain. It is only possible to understand this refusal to learn from the demonstrably proven effectiveness of safer sex education amongst gay men in terms of a larger and prior inability to regard lesbians and gay men as fundamentally ordinary and intrinsically unremarkable members of British society. For that reason anti-gay prejudice continues to make heterosexuals increasingly vulnerable to HIV.

At the same time we should notice the extreme levels of prejudice and ignorance concerning the position of the thousands of gay men living with HIV or AIDS in Britain, in order to understand the full significance of the 'moral standards' that have dominated British public life in the 1980s. If there has been a dramatic resurgence of gay political activity in this period, it is hardly surprising since it has become clear that our very existence is widely regarded as regrettable. It is important to consider the full significance of the government's continuing failure to support community-based health education among the social groups most severely affected by HIV disease since 1981. We read and hear about how well 'the gay community' has done in cutting back the rate of new cases of infection, yet in reality the social relations of gay men in Britain are fragile, and the absence of a powerful model of civil rights politics has tended to undermine the emergence of a confident gay culture in Britain.

In these circumstances, community development is much the most important strategy in HIV/AIDS education, since it is based on the development and reinforcement of the sense of individual and collective worth and responsibility. HIV education among gay men has emphasised the importance of safer sex for all men having sex with men, regardless of their known or perceived antibody status, as opposed to official messages which continue to demonise people living with HIV. A special irony of the current situation is that Section 28 has brought gay men and lesbians together, in opposition to frankly anti-gay legislation, and has stimulated a strengthening of gay community values. Yet through all this, I am not aware of a single statement either from the Prime Minister or the Leader of her Majesty's Opposition that draws attention to the tragedy of an epidemic that has already affected tens of thousands throughout the UK. This resounding silence demonstrates with frightening clarity the full extent of the divorce between British parliamentary politics, and the lives of the actual subjects of Britain.

This grim separation of political priorities from the field of everyday life is still more apparent at the level of biomedical research. In the United States there are currently over 200 ongoing clinical trials of possible new treatment drugs against HIV, and the wide range of opportunistic conditions that collectively make up the Acquired Immune Deficiency Syndrome. In Britain there is only one solitary clinical trial, which largely duplicates American research. The Medical Research Council (MRC) has established a directed programme of research, which its Director has described as having 'the aim of developing vaccines for the prevention, and drugs for the treatment, of HIV infection and AIDS'.[2] Yet if one turns to the back of the MRC's guide to its AIDS Directed Programme, one finds committees supervising vaccine trials and the ethical aspects of vaccine research, but there is no committee supervising treatment research or the medical ethics of treatment-related clinical trials, for the simple reason that treatment research is not taking place. The entire bulk of more than £40 million at the MRC's disposal for HIV/AIDS research has been dedicated to the search for a vaccine for the uninfected: people living with HIV disease have been written off in their entirety. Whilst there are excellent reasons for British scientists to wish to build on previous expertise in the field of vaccine research, it is chilling that this has been posed as an alternative to treatment research. In this context we might consider the statement by one leading MRC microbiologist that treatment research raises 'a moral dilemma', since it would 'run the risk of prolonging the lives of people who would be infectious in the community'.[3] It should be perfectly clear that the lives of people living with HIV disease, and their immediate communities are held very cheap both by official HIV education and the top levels of the MRC.

Unfortunately in Britain we have largely lacked the support of strong advocacy organisations like the American Civil Liberties Union (ACLU) and others, which have played an important role at all levels of the US epidemic, from fighting direct discrimination through the courts, to championing patients' rights in relation to biomedical research. Furthermore, the British Left, which might have been expected to take an active interest in the epidemic has on the contrary largely ignored it. Sadly, we suffer from the long legacy of a tradition of ultra-leftism that seems trapped in its own estimations of radicalism that rarely exceed the field of class-related politics, which is hopelessly inadequate to the complexities of power in the modern world. This is not of course to deny the centrality of class in British society, but to point out the impossibility of trying to understand or intervene in the political struggles around AIDS in class terms alone. Moreover, the Left generally chooses to interpret its refusal or inability to work with other groups and lobbies as evidence of its own purity and correctness, rather than of the bankruptcy of its own self-styled radicalism. A similar puritanical separatism also afflicts many sections of the British women's movement, which has still hardly begun to grasp the wider political significance of AIDS, in relation to longstanding concerns about the management of sexuality and sexual reproduction.

When Health Minister David Mellor observed that perhaps 25 per cent of gay men in London may already be infected, his only comment was that 'people must not breathe a sigh of relief and think it will soon blow over'.[4] Such statements betray a shocking indifference to the actual scale of suffering caused by HIV—shocking, but hardly surprising given the generally abysmal record of British journalism outside the gay press since the beginning of the epidemic. The media continue to pump out prejudice and misinformation that either confuses and alarms readers, or simply denies any possibility of risk to 'decent' people. We may fairly detect two consistent characteristics of such attitudes. On the one hand, the presentation of AIDS as a 'gay plague' continues to articulate deep anxieties about homosexuality. The epidemic may thus become the viral projection of an unconscious desire to kill gay men, and these unconscious attitudes should never be discounted or underestimated.[5] On the

other hand, the 'homosexualising' of AIDS, and the denial of HIV transmission among heterosexuals offers a semi-magical delusion of intrinsic safety which is as potentially threatening to heterosexuals, as their
homophobia is to gay men.[6]

In all this, it should be apparent that fundamental questions about
the meaning of democracy in modern Britain are at stake. We should not
have to struggle against the odds to establish health education which re-
jects scaremongering, victim-blaming, and irrational sexual puritanism.
Effective health education should be a basic and indisputable right, and
never more so than during an epidemic. At the same time, standards of
health-care provision and medical research should never be dependent
upon the individual's sexuality, class, race or ethnicity. The political
management of the British AIDS epidemic demonstrates repeatedly and
at all levels that there are many higher priorities than either preventive
medicine or the saving of lives. It is therefore critically important that
we should be able to identify the leading institutions responsible for
deciding and directing social policies in relation to HIV disease, from
individual departments of government, to the mass media, regional and
district health authorities, the Health Education Authority, the General
Medical Council and so on, in order to lobby them effectively. If such
institutions fail to respond, civil disobedience may well prove necessary,
and ACT UP (London), which was formed early in 1989, has already
organised a number of well-targeted demonstrations in relation to the
cut-backs in social security payments and other issues.

Unfortunately, ACT UP faces formidable problems in Britain. First,
there are the difficulties of 'bandwagoning' and attempts to hijack the
emergent AIDS activist movement by far-left 'interventionists'. Second,
there is no sustained tradition of civil-disobedience politics in Britain,
and British police do not recognise lesbians and gay men as a legitimate
social constituency, unlike many other European countries. Similarly
there is no local tradition of training in nonviolent civil disobedience,
or of the organisation of 'affinity groups' which has been so successful
in ACT UP (New York)—establishing small, close networks of people
who have prepared before a given action to work as a team. Third, there
is little sense in Britain of the possible role of a cultural politics concerned with images and symbols, such as exists in the USA, where the
famous 'Silence = Death' poster from 1986 opened the way for a flood of
incisive and stylish political posters, T-shirts and badges, which provide
AIDS activists with a strong cultural identity and which, in turn, have
raised vital issues of information in the public spaces of New York. Last,

the absence of the sense of constitutional rights that so shapes American oppositional politics makes demonstrators vulnerable to arbitrary arrest and violence, and means that there is not a large and 'ready-made' culture of direct political interventionism on which to draw. This was reflected in the early decision by the 'Frontliners' organisation, which works on behalf of people with AIDS, to dissociate itself from ACT UP (London), on the bizarre grounds that, 'Certain extreme elements have called for demonstrations which would result in people with AIDS/ARC and people with disabilities being arrested.'[7]

Clearly the author of that comment could not imagine a situation in which people with AIDS might decide for themselves whether or not they wanted to take part in organised civil disobedience. Nor do British AIDS service organisations appreciate the full extent to which the influence of ACT UP (New York) and other AIDS activist groups such as AIDS Action Now (Toronto) is already being felt in the UK. For example, the Bristol-Myers corporation has announced plans to make the anti-HIV drug DDI available on the grounds of compassionate usage, largely as a result of North American activist pressure. Bristol-Myers have also included members of AIDS service organisations and the gay press at planning and information meetings, which is previously unheard of in British pharmaceutical industry behaviour.

It is clear then that AIDS can generate political identities which did not precede the epidemic, and draw together groups such as lesbians and gay men, together with black people and the disabled in ways that could not have been anticipated. Such identities and alliances are not natural or inevitable, but have to be forged in collective experience and in shared aims and objectives. For those like myself, who have had direct long-term experience of the American HIV epidemic, personal loss has been a major motivating factor. But this is clearly not the case for most lesbians and gay men in the UK, who are still statistically unlikely to have knowingly had much direct experiences of HIV disease, especially outside London. At the same time it is clear from the consistently low rates of new cases of HIV infection among gay men since 1984 that it has not been direct experience of AIDS that has determined the success of the safer sex revolution in our lives, or the extraordinary growth of non-governmental AIDS service organisations all round the country. On the contrary, it has been the strength of gay culture—from the gay press to theatre and independent film, but most of all in our everyday lives and friendships.

Yet it is precisely gay culture that the present government has consistently targeted, and that the opposition seems unwilling or unable to defend. We constantly hear that straight society has nothing to learn from us, that we are an 'exceptional' case, that we only took up safer sex when we literally saw our friends and lovers dying in front of our very eyes. Such an interpretation is not only ignorant and insulting, it is also profoundly tragic, for it strongly suggests that anti-gay prejudice will continue to prevent many heterosexuals from even trying to learn from our collective cultural experience. This is why the question of entitlement to effective community-based health education and health-care provision, especially in the form of community medicine, is so apparent to so many lesbians and gay men, especially since we are rarely, if ever, identified as a community of need by the National Health Service and other state institutions, regardless of the specific needs relating to AIDS.

Conclusion

Substantial numbers of British lesbians and gay men who have hitherto lacked much sense of a collective identity are now waking up to the direct realities of discrimination and culturally sanctioned prejudice. The deeply engrained sexual conservatism of the labour movement in Britain has effectively abandoned radical sexual politics to the far Left and the women's movement, neither of which have any direct relation to the lives of most gay men. This in effect means that many lesbians and gay men tend to associate the very notion of 'rights' with larger political programmes with which they have little sympathy. At the same time, an articulate but numerically tiny core of professional lobbyists continues a politics in and around the palace of Westminster that has hardly changed since the long years of lobbying that preceded and followed the publication of the Wolfenden Report on homosexual law reform in 1957—in many cases they are the same people. But the assimilationist approach offers few if any real opportunities for the establishment of a broadly-based and effective gay politics in the foreseeable future, for the obvious reason that such an approach is so deeply committed to the parliamentary status quo.

The recently formed lobbying organisation for lesbian and gay rights, the Stonewall Group, has shown considerable imagination in the drafting of a possible Homosexual Equality Bill. This proposes specific legislation to protect lesbians and gay men against discrimination based on sexual orientation, together with the legal recognition of 'domestic partnerships' between same-sex couples, the lowering of the age of consent for gay men to 16 years, and the criminalisation of incitements to violence on the grounds of sexual orientation. Such measures would bring Britain in line with existing laws in many other European countries, and in relation to 'hate crimes', with the USA. Furthermore, they would exemplify the general principle that sexual rights should be above parliamentary party politics. They would also go some way towards the establishment of a *culture of citizenship* among lesbians and gay men, as a constant reminder of constitutional rights, founded upon ethical principles.

We urgently need to establish a far more ethically grounded politics of gender and sexuality, in order to realise what Michel Foucault described in one of his final interviews as 'practices of freedom': 'For what', he asked 'is morality, if not the practice of liberty, the deliberate practice of liberty?'[8] Rather than assuming a natural, inevitable unity among gay men, or between gay men and lesbians, such an approach grounds our experience, in all its diversity and complexity, within a wider ethical context. We need to ensure, constitutionally, that no other social constituencies will ever have to endure what gay men have been through in increasing numbers throughout the course of the 1980s, as if our health and our lives are not as irreducibly valuable as those of other sections of society. The concept and practice of citizenship is one powerful means to this end precisely because citizenship not only involves a discourse of rights, but also of responsibilities. Without such a double emphasis, pluralism quickly descends into a free-for-all competition between rival and conflicting definitions of rights, and difference becomes an identity to be defended by a siege mentality that obscures shared patterns of oppression. AIDS has demonstrated with frightening clarity that lesbians and gay men are not just under-represented within the existing framework of British politics, but are positively excluded from the most basic processes and practices of democracy. This sordid reality has been tacitly or tactically accepted for far too long.

Subjecthood remains the dominant British political identity, founded in the constitutional settlement of 1688. As such, it has protected British politics from what has long been regarded by Westminster as the threat of federalism. It is the ideological cement that holds together the fragile unity of the United Kingdom, but is increasingly vulnerable to the critiques both of competing nationalisms, and the more general cultural pressures that lie behind the emergence of the 'new social movements' of feminism, black politics, environmentalism and gay liberation. Over time, subjecthood has also served to protect the claims and privileges of parliamentarianism, providing a transcendent national political identity, united in allegiance to the Crown in parliament over and above the divisions of class and all other structures of social difference. Furthermore, it encourages the belief that any criticism of either parliamentarianism or the monarchy itself are somehow unpatriotic and anti-democratic. Subjecthood is thus intimately connected to the wider patterns of cultural and class-based deference that are so characteristic of British politics and civil society, by comparison with other European nations.

A whole bundle of major constitutional reforms have recently come under discussion in the wake of the publication of Charter 88. These include electoral reform, freedom of information legislation, the formal incorporation into British law of the European Convention for the Protection of Human Rights and Fundamental Freedoms, a Bill of Rights, the reform of the judiciary and so on. What is now needed is an energetic ideological initiative, to recruit support for these concrete issues of entitlements and responsibilities as they arise for different social constituencies. In its current formulation, the movement for constitutional change in Britain retains the primacy of political and legal institutions which would be empowered to endow or deny rights with the same impunity as the parliamentary traditions that Charter 88 seems unwilling to adequately challenge. This explains the importance of emphasising the ethical dimensions of political and legal reform programmes, and of holding on to questions of power in relation to identity, which is especially important if we accept that identity is not a simple, unitary, and uniformly consistent entity, given from birth. The political culture of subjecthood involves a clear ranking of priorities within our individual and collective identities, a subjection to political, juridical and regal authority in our sense of who we are. Citizenship, however, at least offers the potential for very different processes of identification with one another, founded upon ethical considerations that should always be understood to have precedence and priority over the domain of the legal and the political.

Citizenship emerges as one strategy in what Foucault described as the 'political technology of individuals',[9] who may be brought to recognise and identify themselves through many different aspects and arenas of the social formation, whether through gender, nationalism, religion, health issues, regionalism, race and so on. In one of his later lectures Foucault described his aim to:

> show people that a lot of things that are a part of their landscape— that people think are universal—are the result of some very precise historical changes. All my analyses are against the idea of universal

necessities in human existence. They show the arbitrariness of institutions and show which space of freedom we can still enjoy and how many changes can still be made.[10]

This is especially obvious in his work concerning the conditions of emergence of the modern categories and identities of sexuality. Much of Foucault's later work was taken up with questions of how such historical understanding might be practically applied, and their ethical implications for the constitution of the sense of self. From this perspective, citizenship also offers a concrete alternative to the type of humanism:

> that presents a certain form of ethics as a universal model for any kind of freedom. I think there are more secrets, more possible freedoms, and more inventions in our future than we can imagine in humanism as it is dogmatically represented in every side of the political rainbow.[11]

This is in itself hardly surprising, since humanism has a prior interest in arguing that identity precedes social and political structures, which are seen to work in a purely external way upon a pre-formed rational 'human' subject. Foucault reminds us that:

> In effect, we live in a legal, social, and institutional world where the only relations possible are extremely few, extremely simplified, and extremely poor. Society and the institutions that frame it have limited the possibility of relationships because a rich relational world would be very complex to manage. We should fight against this shrinking of the relational fabric.[12]

One great weakness in the discourse of civil rights in Britain has been its long association with minorities, as if rights were not fundamental for the entire population. Entitlements have similarly been widely regarded primarily as exemptions, such as council housing, free prescriptions, or free school meals, thus limiting the concept to the weak and the disadvantaged. An ethically grounded practice of citizenship has the great initial advantage of being posed to, and on behalf of, the entire population—no longer pictured in crude parliamentary terms as a majority surrounded on all sides by distinct and possibly threatening minorities, but rather as a complex unity of many overlapping and interrelated groups and identities. Citizenship invites such a politics that proceeds from the recognition that our identities are multiply-formed and positioned, rather than fixed rigidly in mechanical dualistic polarities.

Ten long years of Thatcherism have brought home to many the full significance of Foucault's stark observation that:

> The search for a form of morality that would be acceptable for everyone—in the sense that everyone would have to submit to it—strikes me as catastrophic.[13]

It is precisely from our close understanding of the catastrophe to which such a search has led us that the recognition of the need for a common goal of ethical citizenship emerges, and with it the conditions for the emergence of new political identities and forms of social solidarity. In this respect, ethical citizenship anticipates Hannah Arendt's political vision of the republic, dedicated to the overriding principle of freedom, that is quite distinct from familiar notions of popular sovereignty. For Arendt, freedom is incompatible with the democratic politics of majority rule, which ensure that minorities are inevitably oppressed. In her political vision, modern western democracies are at best a 'very imperfect realisation' of the ideal of the free commonwealth, embodied readily in a corresponding concept of *citizenship*.[14] The political history of the AIDS epidemic strongly supports Arendt's explanation of the origins of totalitarianism, which insists that totalising state power starts

> with the *story of the pariah,* and therefore with the 'exception', with the 'politically anomalous' which is then used to explain the rest of society, rather than the other way round.[15]

The experience of countries such as France, Sweden and the United States demonstrates that the status of legal citizenship does not of itself automatically curb excessive state power or the oppression of minorities. But such countries do enjoy the benefits of the culture of citizenship that are almost entirely absent from the UK, where the concept of national sovereignty so frequently steamrollers any respect for cultural diversity within the nation. In this light, citizenship emerges not simply as a political goal, but both as an ethical necessity, in defence of old liberties and as a means for the active encouragement of new practices of freedom, on which the very possibility of a future for Britain as a fully European democracy currently depends.

18. AIDS, The Second Decade:
'Risk', research and modernity

Perceptions of AIDS as an urgent epidemic . . . are waning.
—Lawrence O. Gostin, *Hospitals, Health Care Professionals, and Persons with AIDS*

The problems of the world come down to this: All that we can imagine is more than we want to know.—Allen Barnett, *The Body and Its Dangers and Other Stories*

A recent issue of *Outweek,* the leading US weekly for lesbians and gay men, contained a cartoon by Andrea Natalie, depicting a woman reading a newspaper, alongside a man with the flat-top haircut. The woman is saying: 'Oh, my goodness! In this country every 18 seconds a man assaults a woman. Men rape 4000 women every DAY! Fifty per cent of men batter their wives or lovers. One out of three girls is raped by a man in her family before she is eighteen. Last year men murdered—OH NO! I'd better volunteer some time at the battered women's shelter.'

To which the man replies: 'Good heavens Suzy! You should be spending your volunteer hours taking care of gay men with AIDS! Don't you know there is an epidemic?!'[1]

Although there is a certain risk of seeming overly pedantic, it remains important to be able to unpick the themes that inform such cartoon jokes and anecdotes, since they speak directly and spontaneously of popular perceptions of HIV/AIDS as the first decade of the epidemic draws to a close. The sense of this cartoon, which was selected more or less at random, is based upon a strong sense of distinction between the subject of sexual violence and the subject of AIDS. It draws upon an assumed sense of irony, by which we identify the man ignoring the grim reality of rape as an issue for women. It also forcefully raises the differential status of 'knowledge' as it exists for women and for men. He is revealed as a typical chauvinist, unable to acknowledge the reality of female experience, expecting Suzy automatically to deny her position as a woman in relation to other women, and to knuckle down to the traditional nurturing role allotted to women in patriarchal societies. Yet I would suggest that it is the cartoon itself that is shockingly sexist, drawing on attitudes and assumptions that reveal both a frightening ignorance of HIV/AIDS, and an unacceptable oversimplification of the complex ways in which gender and sexuality articulate with one another and throughout the epidemic.

The latest American AIDS statistics speak baldly of a national catastrophe. Two hundred and twelve new cases of AIDS are diagnosed every day in the USA, where someone dies from AIDS every ten minutes. By the end of 1990 more than 100,000 people had already died from AIDS in the US alone. In 1991 more young Americans will die from AIDS than perished in the entire Vietnam war. Indeed, AIDS is now the leading cause of death for *all* American men aged between 25 and 44, and *all* American women aged between 15 and 33. In February 1990 the Centers for Disease Control reported a cumulative total of 11,189 women with AIDS in the United States, 52 per cent of whom were originally infected through needle-sharing, and a further 19 per cent through unprotected sex with male injecting drug users. Indeed, 28 per cent of *all* people with AIDS in America have been infected through needle-sharing, and it is currently estimated that 70 per cent of injecting drug users in some areas, are already infected. Women with AIDS now make up 9 per cent of the national US total, and heterosexual transmission which accounted for only 1.2 per cent of cases in 1982, is now responsible for 4.9 per cent of the total case-load.

Yet it is clear that such statistics continue to make little impact in relation to the culturally established 'common sense' about AIDS that prevails on both sides of the Atlantic. It has never been more obvious that such 'information', on its own, has little relation to public opinion or public attitudes. From this perspective we may return to the cartoon with which this chapter began. It is initially significant that 'Suzy' is named, whilst her male companion remains an anonymous stereotype of gay masculinity. It is true that AIDS continues to have a terrible, disproportionate impact among the gay communities of the United States, but all too often this obscures the fact that for several years the majority of new cases of HIV infection have been among heterosexuals. Furthermore, gay men are casually portrayed as selfish and insensitive, 'only' concerned with the fate of other gay men. Certainly, at the end of the first decade of AIDS it is almost fashionable to depict gay men in this way, and to overlook the central fact that throughout the entire course of the epidemic it has been gay men who have struggled to alert other social groups to the potential risks of HIV infection. The professional degaying of non-government AIDS service organisations is more than matched by the tendency to minimalise the question of HIV transmission among gay men, and the terrible impact of AIDS throughout the gay communities of the West. It is, therefore, especially depressing, and alarming, that a 'feminist' cartoon, appearing in a lesbian and gay publication in New York City, reveals such ignorance and prejudice. It should not, however, surprise us, for at another level this only serves to draw attention to the continuing uneven effects of marginalisation among the communities most affected by HIV/AIDS. It also draws attention to the long-term effects of conflicting information and misreporting that have so unfortunately prevailed throughout the 1980s. If people are confused, and ignorant, this is hardly their fault, since few have had access to reliable sources of commentary. Nonetheless, this cannot account for the widely held belief that AIDS service organisations are run largely by and for 'white, middle-class gay men', to the deliberate exclusion of other groups. Such attitudes reveal little more than a traditional prejudice against gay men as such, now dressed up in the doubly distasteful rhetoric of supposedly 'progressive' analysis. Furthermore, it matters little whether such prejudice comes from the left or the right, for it is a form of prejudice that continues to put large numbers of people at increased potential risk of HIV infection by persuading them that they themselves could never be directly affected.

Yet the international statistics continue to show a worsening situation. In August 1990 the World Health Organisation reported 'marked increases' of new cases of HIV throughout Asia and Latin America, together with an expanding crisis in sub-Saharan Africa that could lead to a 'dramatic upward revision' of previous estimates.[2] For example, the World Health Organisation had forecast between one and 1.5 million cases of HIV in Asia by the year 2000, but an estimated 500,000 have already been reported. Three million women and children are now expected to die from AIDS around the world in the course of the 1990s. All of this returns us to the vexed question of heterosexual transmission, and the future course of the epidemic.

By June 1990 there had been 3433 cases of AIDS reported in the UK, a figure which the government Chief Medical Officer acknowledges as a serious under-estimate of the real total.[3] There have been 12,370 reported cases of HIV infection in the UK among men, and 1482 among women, with a further 238 ungendered cases recorded by anonymised mass screening. It is always to HIV statistics that we should look to understand the growth of the epidemic, since AIDS figures relate to transmission events that took place, on average, some ten years ago. That this is still rarely appreciated in Britain was demonstrated early in 1990, when a slight fall in the rate of AIDS-related deaths was reported in every non-gay newspaper as if this were a story about HIV transmission. The news was received with widespread relief as if it undermined previous 'exaggerated' estimates. It was indeed good news, for it suggested that treatment and support services for people living with AIDS are slowly improving, as reflected in improved average life expectancy after an AIDS diagnosis. But this point was completely missed by journalists who seem to have very little genuine interest in the long-term prospects of people living with HIV or AIDS. What the story demonstrated was simply that ten years into the epidemic, and six years after the discovery of the Human Immunodeficiency Virus, the significance of the distinction between HIV and AIDS is *still* not recognised outside the discursive field of HIV/AIDS health promotion and direct service provision.

Putting this another way, one might well ask why it is almost impossible to imagine a cartoon depicting a man reading a newspaper alongside a woman in which the man is saying:

Oh, my goodness! In this country there are more than 300 men in prison for sexual 'offences' that don't exist for heterosexuals. Heterosexuals killed 15 gay men in Britain last year. Homosexuality is the leading cause of suicide amongst gay teenagers. There still hasn't been a single safer sex advert for gay men in a national newspaper. Last week Richard Ingrams was still calling in the *Observer* for quarantine for people with HIV! The *Star* calls gay men with AIDS 'human wreckage'. How many gay men have HIV—OH NO! I'd better volunteer to work with the Terrence Higgins Trust.

To which the woman would reply:

Good heavens Mike! You should be spending your time helping out at the black lesbians' creche at the Women's Centre! Don't you know this is a racist, sexist, patriarchal society?

Such an imaginary cartoon is only extremely unlikely because it would run the grave risk of drawing too much attention to the level of prejudice against gay men which is so sadly rife in contemporary Britain, whether among feminists or anti-feminists, racists or anti-racists, Thatcherites or anti-Thatcherites. The point is that we should not be setting up different areas of discrimination as if they were in competition with one another. Rather, we should be trying to articulate the ways in which different types of prejudice and discrimination proliferate in relation to different institutions and different social identities, all with their distinct histories, senses of boundaries and goals.[4]

As a gay man who has been actively involved in HIV/AIDS work in Europe and North America since the mid-1980s it seems clear to me that in an important sense epidemiology is everything when it comes to HIV/AIDS. The single, central issue that has determined policy responses to the epidemic on both sides of the Atlantic has been the fact that our experience in Europe, such as it has been, has been overwhelmingly that of asymptomatic HIV infection. In the United States and Canada, however, experience all along has been largely that of acute care, escalating mortality statistics, and the ensuing cultural responses of mourning, anger and, increasingly, direct activism.[5] AIDS *as such* in Europe remains largely a cultural phenomenon, even for most gay men—mediated above all by the national press and television—for the most part imagined rather than directly known from personal, lived experience. In spite of this major difference, it is clear that throughout the world responses to the epidemic have been concentrated on three broad, primary terrains: first, that of health education, or preventive medicine; second, that of treatment, care and service provision; and third, that of cultural responses, where the 'meanings' of AIDS are determined for most people.

All three terrains have been subject to massive political interference from the very beginning of the epidemic, and all three have been sites of intense contestation and polarisation. Furthermore, all three share a common dependence on such research as is available to them, and hence on research policy and funding agencies. Indeed, it is no exaggeration to say that the single most important factor that will determine the course of the second decade of AIDS will be the quality and quantity of research that will inform local, national and international responses to the epidemic. Yet research does not take place in a social vacuum, and this only underscores the fact that these three areas are rarely entirely distinct from one another. Epidemiology is of use to health educators and service providers alike, just as biomedical research serves care providers, housing workers and many others. And all are, of course, influenced by the wider cultural conditions that frame popular perceptions of personal risk and research priorities alike. This is why research has been and will continue to be the single most important dynamic factor in the future management of all aspects of the epidemic. In this chapter the emphasis is on the first of these terrains—health education.

Health education research

Hans Moerkerk, Secretary of the Dutch Commission on AIDS Control, has distinguished three separate sets of strategies in Europe in relation to HIV/AIDS prevention.[6] First, he identifies the approach based on notions of *behaviour modification,* involving straightforward technical interventions: the provision of condoms and condom education, the establishment of needle exchange projects and so on. Second, he identifies approaches which aim at *lifestyle modification,* and attempt to work at a more sophisticated level, acknowledging the importance of social and psychological factors, community identities and so on. Third, he identifies the aim of *group cultural modification,* which employs frankly repressive techniques to supposedly prevent HIV transmission by punitive means. These might include closing down bars or saunas, harassing prostitutes or criminalising people with HIV. As he concludes, it has been the demonstrable ineffectiveness and even counterproductiveness of this last approach that has led countries such as the Netherlands and Australia to opt for variants and combinations of the first two approaches. With Peter Aggleton, Moerkerk has also outlined the various policies adopted in Europe in some detail, noting that repressive and politically motivated measures have been applied in countries whose social, economic and political structures vary considerably.[7]

In these terms we may distinguish at least three approaches. First, there has been a *pragmatic response* in Norway, Denmark, Switzerland and the Netherlands. These countries may be distinguished by the speed of their national response to the epidemic, and the willingness of state agencies to negotiate with and consult community organisations and non-government AIDS service organisations, preferring to establish consensus rather than impose coercive controls. As in the case of Norway, however, this approach may simply mask an underlying refusal or inability to acknowledge the cultural legitimacy of some groups, especially gay men.

Second, they identify a *political response,* which places political considerations above all others. Such may be found in West Germany, Austria, Iceland and Ireland, as well as the spectacular examples of the

United Kingdom and the United States. In these countries the work of non-government AIDS service organisations preceded state interventions, and the relations between state and non-state HIV/AIDS education have often been fraught. Indeed, much of the work carried out by non-governmental organisations (NGOs) is dedicated to the task of re-education, correcting the mistakes of 'official' campaigns.[8] Funding has long been difficult to obtain, and self-censorship is rife, together with conflicts between different areas of work such as buddying and support services, legal work and telephone counselling. In such circumstances health education often has a low priority since it is acknowledged to be 'risky', especially when any acknowledgement of the needs and rights of gay men or injecting drug users can so easily be interpreted by hostile politicians and others as evidence of the supposed 'promotion' of immorality and 'drug use'. Community groups and NGOs are rarely consulted by state agencies, though lip service may sometimes be paid to the value of their work, just so long as this is not specified.[9]

Third, Moerkerk and Aggleton identify a general *biomedical approach* in countries such as Belgium, France, Spain, Italy and Greece, where governments have had little direct involvement in HIV/AIDS education, preferring to leave this work to state medical institutions, which were never designed to deal with the issues raised by the epidemic.[10] As Moerkerk points out, in this context gay organisations (so far as they exist in the first place) are faced by the combined opposition of the political elite and the medical elite. Policies thus tend to be confused and contradictory, as politicians and doctors struggle to address groups whose very existence they would evidently prefer to forget. This is also the case in the emergent democracies of Eastern and Central Europe, whose nationalist movements are generally distinguished by a strong and explicit homophobia. For example, Poland's first AIDS service organisation was ousted from its office in the Students' Union building in Warsaw by Roman Catholic Solidarity activists within weeks of moving in early in 1990. The biomedical approach still tends to regard HIV antibody testing as if it were the major means of effective prevention, and invariably reflects the well-known social prejudices of the medical professions. Indeed, one of the saddest paradoxes of the European epidemic has concerned the failure of socialised medicine in Europe to acknowledge the complexity of the socities to which it is supposed to be responsible at the level of HIV/AIDS education as much as at the level of actual care.

However, in spite of the importance of such descriptive analysis of differing health education strategies, it is equally important to understand something of the theoretical bases on which they stand. For the different models of HIV/AIDS education reviewed above have their origins in different, and generally conflicting, models of research. We may thus contrast the type of academic epidemiology which speaks confidently of 'risk groups' and 'risk behaviour' to research which attempts to make sense of people's own felt needs, pleasures and identities. For example, one recent survey of risk factors relating to seroconversion among gay and bisexual men who had attended professional education sessions listed variables including:

> age, educational level, occupation, race, type of educational session, the time between the educational session and the conversion visit, age at which volunteers began having sexual intercourse on a regular basis, numbers of all sexual partners, numbers of partners who were anally insertive, percentage of partners with whom condoms were used during receptive intercourse, the greatest amount of alcohol consumed per day, most alcohol consumed on days when drinking, frequency of use of recreational drugs, kinds of recreational drugs used, and depression.[11]

What is so startlingly absent from this long list is any awareness of the possible role of sexual identity and self-confidence (or 'gay zest' as a friend of mine puts it) factors which are on the contrary foregrounded in research conducted from a fuller understanding of the complex, variable relations among information, attitudes, identity and behaviour. In this respect one may immediately contrast research undertaken by researchers who have little or no knowledge or understanding of the social worlds of lesbians and gay men, and research which deliberately employs gay men in order to be effective. One may also distinguish between research conducted in academic departments for publication or conference reports, and research which is specifically designed to answer questions raised by health educators working in the field. Yet in practice, very little HIV/AIDS health education research is conducted in relation to the immediate needs of health educators working in European AIDS service organisations in the voluntary sector. This means that much of their work is essentially ad hoc, and is rarely evaluated. A vicious circle is thus established so that the most effective interventions are the least researched, and therefore are not written up or officially acknowledged. They thus stand little chance of influencing 'official' campaigns, and valuable experience is not communicated nationally or internationally.

Academic AIDS research in Europe still tends to treat its subjects as more or less exotic deviants, and the fluidity and complexity of sexual and drug-using behaviour are not recognised because of the rigid dependence on categories such as prostitution, homosexuality and so on. A visitor from outer space would undoubtedly have the greatest difficulty understanding almost any aspect of sexuality in modern Britain if they had only read the epidemiological literature available in the medical journals. Fortunately, there are some exceptions to the general rule. For example, Hilary Kinnell's work in Birmingham provides important data on risk factors for HIV infection among women in the sex industry because it is especially sensitive to the ways in which 'information' is actually interpreted.[12] Thus while only 4 per cent of her sample of women failed to identify unprotected anal sex as a risk factor for men, 33 per cent failed to identify this as a risk for women. Messages which simply talk about 'anal sex' may be 'understood', and may be reflected in quantitative surveys, but nonetheless there may be little relation between the results of surveys whose questions are ill-conceived and actual risk factors in the lives of those being questioned. Kinnell's work also demonstrates a significant correlation between anti-gay attitudes and risk behaviour, though very few surveys ever include questions about attitudes towards homosexuality on the part of heterosexuals, although this has long been recognised as an important issue by gay health educators.

Kinnell's work similarly calls into question the familiar epidemiological obsession with the issue of numbers of sexual partners, usually understood as an intrinsic independent risk factor. For example, her survey reveals that younger women aged between 17 and 22 tend to have many more clients than older women, but are much better informed and take far fewer risks. Older women, with fewer partners, are often involved in casual work in order to support children, pay the poll-tax and so on. The available sociology of prostitution clearly shows that prostitutes are generally well informed about sexually transmitted diseases, and sexual health, since this relates so directly to their ability to work. Yet as Judith B. Cohen has pointed out, researchers still frequently speak of clients being 'exposed to' prostitutes and thence HIV infection as if they were the sexual equivalent to a leaky nuclear reactor.[13] In this manner moralism interferes with the task of researching strategies for developing effective health promotion. As recently as April 1990 a London magistrate jailed an 18-year-old seropositive mother for loitering, commenting that: 'Any man who takes his chances with a prostitute on the street deserves what he gets.'[14] It seems apparent that one major risk factor for prostitutes continues to be prejudice and the effects of criminalisation, which continue to portray male clients as 'victims' and to disregard the question of how sex industry workers can themselves be protected. In this respect much epidemiology resembles traditional forms of policing and surveillance rather than affording a means of effective health education.[15]

The epidemiological scapegoating of prostitutes is repeated throughout the field of HIV/AIDS research, in relation to the social groups who initially proved most vulnerable to HIV. By reinforcing the ideological categories of 'prostitution', 'homosexuality' and 'drug abuse', the opportunity to call into question the methods of behavioural psychology and statistical sociology has been lost. This is largely because academic methodology is *threatened* by what we learn from the study of the epidemic: that sexual and drug-using behaviours are not immutably fixed and stable within clearly defined and identifiable social groups; that the categories of sexual 'science' constitute a complex biopolitics which is perhaps the most fundamental level at which social life is managed, organised and 'thought'; and that the meaning of 'sex' and sexual categories is not natural but cultural. What is most remarkable in all of this, however, is the extent to which psychosocial resarch has ignored the lived experience and entitlements of those it regards as members of 'risk groups', and how closely such resarch tends to align itself with the interests of those it perceives to be fundamentally *not* at risk from HIV. Researchers themselves are almost invariably inscribed within this latter group. Hence the paradox of the massive degree of individualism that characterises so much 'official' HIV/AIDS education. For it is only as long as HIV can be successfully presented as a risk to be faced by isolated individuals, who are understood to be able to make *moral* choices to protect themselves, independently of all other social or personal factors, that the larger abstract categories of 'sexuality' may be protected. In other words, the unequal power relations between heterosexuality and homosexuality are protected and even reinforced by research that presents heterosexuals with HIV as if they are *exceptions,* or indeed not heterosexual, as in the obvious example of most injecting drug users. It remains intensely significant that the simple message that HIV is *potentially* a risk to everyone, across all social and sexual boundaries, is so frequently heard as if it were being claimed that everyone is *equally* at risk. What is being protected in such examples, and what kinds of defences are in play, remains far from clear. Suffice it to say that the precise mechanisms whereby such reversals and double standards are inscribed throughout the field of psychosocial research remain in urgent need of detailed elaboration and theoretical analysis. The most important question remains the ways in which the findings of research might be promptly translated into effective health education initiatives.

In Britain, as in many other countries, much of the most useful research, especially in relation to safer sex, has long tended to take place in an *ad hoc* fashion, undertaken by health educators themselves who are generally gay men, lesbians or feminists, working far away from the established centres of academic social science, either in Departments of Education or of Cultural Studies, or else entirely outside the formal academic world—either for reasons of choice, or because state funding is still not available to such 'risky' projects.

There is a sad irony in the fact that the explosion of research into 'homosexual behaviour' or the 'homosexual lifestyle' has so very little relevance to the immediate, pressing needs of gay men living in the real world of an epidemic. This is largely because gay men's sexuality is so often abstracted and isolated from the rest of their lives, including all questions of class and the contingent world of anti-gay prejudice. Yet far away from the grim day-to-day realities of the epidemic and of increasing homophobia, the question of the moral responsibility of the social sciences in the AIDS crisis is rarely raised, save by the objects of research who thus reveal themselves as 'non-compliant'. The dangerous myth of value-free research continues to legitimate costly and expensive research that is both scientifically and ethically dubious. This is not to question the need for quantitative research into all aspects of human sexuality. However, in the midst of an epidemic such projects can only be justified if they can demonstrate concrete implications for the development of effective health education strategies. If this is not always the case, social scientists cannot be surprised if they are attacked as academic tourists, thriving professionally as 'scientific' spectators on the misery of others—misery that it should be *their* primary responsibility to attempt to minimise. Nonetheless, as we enter the 1990s there is still precious little evidence that most academic psychosocial HIV/AIDS research concerning gay men or other 'risk groups' has their health or well-being anywhere among its aims or objectives.

Fortunately, there are good examples of research which has been specifically designed in relation to immediate concrete needs. Thus we may distinguish the work of Lavinia Crooks and her colleagues at the University of Woollongong, which is closely tied to the work of the AIDS Council of New South Wales, and the Australian Federation of AIDS Organisations (AFAO). This research project has produced much valuable work on the needs of specialised counselling for carers, and especially on the needs of carers who are themselves HIV antibody-positive. I am not aware of a single research project in Britain which betrays the slightest awareness that such people even exist, let alone that they might have special needs and entitlements in relation to which social scientists might be able to make genuinely helpful contributions. Another impressive research project is located at Macquarie University, also in New South Wales. The work of Gary Dowsett and his colleagues in the Social Aspects of the Prevention of AIDS (SAPA) project has few international parallels in its sensitivity to the changing cultural contexts in which safer sex education takes place, contexts that must be fully appreciated if such education is to be effective rather than merely cosmetic.[16] In a recent paper on 'Unsafe Anal Sexual Practice among Homosexual and Bisexual Men' they conclude that:

> We noted at the start of the paper the symbolic significance of anal intercourse both in repressive laws and in gay men's claims for sexual liberation. So far as gay social life can be understood as a 'sexual community', this is a practice which has had a significant role in creating identities and social links. . . . From this point of view, insisting on a total safe sex regime may be counterproductive. Over rigid rules are impractical; invite blowouts, whose net effect may be greater risk than a more moderate regime from the start.[17]

Such work has especially significant implications for safer sex education, not least by pointing to the special needs of those on low incomes, those who have few friends or who have little access to the types of gay community institutions where safer sex is learned as a cultural, community-based aspect of gay identity and gay pride. Such research points:

> to the need to foster group support for change, to work through existing patterns of interpersonal relationships. This has been the approach of many gay community organisations . . . and it needs to be more widely known that there is social-scientific backing for this approach. We need to move beyond the individualistic approach of much official health education and academic AIDS research, towards collective, social strategies of change. The aim of such work is not so much to change individual 'attitudes' or 'health behaviours' as to move whole networks of people towards safer practice and encourage the social processes among them which can sustain the prevention.[18]

British and American research strongly supports more recent Australian findings that: 'Men who are isolated from others like themselves and are unattached to gay community in any form are those least likely to change.'[19] Moreover, such research also repeatedly demonstrates the change to safer sex outside primary long-term sexual relationships among gay men, within which unsafe sex is far from uncommon. Yet this is not remotely surprising. Nor is it in any way unique to gay men. However, when similar studies were reported at both the Fifth and Sixth International Conferences on AIDS, press reaction outside the gay press spoke uniformly of supposedly irresponsible gay men 'slipping' or 'giving up' safer sex.[20] Yet there is a vast amount of international evidence that demonstrates with frightening clarity how very few sexually active heterosexual men have even considered starting to have safer sex in the first place.

The starkest of double standards are at work here, since it has never for one moment been suggested that heterosexuals might consider giving up penetrative sexual intercourse in the way that is so routinely expected of gay men. For example, the practice of anal sex is still evidently regarded as an intrinsic risk factor in much epidemiological analysis, independently of any question of condom use, although vaginal intercourse as such is never regarded in this manner, and its culturally sanctioned acceptability is entirely taken for granted in official surveys.[21] Excellent research has been conducted in Britain at Bristol Polytechnic, and at South Bank Polytechnic in London, but beyond this there is little evidence of any systematic linkage between academic researchers and the sites in which health education initiatives are developed. Furthermore, by their very nature, British non-government AIDS service organisations are unlikely to be aware of the possibility that social scientific research might be of immediate help in their work, since there are so few professional social scientists involved in the voluntary sector. This highly regrettable situation has been made worse by the policy of the government's main funding agencies, including the Economic and Social Research Council (ESRC), only to fund quantitative research. One leading female researcher working on an ESRC-funded project concerned with attitudes and beliefs among female prostitutes told me recently that although she hoped her work might 'be of some use', she had not stopped even to consider its possible implications for the purposes of health education among the very women with whom she was working. Indeed, she was quite indignant in the face of what she evidently regarded as my vulgar, reductive question. Such studies are typically conducted by interviewing cohorts of subjects attending sexually transmitted disease clinics, who are provided with psychological and information-oriented questionnaires, on the basis of which it is asserted that changes in sexual behaviour may be detected. This type of research is literally obsessed with isolating scientific 'indicators' of sexual behaviour in relation to HIV transmission, but as I have already argued, these usually relate far more to conventions of sociological enquiry than to the actual lived experience of the people being questioned, who are casually dehumanised by being viewed behind the thick protective curtains of orthodox academic deviancy theory. Indeed, such research is often the sociological equivalent to barrier-nursing. It should certainly be recognised that academic sociology is one of the strongest bastions of anti-gay prejudice, rationalised and legitimated within the narrow world of academic life by its own working methods and the beliefs on which they are based. Indeed, there can be few social groups less well equipped to appreciate the needs of health education in relation to the AIDS crisis than British social scientists, especially those coming from backgrounds in 'pure' statistics.

In this context one might well contrast British academic research into safer sex to recent Norwegian work conducted by Annick Prieur and her colleagues at the University of Oslo. What is so rare and impressive about Prieur's work is its commitment to *listening* to what her subjects were telling her, and her willingness to check what she was hearing against her own academic and personal preconceptions. Thus her survey on unsafe sex among young gay men in Oslo ends on a personal note, all too rare in such published research findings: 'a wider understanding of rationality is needed: including longing and love as motives for action.'[22]

Such an approach can only derive from a truly open-minded willingness to try to understand the situation in which so many men who have sex with other men find themselves. Not that the circumlocution 'men who have sex with men' does much more than suggest *something* about the variable social and cultural conditions in which homosexual desire is lived in widely differing circumstances. The ceaseless quest for scientifically verifiable 'indicators' and 'objective correlates' is pointless if these only serve further to blind social scientists to the complex realities of sexual desire, identities and behaviour in grossly puritanical, moralistic and anti-gay societies. Effective HIV prevention can only take place when local factors such as the proximity of gay bars and clubs, the patterns of distribution of gay newspapers and magazines, local policing policies and so on have been adequately researched and their consequences understood and factored into health educational initiatives. Above all, it is the availability of a sense of belonging to some kind of community that will always determine the development of a resilient sense of self-esteem which is demonstrably the *sine qua non* of safer sex education, not just for gay men—though this is a principal lesson from the gay response to AIDS—but for everyone. We await the emergence of the sociology of longing and of love with bated breath.

Conclusions

In the meantime we could do worse than pay close attention to the extraordinary critique of the response of the social sciences to an earlier twentieth century catastrophe, contained in Zygmunt Bauman's book, *Modernity and the Holocaust.* Bauman argues that the Holocaust is either regarded as if it were a discrete incident in the history of the Jews, or else from a more Durkheimian perspective an example of the failure of modernity to contain a universal capacity for evil, which broke through the veneer of German civilisation in the form of Nazism—thus conveniently letting everyone else off the hook. Writing of the complex ways in which soldiers, journalists, statisticians and other functionaries came quite easily to regard Jews as less than human, he observes that:

> Dehumanised objects cannot possibly possess a 'cause', much less a 'just' one; they can have no 'interests' to be considered, indeed no claim to subjectivity. Human objects become therefore a 'nuisance factor'. Their obstreperousness further strengthens the self-esteem and the bonds of comradeship that unite the functionaries. The latter see themselves now as companions in a difficult struggle, calling for courage, self-sacrifice and selfless dedication to the cause. It is not the objects of bureaucratic action, but its subjects who suffer and deserve compassion and moral praise. . . . Dehumanisation of the objects and positive moral self-valuation reinforce each other. The functionaries may faithfully serve any goal while their moral conscience remains unimpaired.[23]

I do not wish to appear to be making casual or impertinent analogies between the treatment of the Jews, gypsies, gay men and others, and the events that have determined the first decade of the AIDS crisis. However, it would be entirely inconsistent and unproductive to argue, with Bauman, that the Holocaust was precisely a result of the conditions that constitute modernity, and then imagine that such an analysis can have nothing to say about the history of the present. Bauman argues that the Holocaust could only have come about as a result of a combination of factors including social and psychological tensions deriving from the new, and rigid boundary-drawing tendencies under the conditions of modernisation and the subjectivities these produced, the breakdown of a sense of traditional order, the hardening of nation states and nationalisms, the role of scientific rhetoric in legitimating the ambitions of political and other would-be social engineers, the emergence of modern forms of racism, and their relation to the possibility of a technology of genocide. This is not to claim for one moment either that the AIDS crisis is in any simple sense 'like' the Holocaust, or that anti-Semitism is in any simple sense 'like' the fears of difference that seemingly fuel much anti-gay prejudice. Nonetheless, it is impossible not to note the growing homologies between social policy in the field of HIV/AIDS related education and policies that determine the direction of biomedical research, epidemiology and popular cultural interpretations of the epidemic which continue to regard people with HIV/AIDS as culpable, and less than human.

Besides, we know that power is not a single, unitary force that merely flows through different sites of struggle creating different forms of oppression in the same way, and by the same means. Our analysis of the forces at work in the many institutions which 'manage' the epidemic must be at least as supple and nimble as Bauman's reading of anti-Semitism, following as it does in the mighty footsteps of Hannah Arendt.[24] Indeed, the categories of sexuality and the identities that they engender, including the steady escalation of anti-gay prejudice in countries like Britain or Poland or the Soviet Union which in important ways have *yet to achieve* modernity in the sense described by Bauman, are themselves a central and indispensable element within the wider, evolving disposition of modernisation.

Anti-gay prejudice is no more *necessary* to modernity than anti-Semitism. It is, however, a characteristic and predictable feature of certain aspects of the changes in domesticity, child-raising, pedagogy in schools, medical practice, and social science, which are themselves not the products but the *means* of centralised, bureaucratic modernity, whatever different forms it may have assumed in the intersection with different national histories. Who, for example, could possibly have predicted the widespread passivity among gay men in relation to the practices of clinical medicine throughout the epidemic in Western Europe that results from the client mentality produced within cradle-to-grave welfare and national health services? Who could have imagined that, on the contrary, the epidemic would stimulate the most urgent confrontation with institutionalised medicine in the modern period in the United States?

Who could have imagined the sheer scale of the failures of governments, national medical research institutes, health education agencies, journalists, religious leaders, politicians and sociologists alike, to acknowledge the enormity of the disaster that confronts gay men and injecting drug users, haemophiliacs and the poor and disadvantaged of the earth?

I sometimes hear the message that 'things could be worse', but this can only come from those who continue to place their faith in the supposedly disinterested forces of social democratic consensus and morality. As we enter the second decade of the epidemic it seems imperative that we find time to consider, in all the necessary sobriety we can muster, the long-term consequences of the categories and identities of 'sexuality' in relation to the lives at stake in the ongoing struggles against state censorship, the unavailability of private or public funding, the continuing design of unethical and thus unscientific protocols for the conduct of clinical trials, the refusal to legislate against HIV/AIDS-related discrimination (however flagrant), the sheer, relentless violence of the response to humane health education, medical research and cultural agencies.

Five years ago I began to write about AIDS on the basis of my own appalled and initially unbelieving perception that the social constituencies associated with AIDS were widely regarded, in their entirety, as disposable. For a long time I found it well nigh impossible to accept the accumulating evidence before me. In the meantime little has changed, and I see no reason to revise my earlier judgement. As we enter the second decade of AIDS, I can see no evidence whatsoever that countries such as Britain and the United States have even begun to grasp what the first decade was really like, and this alone provides no grounds for optimism. As the epidemic worsens, we shall see whether AIDS continues to be accepted as a minor cost of modernity, or whether other moral and ethical forces in our societies will be brought in to challenge this 'morality'. Certainly new battle lines are currently being established between rival pictures of human morality, and these will doubtless be increasingly involved in direct confrontation throughout the 1990s. The great issues of abortion, embryo research, marriage, censorship and sexual morality will continue to intersect with the issues raised by the epidemic in ever more complex conjunctions. But of these, AIDS is likely to prove by far the most controversial, for the simple reason that it has the power to condense almost all the other issues into itself and is thus radically overdetermined as a site on which conflict is likely to take place. We will not know that this struggle for the right to diversity has been won until our respective societies, including our governments and doctors, and teachers, and journalists and social scientists are able to accept, quite casually, that gay men simply like sex just like everyone else. Given the great distance of that ideal, imaginary goal, we cannot afford to be complacent or delude ourselves that 'common sense' will ultimately, inevitably, prevail. Unfortunately, it would appear that the dominant common sense of the United Kingdom has little or no interest in the fate of gay men. This, during an epidemic, guarantees otherwise avoidable increases in HIV infection, and otherwise avoidable human suffering on a dreadful scale. One can only enter the 1990s with profound forebodings, for while we know that the future is not fixed, we also know that the evidence of the 1980s strongly suggests a worsening crisis ahead.

19. Silence Equals Death

I remember first reading about AIDS in New York in 1983. An article in the *New York Native* informed me that if it didn't rouse me 'to anger, fury, rage and action, gay men have no future on this earth'. I dismissed this as another example of American hyperbole, written by some crackpot with an axe to grind. At the time I failed to identify the call to action, which doesn't surprise me retrospectively. Indeed, it's precisely because I am fairly typical of the majority of European gay men for whom AIDS didn't become a reality until the mid 1980s, that I try hard not to judge other people's inability to grasp the full, terrible significance of the epidemic.

I later shared a panel with the writer of that article, Larry Kramer, author of *Faggots* and *The Normal Heart* at a New York conference in 1986. But by that time AIDS had entirely transformed my life, as it had long since transformed the lives of many of my closest American friends. At some time in the 1970s a seemingly new and unknown virus had emerged in the West with, as we now know, an average period of ten years between infection and an AIDS diagnosis. It's hardly surprising that it was widely transmitted at a time when very few people used condoms.

I am also fairly typical of a type of European gay man who quickly became involved in the difficult task of alerting people in Britain to the potential danger that faced us, so far from America, so far from the confident gay culture of the United States with its excellent gay press, radio, cable and collective community values. It is common in British journalism to claim that gay men took up safer sex only as their friends began to drop dead at their feet. Yet in New York and San Francisco, safer sex became the norm long before the escalation of AIDS statistics in the mid-1980s, and even before the discovery of the Human Immunodeficiency

Virus (HIV), which was first made public in 1984. To this day, most gay men in European cities are statistically unlikely to know anyone with AIDS. As the 1980s progressed it became increasingly apparent, however, that the most important difference between the American and the European gay experience of the epidemic lay in the fact that on this side of the Atlantic the overwhelming experience was of asymptomatic HIV infection, while in the US it was acute illness, hospitalisation and death.

Few Europeans, gay or straight, can begin to appreciate the significance of the knowledge among American gay men that at least a million are already infected. For many years most of my friends have known or suspected that they are HIV antibody-positive, that is if they are not already ill. In Europe, on the contrary, the vast majority of gay men know, or more importantly believe, that they are uninfected.

This is why safer sex education has had to draw on the fragile resources of a gay movement which is increasingly beleaguered, at least in the UK. As Douglas Crimp, American art critic and AIDS activist, pointed out:

> Seldom has a society so savaged people during their hour of loss. The violence we encounter is relentless, the violence of silence and omission almost as impossible to endure as the violence of unleashed hatred and outright murder.

AIDS has to be understood both in its local context, and in relation to the particular moment in time. I haven't kept a regular diary during the past ten years. Nonetheless it may help to recall some anecdotes which provide a sense of how things have changed.

The first friend of mine to die from AIDS became sick in 1984, in France. He'd lived in France as a typical gay exile from British homophobia, but didn't tell any of his old friends in London about his diagnosis. This we learned from his grieving, uncomprehending parents, who had nursed him lovingly, but with little understanding of why he had left England in the first place.

At his funeral in the smug, prim twilight zone of the outer suburbs, nobody acknowledged that he was gay, nor did they say what he had died from. His mother and father were terrified that the rest of the family would 'find out', and couldn't even tell their next door neighbours of thirty years' standing the truth.

I remember going to a gay bookstore in New York a few years ago with an old friend, alas no longer alive. There was a pile of calendars on sale, and when I picked one up, he casually quipped, in a typical New York gay way: 'Who'd buy a calendar these days? They ought to try selling them in monthly instalments.' It took me a moment to catch his drift, and I froze. That was when I first truly realised what the epidemic meant in America—the dry, throwaway line that spoke of a population group that had ceased to believe in its own future.

There is a 'natural history' within the American gay communities' experience of AIDS, a move through the course of the decade from an initial sense of shock, to a deeper sense of loss, and beyond that to a growing collective resolve that the epidemic can and must be defeated. It was from this last sense of outrage at the scale of government indifference that the AIDS activist movement was born in the early months of 1987, in the form of the AIDS Coalition to Unleash Power, ACT UP.

Founded by Larry Kramer, ACT UP has become the most significant campaigning group in the US since the anti-war movement of the 1960s. Behind its celebrated slogan 'SILENCE=DEATH', ACT UP combines an astonishingly well-researched critique of the failures of medicine and the biomedical research in the USA, with a policy of confrontation. As their Treatment Data Committee's Report to the Sixth International Conference on AIDS in San Francisco in July 1990 baldly stated:

> There is only so much horror that a people can tolerate. We propose the elements of a rational, comprehensive and coordinated research effort to target systematically all the serious and fatal complications of HIV. If our message is not heeded in the coming year, the rapidly diminishing hopes of our communities will vanish, What will happen then?

ACT UP estimates the likelihood of its proposals being adopted as 'virtually nil'. Nothing could demonstrate more clearly the unevenness and unpredictability of American responses to HIV/AIDS than the recent behaviour of George Bush and his wife Barbara. Back in July, the President refused to address the opening session of the San Francisco conference, preferring instead to attend a fund-raising benefit for Senator Jesse Helms, who has been described as: 'the country's greatest enemy of compassionate AIDS care'. It was Helms who managed to prevent all state funding for safer sex education in the US in the late 1980s, and he remains an implacable opponent of lesbian and gay rights. Bush's decision was widely regarded as callous and insulting by mainstream medical researchers, doctors and activists alike.

A few weeks later, right-wing outrage greeted the publication of a letter from Barbara Bush to Paulette Goodman, president of the Federation of Parents and Friends of Lesbians and Gays, a lobbying organisation better known as P-FLAG. Mrs Bush had been invited to address a few words of encouragement 'to some 24 million gay Americans and their families'. The First Lady wrote back saying that she appreciated 'your encouraging me to help change attitudes', since discrimination 'always brings with it pain and perpetuates hatred and intolerance.'

Needless to say, this was a wild provocation to the Moral Majority, who were still foaming at the mouth about the presence earlier in the summer of lesbian and gay lobbyists in the White House, whence they had been invited to attend the signing of the so-called Hate Crimes Bill. This requires the US government to publish annual statistics on all crimes of violence based on religious or racial hatred, or hatred founded on sexual orientation.

In late July the US Congress also passed the Americans With Disabilities Act, compared in the *New York Times* to the historic Civil Rights Act of 1864. This requires all public facilities in America to be made accessible to the disabled, including people living with AIDS. And on 1 August 1990 the House of Representatives approved the first stage of a major new Housing Bill, which includes the provision of $150 million to help people with AIDS. Described by its supporters as, 'the first comprehensive set of new Government housing initiatives in a decade', the Housing Bill looks set to be vigorously opposed by the White House, which has previously resisted all attempts to establish the notion of rights to housing.

Housing is an especially desperate issue in relation to AIDS, not only because of the visible army of homeless, infected drug users, but because at least 28 per cent of Americans have no adequate health insurance, without which AIDS can quickly lead to destitution as a result of medical costs. It is depressing, if not entirely surprising, to learn that it is becoming ever more difficult to fund-raise around HIV/AIDS issues in America, where the epidemic is no longer 'flavour of the month' with charitable trusts.

In the meantime, the government of California recently announced a 12 per cent cutback in AIDS funding, while Rena Durazzo, director of public policy at the San Francisco AIDS Foundation, reports 'seeing clear indications that corporations want to put their money someplace else'. It is also ominous that not one of the three foundations in Dallas that have hitherto supported local service provision for people living with AIDS is still giving money.

Meanwhile, more young Americans will die as a result of AIDS in

1991 than perished in the Vietnam War. In the USA there are 122 newly diagnosed cases of AIDS every day, and a death every 10 minutes. Of all people with AIDS, 28 per cent were infected via shared needles, and some 70 per cent of injecting drug users in New York, New Jersey and Puerto Rico are thought to be HIV positive, though this figure drops to 5 per cent in other areas.

Recent statistics also reveal 11,989 women with AIDS, who now make up 9 per cent of the total AIDS statistics. Yet some people continue to argue that because most of these women were infected by needle use or as a result of sex with drug users or bisexual men, we can safely disregard the risk of heterosexual transmission.

Of American women with AIDS, 27 per cent are black and 16 per cent are Hispanic, although blacks and Hispanics make up only 12 and 6 per cent respectively of the US population. Such figures speak volumes about the disproportionate impact of HIV on America's minority communities. It is especially ironic that it is the black middle class that has led the crusade against the introduction of needle exchanges, and seems far more concerned by the far-fetched possibility that needle exchanges might 'promote' or encourage drug use.

Fortunately, in Britain the Department of Health has long recognised the vital importance of not confusing the politically motivated and largely cosmetic 'war on drugs' with the higher priority of protecting injecting drug users from HIV.

Things are not looking good on the US medical front either. The government's National Research Council on AIDS recently dismissed any idea that the epidemic is ending, concluding simply that 'ongoing efforts fall far short of the magnitude of intervention needed', comparing the chaotic state of US research to an orchestra without a conductor. Of some 45,000 doctors in Manhattan, Gay Men's Health Crisis lists only 45 able or willing to take on new patients with HIV or AIDS, while shortages are much worse elsewhere.

But at least in America, unlike Britain, there is a strong sense of the responsibility of state-funded researchers to undertake what the profit-motivated private sector pharmaceutical companies cannot or will not do—such as dosage comparisons of new, experimental drugs, or combination trials of drugs that are almost never taken in isolation, since people with AIDS invariably require anti-HIV compounds, as well as medications to prevent or treat individual AIDS conditions to which they are vulnerable because of their weakened immunological defences. Care and types of medical intervention are far from standardised, while whole areas of research continue to go out of the way not to get involved at all.

Today you can literally hear the epidemic in American cities. It takes the form of the familiar, regular electronic messages signalled at four-hourly intervals from tiny, timed bleepers, carried by tens of thousands of people—reminding them to take their AZT, the only treatment currently licensed against HIV—in restaurants, cinemas, offices, everywhere.

A few weeks ago I was staying on Fire Island, a popular resort for New York's lesbians and gay men, about an hour from the city. I was there to visit a number of friends who are ill, and to speak at a fundraising rally for ACT UP. Fire Island is a unique experience since almost everyone there is gay. It is impossible to describe the simple feeling of physical safety that one gets, coming from London. At the same time one is always aware of the epidemic, as people go home to take care of friends and loved ones, and from the sight of young men in the supermarkets and at the discos, looking like Belsen victims, but getting on with their lives with great dignity. I was staying with six other gay men, and one heterosexual woman. Four of the men were HIV positive and one, my oldest and dearest gay friend in America, living with AIDS. He developed the syndrome four years ago, on holiday here in London, and now has a catheter implanted in his chest to deliver the drugs on which his life depends, but which the veins in his limbs can no longer take. Every evening he hooks up his intravenous drip to a couple of coat hangers suspended from a standard lamp, and settles down to watch a video as he takes his medication. Phoning tonight from New York he tells me that he's lost a further 10 pounds in weight in the week since I left, and must now have a daily food drip for 12 hours. But he was out swimming every day, with the little white catheter tube hanging from his chest, like so many others on Fire Island this year.

In America, as in Britain, people often have difficulty in asking questions about medical procedures. Most mean well, and if they say nothing about a catheter this is only because they don't know how to raise the subject, and say nothing for fear of causing offence. It is infinitely moving to see how gay men and their friends support one another through this long, seemingly endless tragedy that we live from day to day, with a kind of etiquette that can have few parallels in the modern world. AIDS involves a decorum, a style of life that includes anxieties about one's own health, and the health of anyone one hasn't seen or heard from in more than, say, six months. In such circumstances the telephone takes on a new and unexpected significance, just as a parting wave at the airport or the train station often means goodbye forever.

All of this is 'difficult' to live with. There can be no compensation for the losses we have known, nor the more dreadful losses that lie ahead, most of which could have been avoided if the fear and hatred of gay men had not been so intense. It strikes me more and more that gay men are vulnerable to HIV almost entirely as a result of heterosexual intolerance and cruelty, from the cradle to the grave—a cruelty so vicious and so pathological that most people could still countenance the total extinction of all gay men before they would contemplate the banal and trivial act of pulling a bit of rubber down a length of macho gristle. This hurts. It also infuriates. We've done all we can to warn our heterosexual friends, and to inform them about our experience in the 1980s. I have now lectured on AIDS at Harvard, Yale, Princeton—the list could go on and on. Yet this is only the third time I have managed to reach the 'straight' press in Britain in all these long, long years. And still our pathetically underfunded and overworked AIDS service organisations are under attack from the virtuous forces of moral probity and public decency. It is exhausting, and sometimes, briefly, one gives in to despair.

Historians will not recall the man who rolls his boyfriend on his side for the three hundredth time to wipe his arse, or the woman who hooks up her husband to his drip every night when she gets home from an office where she cannot possibly afford to tell a soul what she is going through for fear of losing her job . . . I could go on, but I don't want to appear an 'AIDS bore'.

Tonight I am thinking about the time I helped Keith Haring put panstick on the lesions on his face before I interviewed him for the BBC a few months before he died, and how his eyes bored into mine as someone whispered, 'Make him talk about people who are sick'. I am thinking about a friend, a dear friend, a distinguished artist here in London, who lost his sight a few months ago and casually commented how 'awful' this would be for his boyfriend, having to lead him around; and of a dear friend in his late 30s telling me quietly how he killed his lover, who had also been my lover years ago. Most crises have an ending. This one is indefinite.

Why British society continues to have such difficulties in acknowledging and accepting the common humanity (and frailty) of injecting drug users and gay men I cannot tell. Suffice to say that it diminishes us all, but some far, far more than others.

1991 ———————

20. State of Emergency

It is ten years since AIDS was first identified in the United States, although it is clear that the subsequently discovered HIV had been widely transmitted in the course of the late 1970s. Different countries have responded to the epidemic in different ways. Some governments intervened relatively early on to set up health education, and organisations providing a wide range of support services. Other countries left it to the voluntary sector, sometimes funded at arm's length by local or central government, but largely dependent on private charity. This has been the British experience, where there has never been a properly co-ordinated national plan. Not surprisingly therefore the whole situation remains volatile and uneven.

As a result of medical research, and gradually improving patient management, the life-expectancy of people with AIDS has improved dramatically, whilst a great variety of AIDS service organisations now exist to meet the changing needs of the epidemic. Nonetheless Britain is stuck with the legacy of ten years of largely *ad hoc* work: our problems are both local and national.

The British media have depicted AIDS as a form of self-inflicted 'home goal' (to use Princess Anne's distasteful phrase) on the part of the 'immoral'. Indeed, the very possibility of heterosexual transmission of HIV was widely denied until the second half of 1990. Yet in the rush to correct this fundamental misapprehension, it now often seems as if concern is entirely focused on heterosexuals. The perception is that AIDS has, as it were, 'moved on' from gay men. Nothing could be further from the truth, as the most recent statistics demonstrate only too clearly.

Of the total of 4,228 cases of AIDS diagnosed in Britain since 1982, 3,330 have been amongst gay men, compared with 167 cases amongst injecting drug users, 38 cases of infants infected from their mothers, 145 women who claimed to be infected sexually, and 363 men infected by women. Of the 4,098 newly diagnosed cases of HIV in 1990, 3,332 were amongst gay men. It is from this perspective that we must assess the current management of the epidemic, from health education, to medical and social research, and service provision.

First, there is the general crisis of the NHS, which threatens the provision of good standards of treatment across the board. There is practically no acknowledgement of the health needs of lesbians and gay men in the various proposals now being implemented, and hardly any consultation with us. Second, there is a major crisis in relation to the testing of potential treatment drugs for people with HIV or AIDS. In spite of worldwide recommendations that AZT should not be prescribed at levels higher than 600mg, the major 'early intervention' trial in the UK still offers a daily dose of 1000mg to those who are not receiving the placebo against which the drug's effects are being tested. Combination trials of different anti-HIV drugs are nowhere near availability, whilst in any case it is unlikely that those who are already intolerant to AZT will benefit greatly from drugs such as ddl or ddC which work in substantially the same way as AZT. Furthermore, other trials already offer a pessimistic verdict on AZT as 'early intervention'. Third, there are major problems which continue to beset non-government AIDS service organisations ranging from serious shortage of funds, to equally serious shortages of vision and courage.

For example, the Terrence Higgins Trust is evidently failing in its responsibilities to gay men at a time when there is no other leading national organisation which understands or represents our interests. The most recent issue of the *Trust Newsletter* informs its readers that the Board of Directors is now evenly divided between women and men, which 'reflects the role women play in THT—and which stands us in good stead for funding applications'. Whilst gender parity is of course an admirable general principle, it is doubtful how this relates to the indisputable fact that since 1982, 70 per cent of people with AIDS in Britain have been gay men, a figure that remains at 68 per cent in the last two years taken separately. The THT appears to be drifting into a dreamworld which has little or no relation to the actual epidemic we face. Nobody could under-estimate the difficulties faced by the new Executive Director Naomi Wayne, but her tasks will not be made easier as a result of statements like those recently attributed to her in the *Guardian* (6 March) where she claimed that 'AIDS and the spread of HIV infection is not a gay or even a male problem'.

This is not of course to claim that HIV/AIDS are *only* problems for gay men, but that we remain today incomparably worse affected by this epidemic, and more vulnerable to HIV, than any other social constituency in the UK. HIV is not an 'equal opportunity' infection; it has a quite distinctive social profile. The THT was set up to meet the needs of the gay communities in Britain, needs which are still not being met by local authorities around the country. Indeed, the THT only got round to employing a gay men's health educator last autumn! It is also far from obvious that gender parity has anything whatsoever to do with the prospects of state funding, since it is perfectly obvious (or should be) that the Department of Health funds the THT precisely to meet the needs of gay men which cannot be 'officially' acknowledged elsewhere in this most homophobic of European countries.

Fourth, there is the wider problem of the British mass media, which still routinely pumps out prejudice and misinformation about HIV/AIDS. It is relatively easy to knock the tabloid press in this context, but the response of the 'quality' press is at least as troubling.

Fifth, there is the continued refusal to legislate against HIV/AIDS-related discrimination, or to respond to the specific financial needs of people with HIV/AIDS, who are still suffering unnecessarily as a direct result of the 1987 Social Security Act. The situation in British prisons is appalling, and stigmatisation and lack of appropriate medical care abound. Health educators piously inform us about the need to reach men who have sex with men, who don't have any real gay identity. Yet they do this not in order to design anti-homophobic projects which might facilitate the adoption of gay identity amongst such men, but rather to reinforce the same homophobic values and double-standards which make it so hard for many men to accept their homosexuality in the first place!

What then can be done to remedy this emergency? There seem to be three general propositions which need to be urgently considered. The first concerns the voluntary sector as a whole. It is not in the interests of people with HIV or AIDS that they should continue to be seen as distinct groups, either medically or socially. Second, the issue of homophobia in relation to the epidemic must be tackled. It is homophobia which inhibits effective health education for gay men, whose needs in this area are less recognised than those of any other social group in the UK. Furthermore, homophobia continues to blight most aspects of care, support and funding, as well as cultural perceptions and understandings of the whole epidemic. Third, we need to involve far, far more gay men in campaigns for both better treatment drugs and better health education. Care and prevention must not be seen as alternatives.

We live in the worst of all possible worlds: health education for gay men hardly exists, and one would be extremely lucky to find any leaflets, including the Health Education Authority's dismal materials, in a gay bar or club in Britain today. At the same time there seems to be little or no sense of urgency amongst gay men about the extent of HIV and AIDS in our communities, and little awareness of the catastrophe we face later this decade as thousands more gay men with HIV become symptomatic.

We need to be better informed about both treatment issues and health promotion. If organisations such as the Terrence Higgins Trust are unwilling or unable to shoulder the responsibility of effective health education and the provision of up-to-date medical information for gay men, it will mean that increasing numbers of us will no longer feel able or prepared to support it. We must vigorously challenge the widespread assumption that 'the worst' is somehow over. The worst has hardly begun.

21. Perspectives on Testing

Since the passing of the Sexual Offences Act in 1967, no single event has had a greater personal impact on most gay men's lives than the introduction of the HIV antibody test in 1984. The test is a form of poisoned chalice. I frequently hear people say that they haven't taken the test because they 'couldn't live with' a positive result, or words to that effect. Behind this formula there lies an enormous amount of personal anxiety. It would certainly be very insensitive to pretend that HIV antibody testing is not a very frightening subject at a time when one in four gay men taking the test in London STD clinics finds out they are HIV positive. Nor is the situation improved by the types of crusading—either for or against testing—which tend to over-simplify the issues, whilst ignoring the most basic human factors involved.

Unfortunately there has been little serious research about gay men's attitudes to the HIV antibody test in Britain. One recent article considered testing only from the two perspectives of the need to obtain accurate statistics, and the supposed relation between sexual behaviour and known HIV status. There was not so much as a mention of the possible benefits in terms of so-called 'early intervention' medical treatment and care, whilst the history of discussion in the gay media about testing was also entirely ignored.

We are fortunate in Britain that the subject of testing has not so far been subjected to massive political exploitation. In spite of people like the journalist Christopher Monckton who have campaigned for compulsory testing and the carrying of HIV antibody-status cards, it has been widely recognised that testing is a matter for individual choice, on the basis of the most up-to-date social and medical information. In other words it is understood that the test is only meaningful in relation to other kinds of information about discrimination, and possible treatment drugs, etc. Since such information changes over time, it may be perfectly rational to decide that the time has come for an individual to take the test today, or that the time is not yet right.

Nonetheless, there are powerful forces campaigning for testing now. On the one hand epidemiologists want to obtain accurate statistics: on the other, many doctors and community activists argue that knowledge of one's HIV status is of fundamental significance in relation to one's long-term health prospects. It is interesting that both doctors and some gay activists tend to resort to scare-mongering tactics in order to cajole the unwilling or the undecided into testing.

Most pro-testing arguments from doctors tend to be accompanied by exaggerated claims about the supposed benefits of AZT for asymptomatic people with HIV, usually in the context of equally unscientific statements claiming a 100 per cent progress rate from HIV to AIDS, and a 100 per cent mortality rate. The leading US pro-testing gay activist, Martin Delaney, simply states that 'there are profoundly important medical reasons why you must learn your antibody status as soon as possible: if you don't you may needlessly die!'[1] This, to say the least, is highly contentious!

Other voices argue for testing as if it were a form of health education—a way of frightening people into having safer sex. This approach almost invariably stems from heterosexuals who have no understanding of the successful history of safer sex education amongst gay men, with its emphasis on safer sex as a community norm regardless of our known or perceived HIV status. In effect, the pro-testing position poses as an alternative to safer sex education, and as a way to ignore gay men's needs and entitlements.

In the most thorough survey to date of the available literature on testing, David Miller and Tony Pinching conclude that most scientific studies show that most gay men coming forward for testing have already taken up safer sex, and they emphasise the need for caution on the part of counsellors in relation to many doctors' exaggerated claims about available treatment options for people with HIV.[2]

In the absence of community-based safer sex education for heterosexuals it may be the case that HIV antibody testing does indeed work in a primitive way as an incentive to safer sex and safer injecting drug use for heterosexuals. Yet most gay men face a rather different reality. In the absence of anti-discrimination legislation to protect the rights of people with HIV, and with profoundly conflicting evidence about treatment options, it remains wholly unethical to argue that everyone should (or should not) take the test.

The principal issue still concerns individuals who may wish to take part in clinical trials for potential but unproven drug treatments, or who feel they may benefit from a detailed clinical evaluation. In these, as in all other respects, individuals should talk with professional counsellors, before making a final decision. Few are deceived and nobody is helped by the pretence that decisions about testing are any less painful and complex today than they were seven years ago.

22. Perspectives on Treatment

The HIV antibody test is frequently discussed as if it simply told us whether or not one is HIV antibody-positive, especially by the majority of people who have either tested negative, or who have never taken the test. It is not sufficiently recognised that HIV antibody testing involves ways of thinking about ourselves, and one another, that have the profoundest implications for everyone.

Those who test negative often put the experience largely behind them, understandably wanting to forget the stressful suspense of waiting for the result. Yet we should all understand that a positive result is only the first introduction to a whole battery of different tests, which take place over time, the results of which oblige people with HIV to think about what they can best do to protect their health. This involves considering many options with one's doctor and others in the context of what frequently seems a bewildering complex world of medical terms and concepts.

Because our epidemic has so far been largely one of asymptomatic HIV infection, rather than AIDS, it has been easy to neglect the issue of treatments. This attitude has been compounded by the general European experience of socialised medicine, and in this respect gay men are evidently much like everybody else in our respective societies. Most people assume that doctors and scientists are doing everything they can for the sick. Indeed, so entrenched is this belief that any questioning of our generally supine faith in medicine is genuinely frightening to many people, especially when they themselves are ill.

From very early on in the history of the epidemic, regular publications have appeared in the USA summarising the various complex developments in HIV/AIDS research, and the development of potential treatment drugs. These publications, such as *Treatment Issues, Project Inform,*

Perspective, AIDS Clinical Care, and so on, have resulted in a remarkably well-informed readership, which has little or no real equivalent in Europe, although similar community-oriented publications also exist in Canada and Australia.

Anger at what is widely seen as the mismanagement of HIV/AIDS research in the USA culminated in the emergence of the AIDS Coalition to Unleash Power (ACT UP) early in 1987. There can be no doubt that ACT UP's successful targeting of the American institutions that regulate drug research has resulted in the availability of many drugs to people in need, as is recognised by doctors such as Anthony Fauci, who runs the US AIDS Clinical Trial Group (ACTG). Yet here in Europe we have seen little or no community action around medical issues, which tend to be shrouded in secrecy, rather than out in the public domain.

Throughout my personal involvement in the epidemic I have been deeply impressed by the example of friends living with HIV or AIDS who take the view that the only rational way to live with the uncertainties surrounding treatment issues is to believe in the possibility of increasingly effective treatments for and protection against both HIV and the many conditions to which it may make one vulnerable. As people with AIDS live longer, they and their carers are often faced with truly difficult decisions concerning different possible forms of treatment. For example, many drugs cannot be taken in combination, and others have unintended 'side-effects'.

This then is the context in which to view the current situation in medical research, and the message is still evidently mixed. Whilst there can be no doubt about the benefits of AZT to most people with AIDS, evidence concerning its possible efficacy in earlier stages of HIV disease remains conflicting and inconclusive, though many people with HIV report general benefits, including feelings of better health, increased appetite, better skin conditions, and so on. There is also widespread agreement that the circumstances surrounding the original licensing of AZT in America in 1987 were less than properly scientific.[1]

Whilst we must respect the decision of those who decide they don't want to get involved with questions concerning different treatment options, we run the risk in Britain of abdicating all decisions about the direction and conduct of research to scientists who have rarely demonstrated any real or convincing sense of their awareness of the urgency of these issues.

There is not sufficient interest in treatment issues in most British AIDS service organisations, either in the voluntary or statutory sector. There is not sufficient interest in medical issues in the gay press. There is very little community-based research going on; there is also little sense on the part of the BMA or the Medical Research Council of the need for close, constant community liaison, firmly instituted. There are few watchdogs, and no centralised policy for keeping doctors and other carers up to date on ongoing clinical trials.

This is what AIDS activism boils down to—making sure that the huge sums of money set aside for HIV/AIDS research are spent intelligently and to the maximum practical purpose, and to challenge any institution which puts barriers in the way of developing better care in the form of new, improved treatments. AIDS activism is only frightening to those who have something to hide, or who fail to understand the basic principle of the need to maximise information about matters of such profound significance in our communities.

In 1987 most people thought of AZT as a kind of bridge, which might help people with HIV/AIDS over the period until better anti-HIV drugs appeared. Sadly, no such dramatic gains have taken place, and it is therefore hardly surprising if many people, looking at the scientific evidence available, conclude that official medical complacency has set back, rather than hastened, the arrival of unambiguously better drugs.

These cannot, of course, simply be willed into being, but the widespread lack of any real official sense of urgency in these matters suggests that community pressure may need to be imposed on institutions which seem reluctant to do everything possible to justify the faith on which people with HIV/AIDS depend for the prospect of proper, effective treatment, if not a complete cure. This does not necessarily mean spending more money, but it does mean setting up many more clinical trials of potential treatment drugs.

Last month I concluded that the possibility of entering such clinical trials is one of the major incentives to HIV antibody testing. At a time when there is still only one major clinical trial, of AZT at a high dosage, for people with HIV, this is hardly a strong encouragement for anyone to consider testing.

23. Short-Term Companions:
AIDS and 'popular' entertainment

> This new world may be safer, being told
> The dangers and diseases of the old
> —John Donne, *The First Anniversarie*

My purpose is to tell of bodies which have been transformed into shapes of a different kind—Ovid, *The Metamorphoses*

In an important article about the cultural construction of the social meanings of AIDS, Judith Williamson has well observed how:

> while it is relatively easy to counter hysterical conservatism, it is less easy to pin down the wider sense in which AIDS takes its place within the narrative systems along whose tracks events seem to glide quite naturally, whether in news reports, movie plots, or everyday explanations.[1]

Such narrative systems provide the basic structures through which we communicate and make our various senses of ourselves and of the world. They range from the plot-lines of television soap operas, to the conventions of historical fiction, from the logic of jokes to the sequencing of 'events' on the main evening television news show.

Ever since the beginning of the HIV epidemic, a particular range of mass media narratives has been employed in order to 'handle' a topic which was widely regarded as scandalous, drawing attention to the everyday lives of social groups which are generally marginalised in Anglo-American society—gay men, prostitutes, and injecting drug users.[2] The 'scandal' of AIDS however was never publicly recognised in terms of the terrible tragedy of the epidemic as it is lived within these groups. Rather, it was regarded from the ill-informed and frightened perspective of the rest of the population, often described as 'the general public', whom these groups were held to threaten. In such circumstances, it is perhaps hardly surprising that AIDS has generally tended to be represented in the media in terms of older, culturally available narratives concerning the groups with whom the epidemic was initially associated. AIDS has thus been repeatedly dramatised as if it were a side-effect or by-product of homosexuality, or prostitution, of blackness, or injecting drug use. This in turn has led to increased confusion and uncertainty. For example, media attention continues to concentrate on the most obscure possible modes of HIV transmission, rather than on the long-established evidence that HIV is not casually transmissible.

Since most people have never knowingly met anyone living with HIV or AIDS, this epidemic is uniquely mediated by media representations. Indeed, one might conclude that from the mass media's perspective, AIDS remains a hypothetical epidemic, which has not yet affected real people, that is, 'the general public'. This, of course, is an extremely dangerous situation, since it would be only too easy to conclude that HIV is only an issue for those with the virus. However, most people with HIV are not aware that they have been infected, and for the foreseeable future safer sex and safer needle use remain our only demonstrably effective methods for minimising new cases. Sadly, the major narratives which have framed and defined the subject of AIDS throughout the 1980s have rarely contributed much to wider social or medical understanding of the epidemic.

On the contrary, the major narratives through which most readers and viewers have been encouraged to imagine AIDS belong essentially to the orders of pre-modern thought, which have long posed the sick as essentially dangerous individuals. Thus AIDS has tended to be narrated in a heavily over-determined manner, in which highly charged fantasies of gay men and prostitutes and junkies as uniformly predatory seducers of the 'innocent' and 'vulnerable' are woven together with ancient folkloric notions of disease as retribution, and deep cultural fears of contagion.[3] Thus we will all be familiar with a particular range of stories which have been repeated in different forms since the beginning of the epidemic. For example, the story of an imagined 'AIDS carrier' who sets out to deliberately infect other people; or the story of a loving and faithful wife who has contracted HIV from her husband; or the story of the family whose young child has received infected blood during a routine operation. These stories are, as it were, emblematic. That is to say, they condense together strands of fact and fantasy, in such a way that they come to represent what people often think of automatically as both typical, and truthful. Other such scenarios include the familiar image of a deserted African village, all of the inhabitants of which have succumbed to AIDS; the HIV-positive prostitute who claims that she is not having safer sex with her clients; the vengeful HIV-positive rent-boy; the courageous scientific quest for an effective vaccine, and so on and so forth.

It is worth examining such narratives in some detail, since they all make sense in the broader context of the beliefs and expectations generated in audiences by different types of journalism, cinema, television programming, etc. Thus the 'AIDS carrier' narrative belongs to a cluster of similar stories that are well known from a wide variety of cultural sources, involving strange 'mystery' diseases, illicit sex with sinister strangers, vampirism, and so on. These all share a tendency to demonise the ill, and to present illness itself as a symptom of some deeper malaise. Thus there emerges a division between those thought of as maliciously infectious, and those thought of as their hapless victims. According to this scheme of things, people living with HIV or AIDS are represented as menacing figures, agents of disease against whom one is defenceless. This common narrative has played a central role in determining popular perceptions of the meaning of AIDS in such a way that the possibility of audiences or readers making sympathetic identifications with people living with HIV is usually ruled out of the question. Furthermore, this essentially eugenic fantasy also carries with it a strong implication that the only way to defeat the epidemic is to punish the ill, who must at all costs be identified. Not for the sake of their health, in terms of treatment and care, but in order to protect the supposedly 'innocent'. Thus the very concept of the 'AIDS carrier' may be regarded as a product of traditional 'public health' policy, which frequently involved measures such as quarantine regardless of any question of actual medical needs.

In a similar manner the image of the infected wife speaks from a perspective which is above all concerned to firmly attribute blame to the person who infected her, just as recipients of infected blood products are also frequently featured as the 'innocent victims' of malevolent 'AIDS carriers', rather than of bad medical practice in the early years of the epidemic, and the absence of adequate blood-screening facilities. The image of deserted African villages, or gaunt black Africans (rarely dignified with names) dying in bush hospitals is still frequently used to embody the fantasy of a generalised Africa, in which AIDS is supposedly a reflection of 'primitive' social and medical circumstances. The *unconscious* message here seems to be that AIDS is intrinsically symptomatic of

'African Otherness', and need not therefore be taken seriously by white people, especially in the First World. Thus we are also invited to think, by the same dreamlike logic, that the First World can somehow protect itself from AIDS by forcing African visitors to take HIV antibody tests, and by excluding those who are HIV positive, rather than by safer sex and safer injecting needle use. What is most remarkable in this fantasy is its denial of AIDS as a reality in the First World itself for more than ten years. Once again, AIDS appears as a condition closely associated with 'Otherness', whether racial or sexual or rooted in drug use.[4]

This is quite obviously the implication of the huge number of stories and features about prostitution, which is invariably regarded as danger-ous. Yet it is prostitutes who are represented as agents of danger, rather than as people who may themselves be at risk from their clients, with whom they frequently play a major role as face-to-face safer sex educa-tors. Moreover, the blatant stereotyping of prostitutes in such coverage only serves to disguise both the extent and the diversity of prostitution in our societies. Blaming prostitutes for AIDS allows people the false comfort of feeling morally superior, as if this were some kind of magical protection against HIV. It also speaks volumes about still-deeper levels of misogyny and sexual hypocrisy.[5] Male or female, the spectre of the HIV-positive prostitute evidently narrates a wide array of contemporary sexual anxieties about the whole subject of extra-marital sex. Most of these seem to consist of barely disguised feelings of personal guilt and shame, projected onto prostitutes (and gay men) in the form of sadistic fantasies of punishment and death. All of this avoids the central ques-tion, which does not concern the HIV status of prostitutes, but whether or not they and their clients are having safer sex. This is an especially important point, since it helps us understand the way in which com-mentators so frequently depict gay sex, or prostitution, or injecting drug use, as if they were *intrinsically* dangerous and unacceptable. We are not at risk from sexual intercourse, but from a virus with well-known modes of transmission against which we have immediate protection in which we should feel confidence. Yet the subject of safer sex is only rarely dis-cussed in most media commentary with any frankness, and sensational stories about condoms breaking, or so-called 'relapse' only serve to fur-ther undermine many people's belief that there is anything they can do to protect themselves or one another.

Finally, we are all familiar with the formats of documentary and cur-rent affairs programmes and stories about the epidemic, which provide regular, reassuring narratives about ongoing scientific research, always with the promise of a 'breakthrough' just around the corner. This message is also, ultimately, reassuring: we are assured that there are friendly, brilliant boffins out there in their laboratories, doing mysterious things with test-tubes and computers, so that there's nothing really for us to worry about, and nothing we ourselves can or need to do. That is, as long as one doesn't perceive oneself, or one's sexual partners, as being at any possible risk of contracting HIV. By exoticising the whole subject of AIDS, media commentary lulls people into the potentially dangerous delusion that it can never happen to them. God forbid that we should ever question the authority of doctors, or public health officials, or the pharmaceutical industry, in relation to HIV, or any other illness.

This rather arbitrary list suggests something of the underlying complexities that inform narratives concerned with AIDS, on which most people's perceptions of the epidemic are based. Such agenda-setting may be analysed in much greater detail, and doubtless a full taxonomy of AIDS narratives could be established. The most immediate point, however, concerns the way in which, for more than a decade, the mass media has consistently positioned audiences in *contradictory* ways, implying simultaneously that they both *are,* and *are not,* at risk from HIV. On the one hand, heterosexuals are told AIDS is 'only' a problem for exotic minorities, and on the other they are told they can 'catch' it from their dentist or manicurist. Hence, perhaps, the hostility that is so frequently expressed towards people with HIV, who are almost invariably seen as *threatening* rather than *threatened,* and in need of strict, punitive control, rather than support.

Nonetheless, this dominant agenda has not been established without variation or resistance, and many attempts have been made over the years to 'de-sensationalise' coverage of the epidemic, both in the press and on television, most conspicuously in American independent activist videos such as *Testing the Limits,* and on US cable television.[6] Yet most AIDS narratives continue to regard and depict the groups first affected by HIV in the West as if they were uniform subcultures, without individual variation, or any real emotional depth. Thus gay men are almost always seen to share a standard 'gay lifestyle'. Indeed, from watching television one might well imagine that gay men only exist at nightclubs, or in airy, tasteful apartments with wonderful clothes to match the furniture. One might also imagine that *all* gay men share identical sexual needs, pleasures, and identities. Injecting drug users and prostitutes are significantly treated in a markedly similar manner, as if *all* prostitutes and *all* injecting drug users are somehow the same. They are thus made to appear simultaneously as villains ('AIDS carriers', etc.), and as victims (as long as they stay mute or, better still, apologetic), but almost *never* as members of social groups struggling daily to survive and resist the worst natural disaster within most Western societies since the great influenza epidemic of 1918, which killed millions of people. This is especially marked in relation to depictions of gay men in north American and north European countries, who have so far borne the brunt of HIV and its many consequences.

Anti-gay prejudice has been widely mobilised in relation to AIDS by varying institutions, ranging from churches, to individual newspapers, and political parties of both the Left and the Right. In this context, desensationalising strategies have tended to take the form of 'human interest' programmes and features, although these only rarely confront the actual circumstances that make them necessary in the first place. Only a handful of investigative programmes such as Britain's *Hard News,* and *The Media Show* (both on Channel Four), together with BBC-2's *Late Show* have attempted serious, in-depth analysis of the wider biopolitics of mass media representations of AIDS. The great majority of features may best perhaps be regarded as a form of macabre *entertainment,* providing a limited series of heavily moralised *tableaux.* These tell us much about the complex moral and cultural management of modern sexuality and sexual identities, but little or nothing about the complex, shifting realities of the epidemic as it is lived all around the world. In such circumstances AIDS becomes more of a cypher than a syndrome. The epidemic is endlessly staged and enacted as if it were a form of public morality play, about personal guilt, judgement and damnation, rather than as a terrible ongoing catastrophe, to which governments and international institutions including the film and television industries have conspicuously failed to respond in anything like a responsible manner.

AIDS fictions

One strategy intended to correct the relentless homophobia of dominant AIDS commentary has been concentrated in the domain of independent feature films, initiated by the late Arthur J. Bressan's *Buddies* in 1985, and Bill Sherwood's *Parting Glances* in 1986. Both films were set in New York city, and dramatise aspects of the epidemic as lived by gay men. *Buddies* tells the story of a young, successful yuppy, who 'buddies' an older gay man dying from AIDS. The man with AIDS is an ex-hippie, whose outlook and identity had been forged in the early 1970s period of Gay Liberation. The film movingly describes his 'buddie's' gradual recognition of the extent of anti-gay prejudice in the USA, and its baleful influence on the course of the epidemic and his new friend's life-expectancy. It is an extremely ambitious allegory of the difficult social relations between different generations of gay men, and the divisions of class within the gay communities of the USA. *Parting Glances* is less overtly political, and has the rather different, if equally ambitious aim of locating AIDS (and gay men in general) within contemporary Manhattan society. Yet the aim of *Parting Glances* is not simply 'normalisation', but rather a demonstration of the actual diversity of urban New York life, and the centrality of gay men in the social life of the city. Thus the tragedy of AIDS becomes seen as a tragedy for the entire city.

Since 1986 the epidemic has of course deepened and widened in New York, as in most other major Western cities. For example, by the summer of 1987 there had been 1000 diagnosed cases of AIDS in the United Kingdom as a whole, whereas there had been more than 10,000 cases in New York alone.[7] At the time of writing this article there have been approximately 100,000 deaths from AIDS in the USA, and around 2500 deaths in the UK which nonetheless has a fifth of the overall population of the USA. The gradual changes in the demography of the epidemic in the course of the 1980s make it increasingly important to challenge the authority of the mass media's response, which still seems largely frozen in the postures, attitudes and narratives established in the early 1980s. By reducing AIDS to a kind of ghoulish spectacle, media coverage has been responsible for many of the misunderstandings that continue to frame beliefs and behaviour. Thus the recent acknowledgement of the impact of HIV amongst injecting drug users and their sexual partners has frequently been presented in such a way as to imply that the epidemic has somehow 'moved on' from gay men, though nothing could be further from the truth. The same media industry which for many years refused to accept even the *possibility* of heterosexual transmission, now tends to ignore all other modes of transmission, even though the prevalence of HIV amongst gay men means that we are still far more vulnerable than any other social constituency in most First World countries. This is the immediate, pressing context in which the most recent major feature film about AIDS appears.

Like its predecessors, *Longtime Companion* (1990) sets out to realign perceptions of AIDS, and to narrate the history of the epidemic from a gay male perspective. Yet the worsening of the AIDS crisis around the world forces us to consider whether the conventions of Hollywood melodrama, now crossed with the conventions of television soap opera, are sufficiently resilient to effectively undermine the by-now solidly accreted cultural agenda of AIDS which has been established for almost ten years by the Press and television alike, with an unusual and significant degree of unanimity. How does one narrate an epidemic in process? How might one deploy one narrative in order to discredit another? Can a film contest one set of inadequate explanations of an immensely complex social phenomenon, and at the same time establish its own superior explanatory authority? How, in other words, might it be possible to use the narrative forms of the entertainment industry in order to call into question its own stubborn fears and prejudices? In order to answer these questions, it is necessary to consider something of the history of AIDS fictions as they have emerged over time in different media.

By the summer of 1988 AIDS had struck the fictional worlds of three major US network television soap operas—CBS's, *The Young And The Restless,* ABC's, *All My Children,* and NBC's, *Another World.* Yet as *New York Times* critic Deborah Rogers has pointed out: 'All three AIDS plots on these television serials feature patients who are women—and women with no history of drug abuse'.[8]

A year earlier Britain's Central television produced Alma Cullen's four-part mini-series *Intimate Contact,* which four years later is still slated for a possible movie remake. *Intimate Contact* tells the story of a philandering businessman who contracts HIV from a prostitute in New York, and is more concerned with the snobbery and hypocrisy of his family's responses, than with his illness. It is thus rather like a Victorian 'improving' fiction, intended to edify its audience, and to dispel prejudice. Perhaps the most fascinating aspect of *Intimate Contact* lies in its depiction of the sick man's wife, Ruth (played by Claire Bloom). Ruth is totally shut off in her houseproud, middle-class world, and the extent of her inability to deal with her husband's diagnosis is shown as a direct result of her smug, complacent Thatcherite world view and class position. However, as a result of her meeting a gay couple and an HIV-positive haemophiliac boy and his father she learns the lesson of 'compassion'. In other words, *Intimate Contact* finds in AIDS only an example, albeit extreme, of the supposedly universal problems of ignorance and prejudice. The husband with AIDS dies conveniently early on in the series, which finds its closure in the moral 'improvement' (and new likeability) of the heroine. Indeed, one almost comes to regard AIDS as a blessing in disguise, at least from Ruth's point of view. AIDS is not seen to possess any real specificity of its own in *Intimate Contact,* and this to a great extent reflects British liberal opinion to the present day. In narrative and ideological terms this duplicates the problems raised by NBC's 1986 made-for-television movie *An Early Frost*. As Vito Russo pointed out:

> In *An Early Frost* we see how AIDS affects a young man's mother, father, sister, brother-in-law and grandmother. There is no consideration given to the fact that this is happening to him—not them.[9]

An Early Frost narrates the simultaneous coming out of a young gay man to his family, alongside his dilemma of living with AIDS. Yet the extraordinary level of violent prejudice this brings out in his family is understood by the film to be quite natural and inevitable, if ultimately susceptible to reason and 'love'. Prejudice is seen as a kind of free-floating universal, able to be attracted to almost any object in an arbitrary fashion. Thus both *An Early Frost* and *Intimate Contact* were entirely unable to confront the specific, concrete issues raised by homophobia, and by AIDS. The 'problem' of the epidemic is thus posed for heterosexuals as a question of rationality and familial stability, and how 'well' they can behave, rather than the question facing millions of gay men about how long we or our closest friends will manage to stay alive.

Longtime Companion

This is the immediate representational context in which *Longtime Companion* was made, and is viewed. In recent months I have seen the film in New York, London and Melbourne, and differing audience responses provided an especially keen sense of the enormity of the differing experience of the epidemic in these three cities alone. The American television critic in *People* magazine genuinely found *Intimate Contact* shocking in terms of its 'frankness', and 'amazing', because 'the victims are at first unlikeable'. Such issues are not raised by *Longtime Companion*, for the simple reason that its narrative structure is not organised around exemplary victims and *individual change*. Rather, it sets out to narrate a collective experience, and this is its greatest strength. In New York the great majority of gay men have already lost many friends to AIDS, and will know many more who are ill. The lowest estimates suggest that at least 36 per cent of all gay men in New York are HIV positive. In London however, far fewer gay men have had any direct experience of AIDS, though far more will know somebody with HIV. Throughout the 1980s the American urban experience of AIDS has increasingly involved a grim

routine of visits to people in acute hospital care, deaths, and mourning, whereas in Britain the overwhelming experience has been of people
with HIV who are to all extents and purposes (it is widely perceived)
perfectly well. Melbourne, like its sister city of Sydney, has a worse epidemic than London, but the situation is nowhere near as bad as New
York. Yet the internal cohesion of the Australian gay communities means
that the epidemic is felt in a more immediate way than it is in London.
This is largely a result of different political histories.[10]

For example, the Australian government's response to AIDS has been
far more pragmatic and practical than government responses in Britain
or France or the US. More than 80 per cent of Australian AIDS cases
have been amongst gay men, and acknowledging the risk of HIV infection to gay men and others, the government set up community-based
AIDS councils in all Australia's States and Territories, co-ordinated by
the Australian Federation of AIDS Organisations (AFAO), a small organisation based in Canberra. As a result, AIDS education in Australia has
been based on the demonstrably effective principles of community development, and the AIDS Councils have demonstrated a commitment to
the experience and wishes of volunteers. This has resulted in turn in a
much more flexible, pragmatic approach than is generally found in other
countries, where non-government organisations are more traditional in
their structure, with a top-down attitude to volunteers, who rarely get
any opportunity to move upwards through the organisations into paid
jobs. Australian AIDS service organisations also recognise the need to
develop clear policies, with mid- and long-term goals, largely because
they enjoy a financial security which has not been felt in most other
countries. The AIDS Councils have not resorted to the types of crude
scaremongering that have been typical elsewhere in the name of AIDS
'education', and Australia thus has one of the best-educated and serviced
gay communities in the world.

In Australia political struggles for the decriminalisation of homosexuality were waged throughout the 1970s and 1980s on a state-by-state
basis, and this resulted in a highly organised, purposeful sense of gay and
lesbian identity amongst large numbers of people. Moreover, the Australian ideology of multiculturalism traverses racial, ethnic and sexual
boundaries in such a way that gay groups are recognised by the central government as legitimate representatives of a social constituency
with special needs and entitlements in this health emergency. In other
words, Australia has managed to recognise AIDS as a disaster of *national*
proportions, unlike other countries where the epidemic has only been

perceived to affect certain groups who are hardly regarded as national subjects in the first place. In this respect, the sight of ordinary lesbians and gay men getting on with our own lives, usually in ways like everybody else, has a special significance in countries like Britain and the US, where we are generally regarded as strange and exotic.

Multiculturalism has never existed as an official ideology in Britain, and remains distinctly unfashionable. Moreover, the government has not been able to recognise community groups which could represent the interests of lesbians and gay men, so that AIDS service organisations such as the Terrence Higgins Trust are frequently attacked for supposedly 'promoting' homosexuality, or being gay 'conspiracies'. This is simply because the work of such organisations proceeds from a concern for the lives of gay people, and others, which many politicians, journalists and church leaders and journalists evidently do not share. One tragic effect of this has been a timidity on the part of British and American AIDS service organisations in regard to subjects such as gay men's safer sex education, which are thought to be 'controversial', and which might lead to loss of revenue. Thus there are far fewer safer sex leaflets and other materials available to most gay men in Britain than there are to our Australian equivalents. Much more concern was expressed in Britain in the 1980s about the 'decency' or otherwise of safer sex materials than about the actual human tragedy of AIDS for those affected. It is thus hardly surprising that so many British and American gay men are deeply concerned and angry about the representation of AIDS in our television networks and cinemas, since they have so consistently ignored our experience, and our profound losses.

The sheer scale of the American epidemic has resulted in a growing awareness of the terrible consequences of the American model of private medicine, which has stimulated the emergence of AIDS activist organisations such as the AIDS Coalition to Unleash Power (ACT UP), founded by Larry Kramer in New York in 1987.[11] Increasing numbers of Americans have come to question the dismal track record of the US government in all areas of HIV/AIDS policy, from the funding and direction of biomedical research, to housing, or social security benefits, and health education. Community-based responses to AIDS in different countries depend in large measure on the degree of self-confidence and organisation within the communities affected by AIDS in the period *before the epidemic began.* These same factors also contribute to the ways that heterosexuals think about AIDS, according to marked national variations in attitudes towards homosexuality, and levels of homophobia within different national popular cultures. All of this in turn shapes both the production and the reception of 'information' about HIV/AIDS, whether in the form of explicit, targeted health education campaigns, or newspaper reporting, or in feature films.

These are the specific, if shifting conditions, in which cultural producers are obliged to narrate AIDS, either on the terms of dominant popular beliefs and attitudes, or against the grain of narratives on which such attitudes and beliefs are based. In this context, the subject of death has come to acquire a special significance. On the one hand it is frequently erroneously claimed that all gay men have been surrounded by death on a vast scale, whilst at the same time the deaths of gay men are never looked at closely, or regarded as fully *tragic*. Thus the actual diversity of gay experience of the epidemic is obscured, as well as the concrete fact of death as it has affected gay men in so many different, yet aligned, ways. Most public AIDS narratives have depicted the epidemic from the outside, as it were, and almost invariably tend to be organised around the assumption that an HIV diagnosis is an automatic death sentence. What is so infuriating to those of us living inside the epidemic, as it were, is the way that such ruthless fatalism ignores all the most important information concerning different mortality rates in different population groups, differing rates of progression from HIV to AIDS, differing standards of patient management, differing degrees of access to proper medical care and treatment drugs, and so on. For if the subject of deaths from AIDS were taken seriously, these issues would be equally familiar to everyone. Yet AIDS fictions rarely acknowledge the ways in which AIDS activists have contributed directly to the increased life expectancy of people with AIDS, by forcing the US government's medical agencies to release treatment drugs and expand access to clinical trials of experimental treatment drugs, and so on. Hence, the widespread perception from within the cultural field of the epidemic that most AIDS commentary prefers the familiar, and essentially sentimental narrative of long-term chronic illness leading to inevitable death, to other narratives that might refute the logic which requires that everyone with HIV *must* die as a result. Indeed, amongst all the uneven and conflicting public responses to AIDS, it is the widespread indifference to the deaths of tens of thousands of young gay men that is most unacceptable and frightening to AIDS activists. For that same cultural indifference is already in place to anaesthetise 'public opinion' in relation to the many hundreds of thousands of deaths that are likely to occur unless better treatments are found very quickly, and made widely available. Effective treatments cannot be discovered simply by acts of will. But without a real sense of urgency concerning the scale of potential deaths, treatment research is unlikely to receive the funding or the prioritisation it requires.

Longtime Companion is in many important respects a film about the deaths of gay men. It is also a film which attempts to explain something of how gay men live—or, at least, how middle-class white gay men in New York live. Furthermore, we should note that the death of gay men is not entirely new as a topic. On the contrary, the picture of the supposedly lonely, miserable old age and expiration of gay men has long been a central warning trope held up to young gay men throughout the modern period. This projective fantasy evidently overlooks the types of social solidarity and organisation that exist amongst older gay men, who are in fact less likely to experience the types of systematic neglect and isolation that are the increasingly common fate of their heterosexual peers. Nonetheless, homophobic ideology seems to *require* the motif of the pathetic, isolated, ageing gay man as a form of sadistic wish fulfilment. In this respect it appears that there is a close social and psychological relation between the image of the sordid, older gay man, and the parallel cultural picture of the gay 'AIDS victim'. Both are expressions of vengeful emotions, and the policing of the boundaries of individual and collective sexual identities. However, when we talk of homophobia we should not be trying to theorise it solely in relation to the explicit, *conscious* projects developed by those relatively few people who deliberately and maliciously target the lives and happiness of lesbians and gay men. On the contrary, we need to think about the broad mass of perfectly decent people who thoughtlessly and more or less automatically reproduce the values of a culture which identifies homosexuality in an extraordinarily narrow range of ways. Most people are not ogres of homophobic hatred, and there is thus an urgent need to develop cultural interventions which are able to challenge the logic and rhetoric of homophobia, whether it comes from gossip columns, or from governments. In other words, the cultural legitimacy of homophobia must be a central target in effective cultural work concerned with the meaning of AIDS, amongst gay men and heterosexuals alike.

It is entirely understandable that much has been made of the difficulties in getting *Longtime Companion* to the screen in the USA and elsewhere, but this should not lead one to suspend all one's ordinary critical faculties. It is *not*, as we have seen, the first commercial feature film about AIDS, as falsely claimed in some of the publicity surrounding the film's launch. Nor will it be the last. However, for this very reason it is important to try to think about the film's real achievements, as well as its problems and occasional failures. *Longtime Companion* sets out to chronicle how a group of relatively affluent white gay men in Manhattan were effected by AIDS in the course of the 1980s. By the end of the film, most of the central characters have died, whilst the survivors have come to realise the full extent of the failings of the US health care system, which is shown to have put white middle-class men in much the same grim position as the poorest black, injecting drug users from Brooklyn and Harlem. In New York the film was criticised by some gay critics on the grounds that it neglects the experience of AIDS in the city's black and Hispanic populations, whilst one heterosexual critic objected to the absence of heterosexual families. Both complaints strike me as beside the point. For surely there can be no good reason why a film should not be made specifically about the experience of the social group which all along has been worst affected in the USA? Besides, there is a bitter irony in gay criticism that only serves to reinforce the fundamentally homophobic notion that it is wrong to make a film which takes gay lives and feelings seriously for once. The second objection was even stranger, since it so obviously stemmed from an inability to understand why the large numbers of gay men choose to live in cities such as New York and San Francisco, rather than in the small towns and suburbs that refuse to accept them.

Certainly *Longtime Companion* is very good indeed at depicting the level of everyday life during an epidemic, and one could hardly come away without an awareness of the relentlessly accumulating centrality of biomedical issues in the lives of most urban American gay men. By now most gay New Yorkers are only too familiar with the full range of ghastly, life-threatening illnesses to which HIV may make one vulnerable. Toxoplasmosis (toxo); cytomegalovirus (CMV); mycrobacterium avium intracellulare (MAI); pneumocystis carinii pneumonia (PCP); cryptospiridiosis (crypto) . . . the names trip off our tongues like old friends, but old friends from another planet as far as most other people are concerned. We also see and hear about the vast array of treatments with which so many are also increasingly familiar: Acyclovir (against herpes); AZT and ddI and ddC (against HIV); Foscarnet and DHPG (against CMV retinitis); Nebulised Pentamidine (against PCP), and on and on and on. Indeed, the routine nature of care and the casual, routine way in which these men face, discuss, and share appalling illnesses is one of the most striking aspects of the film, together with its depiction of the gradual pauperisation to which AIDS so frequently leads, even for those who are adequately insured. These are not issues that have surfaced elsewhere in the mass media. Way back in 1984 Richard Goldstein wrote an article in the *Village Voice* in New York in which he compared AIDS to the Blitz in London, noting however that AIDS is more like a Blitz taking place in a city where most people are walking around like tourists, as if nothing were happening, utterly unaware of the disaster all around them. This is the sense that *Longtime Companion* never quite manages to achieve, for the simple reason that it doesn't look beyond the world of gay men, save in the person of Lisa, a heterosexual woman played by Mary Louise Parker, in what is much the best performance in the film.

The film's critics also seem to me to have entirely missed the significance of its depiction of gay relationships, love, friendship and sex, and the full extent to which it takes these for granted as facts of life rather than as matters of 'controversy'. *Longtime Companion* ends with a dream sequence as Lisa and her two closest surviving gay friends walk slowly along the beach on Fire Island in 1989, where the beginning of the film had been set eight years earlier. They are discussing a forthcoming ACT UP demonstration which they are going to attend, which is simultaneously a measure of their politicisation and their friendship as men and women, gay and straight. In the dream, all their dead friends come pouring down the tow-path onto the beach, where they embrace and are reunited. At the New York screening I attended, most people seemed unmoved and, if anything, angered at what they saw as a gratuitous determination to give the film some kind of upbeat 'happy ending' at whatever cost. In London and Melbourne however people all around me were in tears and evidently deeply moved. This in itself tells us something about the extent to which New Yorkers have been hardened by AIDS, something about the extent of suffering and the numbing that so frequently goes with loss on this scale. Obviously AIDS has no 'happy ending'. The dead do not come back to life. But I don't think that this is what the filmmakers were trying to pretend. On the contrary, the sequence works precisely on the level of its cathartic release of long pent-up emotions which themselves are frequently in conflict. For example, in one of the film's more powerful yet understated sequences we see how one of the central characters, Willy, is terrified of possible contagion in the early stages of the epidemic, and in consequence neglects a dying friend. This is less a judgement than an observation of how things *were,* and how sometimes they *still are.* For gay men have no automatic or magical access to superior information than that generally available on television and in the same newspapers they, and most other people, read. The dream sequence at the end of *Longtime Companion* seems to me to speak of the rarely stated scale of horror all around us, and the certainty of worse to come. It also speaks of the most simple and passionate wish that none of this had ever happened, that our dearest friends might indeed come back to life again, that we miss them horribly. This is surely not to be dismissed as 'denial' or 'delusion', but should be understood as a necessary catharsis, and moreover a catharsis that binds our communities ever closer in the fight to save lives.

This is not to say the film presents no problems. For example, it is inexplicable to me how a film about AIDS released in 1990 cannot even bring itself to so much as mention safer sex. Yet criticisms that it fails to deal adequately with the rise of AIDS service organisations, or AIDS activism again seem beside the point. This is a film about mainstream, non-political, ambitious young gay New Yorkers, and it seems to me to represent that large population with more than a little insight. If such bright, successful, young white gay men had little opportunity to understand the epidemic, what hope was there for the rest of the population? This seems to me a vitally important underlying theme in *Longtime Companion,* a theme which we neglect at our peril. An old friend of mine in New York reacted furiously to the sight of an ACT UP sticker in the film in a sequence set a year before it actually appeared. At the time, Vito Russo whispered in my ear that the heart of someone who could only care about dates must have shrunk to the size of a pea. Yet at the same time we in other countries have to try to remember what gay New Yorkers have been living through during the past decade. With so little official public concern, and so little material support, it is hardly surprising if many have developed thick protective carapaces around their feelings, simply as a matter of emotional survival. We in Britain may gauge something perhaps of the scale of emotional trauma for those in its midst, from the words of a 23-year-old American gay man recently diagnosed with HIV, who told his therapist:

> I'm sometimes glad to think that in ten years I'll be dead. By then the only gay people left will be those whose lives were ruined by watching the rest of us die.[12]

In the course of the 1980s, American gay men have moved from shock, to grief, to fury at the enormity of the failures of government and mass media responses to the epidemic. This guarantees a heavily over-determined response to any feature film dealing with AIDS. However, our entirely justified anger at the US film industry's homophobia, and its refusal to deal fairly and truthfully with AIDS should not blind us to the achievements of a film which at least begins to redress serious sins of omission. Nor in Britain should we forget the gulf between the US television and film industries, and most Americans, including critics. In 1989 I chaired a public discussion in Montreal on the vexed issue of AIDS and the role of the media, at the SIDART section of the Fifth International AIDS Conference. The panel included actor Tom Hulce, *Longtime Companion*'s producer Lindsay Law, and other professional representatives from the north American film and television industries, together with the producer of Danish television's safer sex slots.

There was however little opportunity for discussion, because of the furious response from many Americans in the audience to the film and television executives. In retrospect, it became clearer to me that the barrage of violent criticism had little or nothing to do with what the speakers actually said. Rather, it reflected the profound sense of alienation American lesbians and gay men feel from the US film and network television industries. As a European, I tend to take for granted the high proportion of independent films made in countries such as Britain and Germany, and the routine access to network television enjoyed by European cultural activists, including lesbians and gay men—access that remains unthinkable in the United States.

There are certain parallels here to the reception of *Longtime Companion*. However bad the epidemic may be in Britain, or Australia, or Canada, we in those countries enjoy advantages that are all but unimaginable in the US, whether in terms of socialised medicine, or government-funded yet independent AIDS service organisations, or regular access to network television audiences on our own terms. Whilst it is far from clear to me what Americans might possibly learn from an out-of-date television mini-series such as *Intimate Contact,* it would appear that *Longtime Companion* does succeed in communicating a specifically American experience of the epidemic to non-American viewers. It also manages to articulate AIDS as a simultaneously personal and national issue in the US, where representations of gay men are so heavily policed, and shaped in the likeness of homophobic fantasy rather than the actual sexual diversity of the television-watching and cinema-going population. In this respect there are significant parallels between debates about *Longtime Companion* and the issues raised by television fund-raiser *Red Hot & Blue,* which was broadcast on ABC television in the US on World AIDS Day, 1990, in a version which was heavily censored compared to the full-length version shown in all other countries, including Australia and the UK.

Red Hot & Blue had been the first attempt to combine fundraising with health education in a single network television programme. Nineteen different artists recorded different Cole Porter standards, and were filmed in turn by nineteen well-known directors, including Percy Adlon, Jim Jarmusch, Jonathan Demme, Wim Wenders and Alex Cox. Interspersed between the songs were health education 'shorts', including one made by the Gran Fury Collective. More activist information was also contained within some of the individual videos, especially the film by Adelle Lutz and Sandy McLeod of the British group Erasure, singing 'Too Darn Hot', against a background of ACT UP demonstration footage, statistics, and so on. The record sleeve and CD also contain lengthy information about HIV/AIDS including a list of twelve things everyone can do in their own lives about the epidemic. These include fighting 'for legislation to protect the ordinary human rights of people living with HIV and AIDS', making sure 'we have reliable information that is up to date', 'fighting prejudice' and so on.[13]

Yet in Britain *Red Hot & Blue* received a very hostile response, which often included the criticism that Cole Porter's songs had somehow been sullied or contaminated by association with hip-hop music, or rap groups such as The Jungle Brothers. Thus Julie Burchill grizzled in the *Mail on Sunday* that 'the songs of Cole Porter are part of our heritage . . . and the HIV hit squad have no right to vandalize it'. The fantasy seems to be that contemporary remakes will somehow damage all previous recordings by singers such as Ella Fitzgerald or Frank Sinatra. The impression that some kind of displacement is going on in such comments is reinforced by Burchill's claim that:

> With AIDS has come a new sort of clod-hopping authoritarianism from those who work for its charities—a shrill, smug insistence that any sort of behaviour is acceptable from homosexuals now that the chips are down, whether it is 'outing' reluctant gays, or orgying in Piccadilly Circus.[14]

Red Hot & Blue, concludes Burchill, is a form of 'grave-robbing'. It is, however, far from clear what she means by a 'clod-hopping authoritarianism' from AIDS charities which have nothing to do with 'outing', whilst her reference to 'orgying in Piccadilly Circus' implies her awareness of a demonstration organised by the queer activist organisation *OutRage* calling for the repeal of discriminatory laws which prevent lesbians and gay men from showing any kind of physical affection in public. What Julie Burchill truly hates is gay men, and like so many of her kind she reads AIDS as some kind of reflection on homosexuality. The only authoritarianism apparent is her own.

This is not dissimilar to the attitude of a commissioning editor from Britain's Channel 4 television, who found the sight of a white man and a black man rolling around rather suggestively on the floor in Jimmy Somerville's video as 'a little too specific . . . a touch of the "Shock-Horror" syndrome'.[15] Since both men were fully clothed from the waist down, this sounds a rather remarkable verdict. I suspect however the key word here is 'syndrome', which again speaks of unconscious anxieties and defences. Together with Neneh Cherry's video including messages about the need to avoid sharing needles, and several others, it was removed by the ABC network bosses. One ABC director explained on Channel 4's *The Media Show* how *Red Hot & Blue* was good television insofar as it allowed Cole Porter's songs to reach an audience aged from 2 to 90. She didn't regard the show as being about HIV/AIDS at all. As she explained:

> I'm in the Entertainment Division, not in the News Division; I'm not in the Documentary Division, not in the News Division. I'm in the Entertainment Division, and that is our mandate—to entertain.[16]

Here 'entertainment' is defined in strict opposition to news values, or any other claims to informational significance. 'Entertainment' is thus pictured as a wholly autonomous domain, whose values must not be confused with those of 'real life'. This is still more apparent from an ABC Broadcast Standards and Practice executive, Susan Futtman, who described television as 'a free market-place' for 'a range of ideas'. However, she found problems with the use of stars:

> whom people look up to, taking a very particular stand, without the chance for any other side having any rebuttal . . . I don't think any network would want to take an advocacy position on a subject like that (e.g. needle exchanges, and safer sex). You have to take the larger issue. . . . If you support one, you have to support them all.[17]

In other words, Ms Futtman argued that there is an intrinsic 'balance' on television that needs to be maintained, regardless of the fact that the only kind of condom education that can be broadcast on US Network television consists of short films in the *America Responds to AIDS* series, whose prime concern is the need to avoid any possible offence to anyone, rather than people's entitlement to information on which their lives may well depend. One such US television advertisement shows a man pulling a sock onto one of his feet, explaining that:

> If I told you I could save my life just by putting on my socks you wouldn't believe me, because life is never that simple.

Having successfully managed to put on his sock, he sinks back into shadow and informs us that there is however 'something' we can do. The word 'condom' is never used. The whole message depends upon an understood and taken-for-granted association between the sight of pulling on a sock, and the *idea* of rolling on a condom. The reality of this last dreadful act is however, of course, too awful to name, let alone to illustrate.

When asked directly whether she thought there can be an 'opposite view' on safer sex, Ms Futtman readily agreed:

> Yes, I think there is. Very simple: 'Don't Have Sex'. That's a real opposite view. . . . We must respect those are ideas that people have.[18]

Yet the fact remains that it is the thinking of the far right and Christian fundamentalists which has consistently set the AIDS agenda on US network television. Audiences have thus been systematically denied access to information about HIV which does not simply equate safer sex with either monogamy or chastity. These are decisions which some will reach, but they are hardly realistic in relation to most people's emotional or physical needs. Anyone who has more than one sexual partner in a lifetime is more or less ignored by the moralistic interpretation of safer sex. Indeed, it is precisely this kind of narrow, negative message about how to have sex in an epidemic that may actually put audiences at *increased* risk of HIV infection, by undermining the one, central message about the need to use a condom when fucking. In this crisis, it is euphemism that costs lives. Susan Futtman explicitly compared the role of Network television companies to that of parents, arguing that television is 'in the place of the parent', for 'other people's children'.[19] This, I suspect, goes to the very heart of the problems so much network television and cinema has in dealing with the epidemic. For it would appear that entire, complex institutions can come to identify with a parenting role, based on so-called 'family values'. This amounts to an essentially punitive form of parenting, which aims to mould the young into the likeness of their parents. Thus the 'influence' of television is imagined by analogy with the direct influence of supposedly good parenting.

Television network executives evidently think of their audience as if it consisted primarily, if not exclusively, of children and, furthermore, as if children must be protected at all costs from any acknowledgement whatsoever of sex. The very concept of 'audience' is thus infantilised, and unable to address viewers able to exercise choices about what they watch. In this manner television can ignore the fact that millions of American lesbians and gay men watch Network television, together with many hundreds of thousands of other people already directly affected by the epidemic every day of their lives. Yet the networks feel that they don't have a 'position' on AIDS, because they have never permitted any oppositional voices that would conflict with 'family values'. However, the model of parenting that television exercises over its audiences is hardly of a kind to encourage the development of emotional growth from dependence to independence. Moreover, by 'protecting' its imaginary child-audience, television ensures that it can never, ever grow up. This is not, presumably, most people's idea of 'good parenting'.

Conclusion

Throughout the history of the epidemic, the mass media have tended to actively collude with government policies, just as television generally follows a governmental line in regarding the population primarily in terms of reproductive sexuality, rather than people's actual sexual wishes, pleasures and identities. In this respect television routinely turns a homophobic gaze onto the epidemic. Thus AIDS fictions produced for a homophobically imagined 'general public' are usually limited to a strict set of permissable narratives. We may witness the protracted deaths of 'innocent' children, who make up less than 1 per cent of total AIDS cases in the UK, but we may not enquire why so many of them do not necessarily seem to be getting the best treatment. We may feel angry on behalf of a young woman who appears to have been infected by her dentist, but we are not encouraged to note that this is the only known such example, and that it almost certainly resulted from the dentist's unhygienic working practices, if indeed, it ever really took place.

Throughout the range of AIDS fictions, exceptional situations are routinely presented as if they were typical, whilst the actual routine experience of the vast majority of people living with HIV and AIDS is studiously ignored. In this respect AIDS fictions tend to faithfully duplicate older cultural narratives concerning the brave sufferings of 'victims' of long-term chronic illness, as well as older homophobic and misogynistic narratives of sexual corruption, degradation, guilt, psychotic killers, molestation, and so on. Thus AIDS has come to constitute the latest in a long line of plot devices used to hold women, gay men, and young people in line if they demonstrate any signs of sexual independence or self-confidence. It is precisely these aspects of lesbian and gay culture that network television finds unacceptable, whilst delegating responsibility for its prejudices to the imagined Higher Authority of supposedly unquestionable and universal 'family values'. This dire situation is far more extreme in the US, but it is much too soon to say to what extent recent changes in the franchising of commercial national television networks in Britain are likely to affect the look of British television. At least in Britain, unlike the US, news and current affairs broadcasting has generally provided a regular place for community AIDS workers to oppose those who seek to exploit the epidemic for their own political or religious ends. Although the extreme moralism and prudery of the Thatcher years is evidently in the decline, both culturally and politically, it is also far too early to say how television and cinema may respond to AIDS as the case-loads rise in the coming years. There is certainly an imbalance in contemporary Britain in the early 1990s between a generally liberalising discourse of social and sexual pluralism at Westminster, and a hardening of the ideological arteries within the British print media, where aggressively uninhibited anti-gay prejudice continues to flourish unabated.[20]

In both Britain and Australia, the original American poster used to publicise *Longtime Companion* had the ACT UP slogan 'Read My Lips' removed from the T-shirt worn by a central character in the film-still from which the poster was taken. In the US, Safer Sex posters produced by *Red Hot & Blue* have been ripped down by the police because they show two gay men holding one another lovingly. Such things simply could not happen if homophobia were not so widely culturally sanctioned and accepted throughout the First World, over and above all differences of party politics and national histories. Homophobia has been *constitutive* of modernity, and it remains one of the most degrading and disfiguring aspects of our civilisation. As long as the very concept of the nation-state is founded upon the uniform assumption that reproductive sexuality is the central goal and aim of *all* human sexuality, we will all continue to be damaged by a brutally reductive vision of what it means to be human. This vision requires and sustains the fatalism of countless AIDS fictions, which effortlessly lull audiences into accepting the primary homophobic fantasy that gay men's lives are fundamentally worthless. AIDS can only be understood in its full reality as a *national tragedy* when the lives of those whom it has devastated first, and worst, are recognised as being as valuable as those of everybody else. AIDS will remain a hypothetical epidemic as far as most people are concerned only as long as we are unable to find better narratives, which can successfully articulate the epidemic in terms of the life of the nation, understood as a complex entity, composed of many different social groups. For we are vulnerable to HIV in areas of our lives that the law and the State have never understood or acknowledged: in our common need for love, in our struggles to achieve self-esteem, in our ability to give and receive sexual pleasure, in our ability to recognise that sexual needs differ between individuals, and over time within the lives of individuals, and so on.

In the course of the 1980s national cultural institutions such as the press have successfully presented AIDS as either an external threat to be repulsed at our borders, or else as an internal threat posed by hidden, subversive aliens in our midst. Such metaphors of risk are always highly significant in island nations, such as Britain, Cuba, and Japan, which are marked by extremes of xenophobia and insularity, reflected in attitudes to HIV. Notions of moral superiority play a special part in such narratives of national identity, and have been evident for centuries, in British notions of the 'loose' and 'lascivious' French; the Spanish pox; and so on. Seeking uniformity, nationalism has long tended to interpret sexual diversity as if it were evidence of 'foreignness', a result of external corruption and vice. From the perspective of the state, homosexuality can only be thought of as a threat from outside the family, rather than something which should properly be regarded as an extremely widespread fact of most families' lives. Denial on such a massive scale is suggestive of the social and psychic role that homophobia plays in the construction and maintenance of compliant national identities. The issue is not whether HIV is 'a gay disease' or 'a heterosexual disease', but of acknowledging that whoever it affects in different national contexts, it is always a *national disaster.* Hence the significance of Derek Jarman's explicit use of analogies between AIDS and the wider impact of Thatcherism in films such as *The Last Of England* and *The Garden,* as well as in his visualisation of Benjamin Britten's *War Requiem,* in which he underscores the significance of the composer's choice of poets, Wilfred Owen and Siegfried Sassoon (all three 'closet' homosexuals), to articulate British post-war national reconstruction. Together with the work of Stuart Marshall, Jarman's films offer us an opportunity to think about how the epidemic might be re-imagined in more truthfully national terms than those which have dictated most public AIDS fictions up till now.[21] I believe that narratives which show how gay men have actually lived through the last decade would contribute mightily to our better understanding of who we are as individuals, and what the nation really is. Such knowledge is probably a *necessary precondition* if heterosexuals are going to be able to learn in time from our ghastly experience of the epidemic within the gay communities of the UK. However, it may well be the case that British homophobia proves to be so intractable and indispensable to the national culture, that nothing will be learned, and an otherwise avoidable epidemic of heterosexually transmitted HIV will ensue as surely as night follows day. This is a terrible and sobering thought, for it means that fear of gay men may ultimately triumph over fear of HIV, by preventing heterosexuals ever asking themselves the simple question of what life might be like these days for gay men. With the honourable exception of *Longtime Companion,* this is the one thing no feature-length AIDS fiction had previously been able to bring off. At this moment, it seems that apart from a handful of independent film-makers and a few script writers for television soaps such as *Eastenders,* the only person in Britain who seems to fully understand the significance of re-narrating AIDS as a national issue is Princess Diana, no less. And after all, who could be better placed to expand popular notions of national identity than the most glamorous and popular embodiment of British nationalism? Such are the contradictions of our times.

24. AIDS and Social Science:
Taking the scenic route through
an emergency

Because the social sciences are rarely viewed as responsible for real harm, they attract comparatively little ethical attention. Yet the consistently low quality of social science research
on display at the 1991 International AIDS Conference prompts concern
about the general critical neglect of sociological research about gay men
and HIV/AIDS when compared to the attention paid to the results of
biomedical research.

In theory, social science can help us design more effective AIDS prevention campaigns and it has much to contribute to the improvement
of standards of care and service provision to people living with HIV or
AIDS. It can help us to better understand behaviour that may put people
at risk of infection. It can also help explain the many conflicting cultural
and political responses to the epidemic, and help us to make more effective interventions. Yet precious little of the vast amount of sociological
research presented at the 1991 Conference in Florence seemed to have
any sense of HIV/AIDS as an emergency within our gay communities, let
alone as an emergency in which sociologists may have particular ethical
responsibilities. The selection of papers was made long in advance by
a small and evidently conservative group of Italian medical scientists,
which serves to highlight the problems that arise when agendas are set
by doctors in areas where they have no expertise. Hence, there is rarely
very much research about nursing, for example, or about clients' views
on the care and services they receive.

In a poster presentation by Laura Spizzichino and others, on 'Prevalence of HIV antibody and risk behaviour among male prostitutes in
Rome', survey results revealed a 76 per cent rate of HIV positivity among
male transvestite prostitutes. Thirty-nine per cent reported television as
their main source of information about the epidemic; 27 per cent said

they would 'change their behaviour' upon learning of their seropositivity. The study concluded with the pious observation that this group
'requires further outreach efforts, since they may constitute a major
source of infection among their clients.'

This attitude is more-or-less typical of the behavioural research dominating the field, and should be a serious cause for both anxiety and anger.
For example, such research automatically regards people with HIV as
'the problem', supposedly threatening the rest of the population; there
is rarely acknowledgement that they have not received effective health
education, and no concern for their welfare. The primary aim of such
research should be the design of the very outreach programmes that the
researchers conclude are necessary.

This presentation was especially revealing because it included a large,
colour photograph as an illustration. This showed a man's hand, with
short (but brightly varnished) fingernails, resting just above the knee
of a stockinged leg, with a black, high-heeled shoe on the suspiciously
large foot and a glimpse of lacy black skirt riding high on the thigh.
If ever one wanted an example of the unconscious of mainstream HIV/
AIDS social science, this was it. Here is the dreaded object, the devious
'AIDS carrier'. It is clear that the researchers regard him/her in the same
way that they intend us to, as both exotic and seductive, perverse and
menacing. From such a perspective it is, of course, highly unlikely that
we will waste much time thinking about the story from the point of view
of an HIV-positive prostitute. Yet this is precisely what social science
should be doing. After all, who else is going to reveal their plight, or that
of male prostitutes in other cities in equally urgent need of outreach
projects and support?

In effect, most of the social science research ostensibly concerned
with gay men and HIV amounts to little more than a kind of academic
'scenic tour' through the worst-hit areas of the epidemic. Most of the
time it simply tells us what we already know, as is most obvious in relation to sex. There have been countless surveys around the world aiming
to demonstrate the supposed links between unsafe sex and the use of
alcohol and drugs. But if alcohol and drugs are the only risk factors for
which sociologists are looking, it is somewhat unlikely that others will
emerge. The 'addiction model' of unsafe sex is especially dominant in
American sociology. Yet none of the researchers seems to have stopped
to ask whether drinking a few beers or smoking a joint might actually
help many people to relax and negotiate safer sex. Nobody seems to be
asking what drives many lesbians and gay men into alcoholism or drug

addiction in the first place, and what this may have to do with social experience. For example, in the Italian research it was clear that television had evidently not helped male prostitutes in Rome understand how and why they might need to protect themselves from HIV. Yet I have never seen the question of which television channel people watch listed as a 'risk factor' for HIV, or one's choice of daily newspaper considered as an indicator of potential risk. Thus, while a CDC (Centers for Disease Control) survey of differing perceptions of the need to use condoms between white and non-white gay men suggested much higher levels of community support among whites, there was no way of telling why this was the case. It is usually stated that 'further research' is needed to design improved and more accurately targeted education. But we don't have time for such delays. We need fast surveys, done in weeks, not years. Moreover, the surveys we need should reflect the priorities raised by AIDS service organisations on the front lines of the epidemic, who have the best and most pragmatic sense of what is required. Sadly, however, such qualitative research doesn't 'butter any parsnips', as we say in England. In other words, it isn't professionally advantageous for sociologists, and doesn't give them prestigious qualifications. Thus, as is so often the case, careerism tends to motivate academics involved in HIV/AIDS research, rather than any sense of personal involvement or responsibility. And guess who suffers?

One sign of the problem that social science has making sense of AIDS was apparent in Florence in the form of a kind of 'parallel track' of community discussions entitled 'Communities Challenging AIDS'. These brought together international community representatives working on prison issues, women and children, and so on. Yet there was not even a single panel explicitly concerned with gay men's issues. This type of obliterative homophobia is far from uncommon at the larger AIDS conferences these days. 'Communities Challenging AIDS' was also the only place in the entire conference where the directions of medical research were put under any kind of critical sociological scrutiny. Yet the abstracts of papers by such distinguished speakers as Mark Harrington and Martin Delaney were not even included in the 'official' volumes of record. Nor were the sessions tape-recorded, unlike the rest of the conference, until protests were made.

These sessions were particularly important since they provided the only opportunity to discuss the medical ethics of research and clinical trials. Such discussions are of vital importance, as may be seen in two recent articles in both the *New England Journal of Medicine* (30 May

1991) and the *British Medical Journal* (11 May 1991). The former, by epidemiologist Ronald Bayer, carried worrisome implications of a new conservatism in the US medical establishment, eager to get back to 'traditional' public health policies—the very policies, one must point out, that are responsible for the systematic denial of effective HIV/AIDS education to gay men in the US and in many other countries. Indeed, the majority of social science presentations at Florence seemed to go out of their way to avoid any danger of considering the vulgar, pragmatic needs of people living with HIV/AIDS or their carers and advocates. The issue of designing more effective protocols for clinical trials was underlined by the *BMJ* report, which noted that 81 per cent of doctors in one survey reported that they themselves would not enter a trial for the treatment of lung cancer which they themselves were supervising. In this respect, the whole question of doctor/patient relations remains one of the most important areas of genuine innovation in contemporary medicine, but the VII International Conference on AIDS was evidently pleased to ignore it. If the experience of AIDS service organisations working with gay men around the world is not to be ignored forever, future conference organisers must recognise their responsibility to actively recruit presentations from those working outside the academic establishment.

Slip-sliding through the AIDS crisis

Another paper given at last year's HIV Conference on AIDS in Florence by the eminent French sociologist Michel Pollak was typical of the conference's mainstream social science presentations. It was entitled 'Changing determinants of risk behaviour in the French gay community'. The use of a concept like 'the gay community' to characterise an entire national population of lesbian and gay individuals generally does not bode well for sensitive research or useful conclusions. Are we meant to conclude that all French gay men are the same and that they respond like automatons to 'changing determinants'? In his 1985 surveys, Pollak distinguishes between two types of HIV prevention education in the 1980s: 'selective strategies', in which people reduce the number of their sexual partners, consider monogamy or celibacy or 'choose carefully', and 'protective strategies', which include use of condoms for fucking and stress the importance of non-penetrative sex and learning to negotiate safer sex with confidence. Pollak found that 30 per cent of the men in his survey had adopted so-called selective strategies, while only 5 per cent were using condoms regularly. Five years later, in a 1990 follow-up,

Pollak discovered that 58 per cent were using both strategies, although 26 per cent reported that they never used condoms.

In his analysis Pollak referred blithely to 'denial' among young gay men. Yet his own figures tell a rather different story. In France, 'official', state-funded, HIV prevention education consisted almost entirely of recommendations concerned with selective strategies. These were effectively *in conflict* with the protective strategies devised by the non-government AIDS service organisations rooted in the Anglo-American principles of community development. (Such organisations emerged belatedly in France as in many other European countries.) In other words, people were told either to 'choose carefully' *or* to always use condoms. The familiar public-health style of HIV prevention education in the 1980s, designed to keep HIV from becoming prevalent among heterosexuals, may thus have had the unintended consequence of putting gay men at *increased* risk of HIV infection. Cutting the number of one's sexual partners or 'choosing carefully' do not seem effective strategies for a population among whom the virus is already widely prevalent.

Pollak's (and others') use of terms such as 'denial' and 'relapse' speaks volumes about their assumptions. They evidently imagine that gay men had vast amounts of HIV prevention education throughout the 1980s rather than *very little indeed*. It is significant that such tacit value judgements are rarely, if ever, made of heterosexuals. In this way a double standard is instituted throughout social science research that fails to establish anything at all about the changing historical context in which different forms of health education emerged. If there is a question of 'denial' to be explored, it is not denial on the part of gay men, who have always depended on the same polluted sources of information (the mass media) as everyone else, but denial practised by the state, especially in coutries such as France, which conspicuously lacks traditions of community-based politics, whether for gay men, women, drug users or racial minorities. This is a particularly urgent, tragic issue since statistics on seroprevalence among young gay men are almost universally met with statements of surprise and condemnation, often by the same public health professionals who for the past decade have denied information and outreach projects to many who now have HIV. Moreover, another conference paper strongly suggested that high self-esteem among young gay men does not necessarily lead to safer sex; on the contrary, such self-esteem may be used as a talisman, a kind of magical prophylaxis against HIV.

The survey also implied that many 'out and proud' young gay men may regard the epidemic as a problem for older men, not for them. This situation raises profound questions about the future of HIV prevention education, especially when it is thought of as a kind of one-off business, like a religious conversion, rather than an ongoing process. It is significant that the only explicit criticism of the use of terms such as 'relapse' came from members of the British Sigma Project, an ongoing national survey of gay male sexual behaviour and attitudes. Most problems in the social science of HIV derive from naivety and confusion, especially among statisticians and behaviourists. This is nowhere more apparent than in research of sexual behaviour within the so-called 'gay community'. Media coverage of the epidemic has resulted in unprecedented publicity about gay men, but acknowledgement of our existence as a social constituency has been accompanied by a widespread fantasy that all gay men are somehow alike. A vast amount of nonsensical research continues to be conducted into 'the gay lifestyle' by people who would presumably scoff at the notion that all heterosexuals share an identical way of life. In reality, gay men experience sex in as many ways as everyone else, ways which change over time.

Only a handful of projects, such as Project Sigma and the teams working at Goldsmith's College in London and at Macquarie University in Sydney, design and conduct research with a sense of the urgent need for new interventions and a desire to learn from the hard-won experience of those actually working in AIDS service organisations, hospitals, clinics and elsewhere. Yet universities and state agencies continue to lavishly fund second-rate projects. It must be recognised that bad research conducted by social scientists causes real harm, both by delaying the implementation of the type of work that leads to more effective social policies, and more simply, by squandering precious resources, human and financial. It is high time that we—AIDS activists and advocates for the PWA community—paid as much attention to social science as to biomedical research.

For example, it should be perfectly obvious to researchers that the factors determining sexual behaviour are not adequately explained by 'addiction models' which reduce complex social phenomena to the status of personal problems. This is victim-blaming of a particularly elevated and distasteful kind. There is no such thing as a 'scientific' indicator that accurately predicts who is likely to have unsafe sex, not is there a distinct minority of recalcitrant 'AIDS carriers' at large in society who must be detected at all costs and forcibly 'educated'.

Virtually all evidence suggests the main factors involved in unsafe sex continue to be censorship and the prejudice of the mass media, regardless of national and cultural boundaries. Who is working to establish supportive health promotion for men having sex with men in countries such as India or Brazil? More than ever, we need activism that confidently targets the institutions determining social research of HIV. The consequence of years of lazy and dangerously homophobic research become daily more plain in the levels of new cases of HIV in our communities. Prevention and treatment are not separate issues, and we must confront bad health education, and the research from which it stems, as energetically as we tackle bad medical practice and research. How about an AIDS Coalition to Unleash Pragmatism?

1992 ————

25. Muddling Through:
The UK responses to AIDS

On 17 May 1991, Junior Health Minister Virginia Bottomley announced the first results from a national programme of anonymised HIV screening. This was carried out on some 44,000 people using blood taken for other purposes at 27 selected ante-natal and sexually transmitted disease clinics. As the *Guardian* reported, figures for pregnant women revealed an infection rate:

> varying from one in 220 to one in 1000, with an average of one in 500. In clinics in Outer London infection rates varied from one in 300 to one in 2500, although in Surrey, Essex, and Sussex no positive results were found.[1]

At the press conference at which these figures were announced, Mrs Bottomley argued for the greater focusing of HIV education on the most seriously affected areas of the country. 'To have major campaigns in areas with infection rates of one in 16,000 is not the best use of resources', she concluded. The government's then Chief Medical Officer commented that people 'have not listened' to messages about HIV/AIDS, and repeated the call for educational reinforcement 'where the risk is highest'.[2]

Commenting later in the day on Radio Four, Mrs Bottomley said she hoped that heterosexuals would learn to take AIDS seriously before they begin to see their friends dying from AIDS. Yet neither she nor any other Government Minister has ever called for greater support for gay men, who remain by far the most badly affected social group in the UK. Tucked away in this story was a comparison between HIV prevalence statistics from the same anonymised screening survey for gay men, and for heterosexuals. These revealed that no less than one in five gay men attending STD clinics are already seropositive, compared to one in 91 heterosexual men, and one in 436 heterosexual women. However the frighteningly disproportionate impact of HIV infection amongst gay men went largely unnoticed and unremarked, for this was a story about heterosexual transmission, in a country where the very possibility of HIV transmission via heterosexual intercourse has been widely and routinely denied in substantial sections of the British press. Moreover, the terms in which this particular story were narrated tell us much about conflicting and muddled attitudes to HIV/AIDS in Britain.

For example, 'official' AIDS commentary in Britain has repeatedly stated that gay men only took up safer sex when we saw our friends literally dropping dead all around us. Behaviour change amongst gay men is also frequently attributed to the government's first public intervention in the form of full-page newspaper advertisements late in 1986. Yet all the available epidemiological evidence plainly demonstrates that safer sex was largely adopted by British gay men in the years before the government made any move whatsoever. Furthermore, it is still statistically unlikely that even in inner London the average gay man will knowingly have met someone living with AIDS, let alone been affected by death on a large scale. Two main factors account for the comparatively small epidemic amongst British gay men. First, and deeply ironically, police and state interference in British 'public' life has meant that Britain never had the types of back-room bars or saunas in which the epidemic was evidently spread in cities such as Paris and New York before anyone knew of the existence of HIV. Second, Britain has an unbroken history of gay organisations and institutions: from the 24-hour London Lesbian and Gay Switchboard, founded in 1973, to a thriving national lesbian and gay press. Indeed, it was Lesbian and Gay Switchboard which organised the first UK conference about AIDS early in 1983. In this context gay identity provided the basis for a strong sense of collective response to the epidemic, as has been the case in all Anglophone societies in which gay culture and identity were in place and flourishing before the epidemic. Moreover, most of the individuals who conceived, set up and staffed the early Non-government AIDS Service Organisations (NGOs), such as the Terrence Higgins Trust, came from a shared social and personal background, a rich world of Anglo-American lesbian and gay culture and politics which had emerged in the wake of the Gay Liberation Front (GLF) movement of the late 1960s and early 1970s.

It was from this community that the first safer sex campaigns for gay men were developed in the early 1980s.[3] Yet throughout the course of the epidemic, the world of gay culture and of the NGOs has had the greatest difficulty in communicating with a government which was explicitly anti-gay. This has led to many wholly avoidable problems and difficulties. Indeed, one way of thinking about the UK response to AIDS is simply in terms of a massive dualism. On the one hand there is the history of community responses to the epidemic, and on the other the belated response of the government and its many agencies. In between these two groupings must be located the medical profession, and the whole world of British popular culture, in particular the press and television, which continue to provide most people in Britain with the information and, more often, misinformation, which frame popular perceptions about all aspects of the epidemic, from notions of personal risk, to opinions about social policy.

These two worlds do not even speak the same language about HIV and AIDS. For example, in the world of the NGOs and the gay press, it has long been the practice to distinguish clearly between HIV, a virus with well-established modes of transmission, and AIDS, a syndrome of many different maladies that may occur in many different combinations and sequences. This distinction is usually used in order to clarify understanding of many other issues, from insurance and social security to decisions about HIV antibody testing. In the world of state discourse and in the national non-gay press, however, one still finds frequent reference to 'the AIDS virus' or 'AIDS testing', and such careless use of language is frequently taken as evidence of deeper misunderstandings and lack of concern. This was clearly evident in the reporting of the May 1991 survey findings, which spoke repeatedly of 'the AIDS virus' and exaggerated the increase in so-called 'heterosexual AIDS' in a manner entirely typical of British national cultural responses to the epidemic. Thus it is routine in Britain to find wholly misleading analogies being made in the press and elsewhere, between percentage increases in HIV or AIDS cases amongst heterosexuals, and the overall cumulative statistics, with the false implication that HIV is being more widely transmitted amongst heterosexuals than amongst gay men or injecting drug users. It now seems that an earlier ideological tendency to deny *any* risk to heterosexuals has been replaced by a regular tendency to *overstate* risk from unprotected vaginal intercourse. At the same time it is often assumed that HIV has, as it were, 'moved on' from gay men. Whilst ministers and others often congratulate the NGOs for their good work, resources for gay men's health education remain sorely inadequate, and the whole subject remains highly controversial. As in many other European countries, the government has not wanted to be seen by the press or the electorate to be 'condoning' homosexuality or injecting drug use. In reality, the government response has been patchy and uneven.

As is well known, the Thatcher epoch in Britain was characterised by a strong current of legal moralism, frequently directed explicitly at lesbians and gay men in such measures as the notorious Section 28 of the Local Government Act (1988), which established in British law the truly bizarre distinction between supposedly 'real' and 'pretend' families, the former being heterosexual, the latter being lesbian or gay.[4] Yet it is vitally important to be able to distinguish between homophobia by *commission*, which directly targets lesbians and gay men as 'deviants' or 'perverts', etc., and homophobia by *omission*, which simply ignores our existence altogether. Such patterns of social and ideological policing, and the identities they generate, are of course uneven and unpredictable. Nonetheless, if the homophobia-by-commission which so typified Thatcherite political culture was intended, consciously or unconsciously, to bolster some nationalistic sense of Britishness, it certainly had unintended consequences. For the dramatically increased police harassment of lesbians and gay men, together with homophobic government policies, and a marked increase in crimes of violence against individuals has only served to result in a marked strengthening of gay community-based identities and a sense of solidarity in resistance to the widespread legitimation of anti-gay prejudice and discrimination. Indeed, there could be few better or clearer examples of Michel Foucault's celebrated concept of sexual politics as 'movements of affirmation', than that of British lesbian and gay politics in the 1980s and 1990s which have seen many new organisations coming into being in resistance to the workings of power.[5] For example, 'OutRage' emerged early in 1990 as an influential activist organisation, and the Stonewall Group, founded in 1989, has also played an important role as a parliamentary lobby group, following an American model of 'respectable' gay politics.

The pattern of European response to AIDS has been set out elsewhere,[6] but much remains to be said about the specifics of different national reactions. In this respect it is instructive to briefly compare the French and UK experiences, especially in the light of the tragic impact of HIV amongst men who have sex with men in France, where the overall epidemic is approximately 400 per cent more severe than in Britain. It is therefore important to understand that in Britain the terms 'homosexual' and 'gay' are only used as if they were synonymous by those who are ignorant, or prejudiced, or both. To describe oneself as 'a homosexual' in Britain is to subscribe to a low sense of self-esteem, and marks one immediately as either a much older man, or else as someone extremely conservative. The term 'gay' has established a particular, local cultural hegemony, implying that women and men whose object-choice is homosexual share the social experience of prejudice and discrimination based on our sexuality. To 'come out' as gay is to refuse such prejudice and discrimination, and to recognise the reality of sexual diversity. Gayness thus provides both an individual and a collective identity, quite unlike the more individualistic term 'homosexual', or for that matter 'heterosexual'. It was without doubt the tenacity of British gay culture in all its myriad forms, that has provided our best defence against HIV.

From this side of the Channel it has been deeply saddening to watch the way in which French homophobia has, by omission, had such a tragic impact on the management of the epidemic amongst 'homosexuals'. It is often argued in France that Britain is a more collectivist society, in relation to French individualism. There is undoubtedly more than a grain of descriptive accuracy here, but is it more than a grain? In Britain we lack a written Constitution, or any statement of ethical principles which remotely resembles the symbolic role played in France by the Rights of Man. Yet French citizenship often seems from a British perspective to be curiously selective, and conceived in rather narrow terms of equality in law. Hence it may be claimed that there is no explicit anti-gay discrimination in France, because existing legislation could, in theory, be used to protect the rights of individual lesbians and gay men. In practice however, it is hard to imagine an openly lesbian or gay public figure in French society, even in the supposedly liberal domain of the arts. Lacking any real equivalent to Anglophone gay identity, French 'homosexuals' have also lacked the kind of community-based institutions which have proved to be the *sine qua non* of the British gay response to the epidemic. One might only begin to compare the scale of the French government's response to the political troubles in Corsica, affecting in all some 200,000 French citizens, to the pitifully inadequate response to the needs of French homosexuals in this epidemic, to be aware of something on the scale of French homophobia by omission, the socialist equivalent to Thatcherite moralism.

Furthermore, French homosexual culture was always more cut off from American, community-based responses (largely for reasons of language) than its British equivalent. For example, writing in 1991 in *Gai Pied,* the only regular national publication for French homosexuals, the founder of France's leading French AIDS service organisation, M. Daniel Defert described a so-called 'bomb effect' in New York in 1981, caused by a single article in the *New York Times*.[7] As evidence he cited the 1990 fiction film *Longtime Companion*. In reality, however, people's understanding of AIDS did not of course emerge quite so suddenly, but depended on a host of complex cultural factors, the most important of which were undoubtedly closely connected to local gay community values, institutions, and identities. Defert claimed that the US NGOs were founded largely by gay men who had not been involved in gay politics, but this does not accord with my own memory of the years 1981–85 in either Boston or New York City, let alone in London or Manchester. His distinction between supposedly communitarian societies such as Britain and the USA, and the French 'tradition assimilatrice' unhelpfully oversimplifies the complex ways in which sexual categories and classifications are inhabited and contested in different societies.

In Britain, as in much of the US, NGOs have struggled against considerable odds to communicate the relatively simple message that everyone may be *potentially* at risk from HIV, but that risk varies according to behaviour and the local levels of HIV prevalence. In France, Defert and others have argued against the so-called 'homosexualisation' of AIDS, in order to 'normalise' perceptions, perhaps with the aim of avoiding a possible anti-homosexual backlash. The result, however, has been the wholesale denial of the types of aggressive community development amongst French homosexuals which alone might have prevented the present catastrophe. In Britain, by contrast, community leaders such as myself were warning precisely against the 'de-gaying' of AIDS many years ago.[8] It is an especially tragic irony that gay identity in its wider northern European and American sense is only now being forged in the ghastly crucible of death on a vast scale, death moreover which might have been largely averted if other models of safer sex education had been energetically researched and implemented.[9]

The model of health education developed within British gay culture in the early 1980s derived from the assumption that safer sex had to be promoted as an issue for all gay men, regardless of our known or perceived HIV status. This was of course extremely significant in a country where the great majority of gay men were, and remain, seronegative. HIV awareness was and is largely dependent on the work of the gay press, and the establishment of safer sex as a cultural norm across boundaries of class, regionality, race, age, and so on. This position preceded the widespread availability of HIV antibody testing in 1985, and has continued to determine social policy on testing. Indeed, we have been fortunate in the UK that debates about testing have been firmly grounded on the principle of informed consent, in such a way that the HIV antibody test is recognised by the Department of Health as well as amongst most gay men as a means of access to treatment and care, rather than as a form of primary HIV prevention. We have therefore largely managed to avoid distracting arguments either for or against testing in the UK. Instead it has been repeatedly emphasised that all decisions about testing should have the benefit of professional counselling, and that personal decisions are likely to vary over time, in line with changing medical information, the availability (or otherwise) of access to clinical trials and treatment drugs, and so on. Indeed, the UK response to HIV testing demonstrates very clearly the unpredictable relations between government politics and actual policy put into practice. In Conservative Britain we enjoy the advantage of high levels of counselling before and after HIV testing, whilst under a socialist government in France this is evidently not the case. Likewise in Britain we have witnessed the widespread introduction of needle-exchanges, quietly encouraged by the Department of Health and expert advisors, in spite of an 'overhead' political rhetoric which borrows much from the Reaganite US policy of a 'war on drugs'. In retrospect it is only too tragically obvious that such a rhetoric turns out in effect to be a war against injecting drug users, and a major factor determining the high levels of seroprevalence amongst injecting drug users in countries such as France and the USA. Nonetheless it should be recognised that British policies concerning HIV testing and needle-exchanges were as much determined by economic cost-benefit analysis as by ethical factors. The continuing under-resourcing of health education for gay men suggests, however, that economic considerations do not necessarily win out in the face of other determining factors. Aggressively politicised hostility towards gay men in parliament and the press has played a major role in shaping the response to our needs, and has also played a direct role in determining otherwise avoidable high levels of homophobia against British gay men. Whilst governments and newspapers do not necessarily consciously intend that a high proportion of gay men should contract HIV, this is the inescapable and inevitable consequence of their policies, aided and abetted by passively acquiescent civil servants and other bureaucrats and administrators, including epidemiologists and social scientists. Such murderous homophobia is deeply inscribed within both French and British national politics and popular culture, however differently they may be articulated and expressed either in concrete action, or the absence of action. For example, as recently as May 1991 leading British newspapers were calling for the complete state defunding of the Terrence Higgins Trust, on the grounds that in promoting safer sex it promotes homosexuality as such, and threatens 'the family'.[10] It is therefore vitally important that we are able to understand and challenge the crudely mechanical theories of sexuality, and sexual object-choice which underpin such calls. For at the end of the day it is clear that were such policies to be implemented, this would lead directly to a catastrophe in Britain on a par with the tragic situation in France. I began my involvement in HIV/AIDS work in the early 1980s on the basis of the gradual recognition that substantial sections of British society regarded gay men as a disposable social constituency. Nothing has subsequently persuaded me to change my mind on this grim point.

One of the most dramatic consequences of Anglophone gay culture has been the emergence of at least three generations of gay men who have not thought of themselves primarily, if at all, in terms of the roles they prefer in particular sexual acts, and especially in anal intercourse. This has profound consquences in relation to HIV education in countries such as France, or Italy, where sexual role stills plays a major role in individual homosexual identities. As Eve Kosofsky Sedgwick points out:

> many Mediterranean and Latin American cultures distinguish sharply between insertive and receptive sexual roles, in assessing the masculinity/femininity of men involved in male-male sex; the concept of homosexual identity *per se* tends not to make sense in these cultural contexts, or tends to make sense to self-identified *jotos* or *passivos* but not *machos* or *activos*.[11]

In such cultures effective safer sex education must both respect and address the identities of men who think of themselves in such terms, but it must also recognise the need to promote gay identity as a form of HIV prevention. It is not homosexuality per se that puts many men at risk from HIV, but homophobia, and the role-defined 'homosexual' identity it tends to encourage—men who expect nothing more than a 'right to privacy', and 'equal rights in law'. Such a situation is always a recipe for marginalisation, prejudice, inequality, and human misery on a vast scale, quite independently of any health hazards.

In Britain the government has actively censored health education materials considered too explicit, or 'pro-gay'. In this respect it should be understood that from the point of view of homophobia, whether of the Left or the Right, any mention of gay sex and gay relationships which puts them on an equal ideological and cultural footing with heterosexuality is likely to be regarded, and criticised, as 'pro-gay'. Indeed, the use of this phrase in English is a reliable indicator of homophobic attitudes and beliefs. The government has not designed or implemented a coherent national HIV/AIDS strategy, and policies have until recently tended to be *ad hoc*. The government's Health Education Authority (HEA) has squandered millions of pounds on advertising designed by expensive advertising agencies which steadfastly refuse to listen to the advice of the HEA's expert gay men's advisory group, which has recently resigned *en bloc*. The HEA's work has largely proceeded from the dubious proposition that 'AIDS doesn't discriminate'.[12] It has never tried to explain the difference between campaigns aiming to *prevent* an HIV epidemic amongst heterosexuals, and campaigns confronting an epidemic amongst gay men which is already of major proportions, because it does not itself recognise or understand the full significance of the distinction. Of course AIDS does not discriminate, in the sense of purposive activity. However, the patterns of HIV infection are extremely obvious, and are largely determined by discrimination, as a result of the denial of adequate HIV education to those most at risk. For example, it is frequently argued by the HEA, and others, that we should not talk about 'risk groups' but about 'risk behaviour', in order to make it clear that everyone having unsafe sex is potentially at risk. However, such an approach also makes it more or less impossible to identify and name those who are indeed at *greatest* risk. This results directly in the neglect of the needs of gay men, who should be recognised as having the greatest entitlement to well-researched, targeted, and evaluated health education. The HEA has used up vast sums of money in its campaigns, which should have gone to NGOs able to design and implement effective HIV prevention programmes amongst gay men without being inhibited by 'political' anxieties concerning possible cuts in funding if the government becomes offended by sexually explicit safer sex campaigns.

Likewise the National AIDS Trust, set up in 1987 to raise funds and awareness, has not been able to identify many of the most urgent ongoing needs of the epidemic because it was never given an independent policy-making role. Whilst the National AIDS Trust (NAT) has done valuable work, helping fund such groups as Positively Women, and drawing attention to the difficulties surrounding sex education in British schools, it has not been able to articulate the epidemic on the national terms that its name might imply. Since the late 1980s, the National Health Service (NHS) and Local Authorities (LAs) have employed increasing numbers of full-time HIV/AIDS workers, both in relation to health promotion and support services. Many of these workers gained their original experience in the voluntary sector, as volunteers, but have found it extremely difficult to work effectively because of the forces of homophobia at work throughout local government and the NHS. Two national organisations have been set up to try to coordinate the work of HIV/AIDS volunteers and full-time workers, but neither have been successful, largely because they were themselves inadequately funded. At the same time, the threat of defunding to NGOs that 'offend' the government, or individual ministries, has led to regrettable levels of self-censorship within the older AIDS service organisations. For example, although the Terrence Higgins Trust is widely regarded in Britain as a largely gay organisation, it should be realised that it employs only one gay man to undertake health education for all gay men, from a total staff of sixty, and that this job only came into being as recently as 1990. Furthermore, safer sex materials for gay men have had to be financed entirely from private charitable funds, in order to forestall any accusations that government money is being spent on 'pornography'. In Britain the bulk of the most important HIV education work amongst those most in need has had to be done by unpaid volunteers, and this is not a prudent or more importantly an *effective* way to conduct such vital work.

Nor has it been easy to draw attention to questions concerning standards of care or medical research in a society where socialised medicine is widely accompanied by a mentality of more or less supine passivity in relation to medical authority. Whilst medical care for people with HIV/AIDS in Britain is almost certainly as good as anywhere on earth, this is largely because our overall epidemic has until now been so disproportionately small. In practice, standards of care are uneven, and vary from region to region, and between hospitals and hospital departments. At the same time, the quality of social science research coordinated by the Economic and Social Research Council (ESRC) has tended to be dominated by behaviourism, which is unable to deal with any questions of sexual desire or sexual identity because its methods are almost exclusively quantitative rather than qualitative. Nonetheless the work of Dr Peter Aggleton and others has contributed much of practical use to HIV/AIDS workers and policy-makers in both the voluntary and statutory sectors.[13] Much of the most useful research on such important questions as sexual fantasy, ambivalence, and sexual identity has taken place *outside* the Academy, with little or no state funding or support. It is in this context that we may begin to understand the emergence of a new generation of British NGOs in recent years, that are much more explicitly task-led than those which survive from the earliest years of the epidemic. For example, since 1988 the *National AIDS Manual* has been a private, non-profit-making company, which now produces three volumes of HIV/AIDS information, updated every ninety or so days. This involves a vast amount of work, and it can only survive as the result of sales. It is the single most important resource in the British HIV/AIDS field, yet it could not receive State funds because of its non-judgemental, non-moralistic tone and contents. Such are the paradoxes of the HIV/AIDS situation on the UK. If we have excellent services, these have often been produced in the teeth of political opposition, whilst useless and demonstrably ineffective projects are frequently lavishly funded from government money. As we move further into the 1990s there is a growing recognition amongst long-term HIV/AIDS workers that we face a real crisis in relation to HIV prevention work for gay men in Britain. In the currently unpredictable political climate it seems very likely that new, and more aggressive NGOs are likely to emerge, in open opposition to what is increasingly regarded as the unacceptable complacency of the older NGOs and the statutory sector alike. At the same time new initiatives are also likely to continue to emerge from people living with HIV and AIDS, as well as from younger lesbians and gay men, many of whom already show signs of reacting against what they regard as the more fuddy-duddy aspects of older gay culture.

In conclusion, one may say that in order to understand the UK response to HIV/AIDS one must consider separately, and in relation to one another: the emergence of the initial voluntary-sector NGO response and its subsequent history; the belated, grudging state interventions since 1986 which have been unpredictable and often inconsistent; the domain of public-sector service provision and care; the world of research, both social and pharmaceutical; and the rampant sensationalism of the mass media, which remains the principle source of most people's information. Thatcherism is over, in the sense of a viable economic and ideological project, but survives by other means in the national daily press. Yet it remains far from clear how the future management of the epidemic will be co-ordinated or planned. The voluntary sector has achieved a remarkable amount in a very short space of time, but there are powerful voices arguing that it is time for the statutory sector to 'take over', claiming that the voluntary sector is largely redundant. There is encouraging evidence of an aggressive new attention to treatment issues on the part of NGOs, and an awareness that far more needs to be done in the field of HIV prevention for gay and bisexual men, whose needs have been largely submerged in 'generalist' HIV education campaigns.

An early and easily understandable emphasis on securing high levels of care and services doubtless distracted attention away from HIV education and treatment research in the late 1980s, but this situation appears to be improving. In the meantime Britain remains a country notorious for confusion and the tradition of 'muddling through'. At this time it seems that a terrifyingly high proportion of gay men and others seem likely to develop AIDS, and those who consequently die will be largely unremarked, and unlamented, as if they had never existed. There has been a similar, yet still more chilly indifference in France, to an even more terrible tragedy than ours in Britain. We all hope for an effective vaccine, an effective anti-viral, ways to restore immunological competence to those with HIV, and so on. Yet in the meantime HIV prevention should be recognised as our highest priority: the only way to combat HIV in the mid- and long-term is by insisting on the entitlements of all gay men, and especially the young, to adequate funding for effective, community-based HIV education which respects and affirms our sexual identities and our rights to our sexual and emotional pleasures. In a most profound sense, the fight against homophobia *is* a fight against HIV, just as the fight against HIV is also, always, a fight against homophobia.

Coda, January 1992

This article is a redrafted version of an essay first written in the summer of 1991. Deep confusion about heterosexual transmission still dominates the UK press agenda. For example, it was reported in the *Independent* in January that the rate of increase of AIDS in Britain among heterosexual men and women 'continues to be faster than in any other group. While homosexuals still account for about 70 per cent of new reports of AIDS cases, the rate of increase in this group was much lower than for those infected through heterosexual sex'.[14] In this manner a rise from 121 to 180 cases amongst heterosexuals is allowed to eclipse more than 1,000 new cases amongst gay men. By focussing exclusively on percentage increases in new cases of HIV or AIDS amongst heterosexuals, a seroprevalence rate of one in five amongst all gay men in London is made to look small by false comparison with heterosexuals, amongst whom the actual rate of overall seroprevalence remains almost undetectable at well below 1 per cent of the population. Meanwhile it has recently been revealed that a very high proportion of the women found to have been seropositive in the 1991 anonymised screening also carried antibodies to malaria, indicating a strong connection with Africa as the probable site of their infection. There ensued a rather absurd debate, in which the Royal College of Nurses claimed that the publication of this new reading of the statistics would spread 'alarm and prejudice rather than help reduce the spread of AIDS'.[15] Yet it is surely the responsibility of epidemiologists to direct our attention to the changing profiles of HIV prevalence and incidence? If African women resident in Britain are indeed at increased statistical risk from HIV, they have an entitlement to properly targeted support. Yet many commentators used the newly available information to claim that white heterosexuals are thus at *no* risk. *The Times* concluded that the entire history of HIV education in Britain amounts only to a 'Pointless panic on AIDS'.[16] Such a view, however, has two profoundly disturbing implications. First, that heterosexuals still don't begin to recognise how fortunate they are in potentially being able to prevent a possible epidemic. Second, that concern about HIV/AIDS is thought to be 'pointless', because they only affect queers and junkies. With such attitudes dominating popular perceptions of the epidemic it is clear that the future course and management of HIV/AIDS in Britain remains largely unpredictable on almost every front, apart from the certainty of yet more avoidable confusion and unnecessary muddle, and escalating levels of death, grief, and anger.

26. Duesberg's Dangerous Dogma

In 1990, Channel 4 broadcast an extremely controversial
television documentary in its *Dispatches* slot which claimed
that HIV is not, after all, the cause of AIDS. The case against HIV
was led by Professor Peter Duesberg, a molecular biologist from the
University of California, Berkeley.

In June 1992, Professor Duesberg popped up again, at a conference
in Amsterdam, repeating his earlier claims which were widely ventilated
in the UK press. These may be summarised into five basic points. First,
he argues, the shortcomings of existing anti-HIV drugs implies that HIV
does not cause AIDS. This entirely ignores the fact that currently available anti-retroviral drugs do indeed demonstrably prolong the life of
people with AIDS. Second, he argues that epidemiological predictions
concerning the future pattern of the epidemic are inaccurate, and that
AIDS has not followed the original predictions. This is simply incorrect.
In most cases, predictions about the future course of the epidemic have
been largely accurate.

He argues that AIDS is too 'selective' to be the result of an infectious
agent—it must be a result of specific social or behavioural factors. This
entirely ignores the fact that HIV has had different effects in different
parts of the world, according to different available routes of transmission. He argues that there has been a 'medical establishment conspiracy',
which has marginalised or suppressed all other explanations. This again
is wildly misleading.

Finally, Professor Duesberg insists that AIDS is the result of the widespread misuse of 'psychoactive drugs' since the 1960s. Hence his conclusion that 'AIDS is caused by noninfectious agents', for example, social
factors, or 'lifestyle'.

Duesberg is able to pass himself off as a beleaguered, isolated radical, struggling against a monolithic scientific establishment that refuses to listen. The truth is quite the reverse. Duesberg has had vast amounts of media coverage, largely because the mass media is only too happy to promote the view that AIDS is caused by deviant lifestyles rather than an infectious agent. If Duesberg were correct, one would only have to prevent drug use, to prevent AIDS.

Of course, such a view overlooks the situation of heterosexuals with HIV, haemophiliacs infected via blood products, and vertical transmission from mothers to babies! The fact that the *Sunday Times* has also campaigned vigorously on behalf of 'compensation' for haemophiliacs with AIDS does not seem to deter the paper from simultaneously denying the existence of an underlying infectious agent, responsible for the epidemic. So much for their serious 'concern'!

Even more sinister than Duesberg is his friend and colleague Gordon Stewart, Emeritus Professor of Public Health at the University of Glasgow, who was an advisor to Channel 4's *Dispatches* programme, in which he also appeared. According to Professor Stewart:

> AIDS is almost exclusively confined to certain groups that engage in some very specific behaviours that put them continuously at risk of various infections. These infections are then manifested in potent form as the diseases we call AIDS. (*Sunday Times*, 7 June 1992)

For Stewart, HIV is merely a 'marker' of behaviour which, in itself, carries high risk of disease. We should scrutinise the 'anti-HIV' theorists very seriously indeed, for they consistently provide a gloss of pseudo-scientific respectability to profoundly irrational and usually homophobic forces.

Just as Duesberg argues that preventing drug use would prevent AIDS, so Stewart argues that preventing gay sex would prevent AIDS. Both men miss the single, fundamental point. It is not injecting drug use, or anal intercourse *per se,* that 'cause' AIDS. Rather, AIDS is caused by a virus which may easily be transmitted if precautions are not taken against it.

Certainly Duesberg's underlying indifference to the ghastly realities of this epidemic was apparent in his recent broadcast advice on London's Capital Radio that safer sex is a waste of time. Even the makers of Channel 4's *Dispatches* in 1990 felt obliged to preface their wretched programme with the hypocritical advice that it was not intended to undermine the practice of safer sex.

As Peter Scott and I wrote in the *National AIDS Manual* two years ago:

'Homosexuality has always existed. Yet gay men only began to develop AIDS in significant numbers in the 1980s. The "lifestyle" lobby claims that this is due to the massive use of recreational drugs in the gay community. There are two clear objections to this view. First, studies of gay men who did and did not use recreational (non-injecting) drugs have shown no correlation between recreational drug use and AIDS. Second, we know that the patterns of recreational drug use are much the same for gay men as for heterosexuals.'

They also claim that every woman with AIDS has developed it as a result of drug use. This is nonsense, and a profound insult to the thousands of women with AIDS who have contracted HIV through unprotected sexual intercourse. The lifestyle lobby also chooses cynically to dismiss all the evidence for AIDS resulting from heterosexual transmission in the developing world. They try to dismiss the overwhelming evidence of people with haemophilia who have developed AIDS by arguing that haemophilia is itself immunosuppressive. This ignores the fact that no one with haemophilia who did not receive infected blood products has ever developed AIDS.

The lifestyle-leads-to-AIDS argument is immensely convenient to those who wish to believe that because they are not gay men and because they have never used drugs, they are at no risk whatsoever of developing AIDS.

The lifestyle argument effectively substitutes semi-magical explanations for hard science.

The underlying situation today is unchanged: in population groups where there is no HIV, there is no AIDS. Sadly, many journalists and commissioning editors still prefer semi-magical explanations of AIDS, usually harnessed to visceral homophobia and prejudice against drug users, rather than hard science, or ordinary human decency and common sense.

27. Bad, Mad and Dangerous

On 31 August, the *Independent* published an extremely disturbing story concerning James Segawa, a 28-year-old Ugandan who had arrived on 22 August at Gatwick Airport, asking for political refugee status. It is alleged that doctors said he was faking his illness upon arrival, and he was moved to the hospital wing of Belmarsh Prison, in southeast London.

On 28 August, Mr Segawa died of meningitis and tuberculosis at the Mayday Hospital, Croydon. Mr Segawa had been HIV positive. He died of AIDS. The *Independent* noted reassuringly that 'Gatwick's interrogation rooms were also "thoroughly cleaned"'. One begins to wonder about what they put the poor man through . . . A spokesman added: 'We do not expect any problems, our staff were warned and they are not in any danger.' Not a word of concern or regret about the death in a strange country of a 28-year-old man. Only the mean, selfish reassurance that nobody had been contaminated.

For several months now the UK press has been having something of a field day with AIDS. The moralism of the tabloids has never been brandished with such sanctimonious arrogance. Newly confident that 'normal' heterosexuals are not at risk, the tabloids have created Frankenstein monsters out of an unfortunate young haemophiliac man from Birmingham, and a London eye doctor. Although it seems that the latter had never even had an HIV test, it was enough for the newspapers that he was both gay, and a surgeon.

Still more loathsome was an article on 26 June by Raj Persaud in the *Guardian* under the jolly headline 'On being loved to death'. According to Mr Persuad:

> Medical research has shown that even after vigorous health education, 60 per cent of those who become HIV positive continue to have sex with strangers.

Furthermore:

> There is another group of 'spreaders' who seem malevolent in their intent . . . People might find they were depressed . . . and might seek sex for comfort. Others have a history of extreme promiscuity before contracting HIV and seem to have difficulty stopping what appears to be a sex addiction . . . The current psychiatric label is compulsive promiscuity disorder.

According to Persaud, 'some will suffer from mental illness' with 'increased sexual appetite'. Others: 'may have physical diseases where those parts of the brain controlling sexual impulses are damaged by tumours or infections leading to hypersexuality. AIDS itself is known to affect the brain and produces an intellectual decline termed AIDS dementia. This condition exists in 15 per cent of those who are HIV positive, suggesting that many may continue with unprotected sex because of lowered intelligence due to the disease itself. . . . A common theme seems to be an equation of danger with pleasure. . . . It may be that some partners collude with the sex and death tryst.'

I quote all this garbage at length because it seems to me to be one example of an extremely serious problem, namely the re-demonisation of peole with HIV and AIDS within the field of British journalism. Two days after the *Guardian* printed this farrago of make-believe nonsense, *Scotland on Sunday* informed its readers that:

> Some studies show 60 per cent of people who are HIV positive carry on having sex with strangers . . . there is also a condition which reduces reasoning capability.

Thus Mr Persaud's ravings pass into the anonymous, general world of supposedly 'expert' opinion, and feed into the rivers of gossip and hearsay and make up the social world with which people with HIV and AIDS are obliged to deal constantly. HIV is evidently being reconstituted for popular consumption as a form of madness, now that the papers realise that the great majority of people with HIV are merely gay men, and therefore mad in some sense anyway. It is precisely stories like this, or the actual persecution of the young Birmingham haemophiliac who, after all is said and done, had received no counselling about the risk of sexual transmission of HIV, which encourage people to regard people with HIV or AIDS as if they were monsters.

Like most journalists, Persaud immediately concludes that it is a terrible thing to have many sexual partners. Furthermore, he seems quite unable to imagine that people with HIV and AIDS can and do have safer sex just like other people.

Evidently most journalists find the concept of solidarity in the face of a tragedy more or less unthinkable. So it is people with HIV or AIDS who must be seen to be 'responsible' both for their own, and another's condition. Not far behind this is the actual wish that all gay men and bisexuals were dead.

Between two and three people die from AIDS every day in Britain. Yet our epidemic is small by European standards of comparison. There are clear, predictable problems that are likely to occur in such situations, where HIV and AIDS are most concentrated within a previously marginalised group. As the threat of a major heterosexual epidemic recedes, it becomes permissable once more to abuse those originally felt to be the 'source' of infection, as if they were the 'cause' of their own destruction. This kind of logic, which was very widespread in the early years of the epidemic, has never entirely gone away. Moreover, there are ominous signs that it is returning with some force.

The situation in which James Segawa found himself last month, dying from AIDS, being shunted from airports to prisons and eventually to hospital, in a completely foreign and profoundly racist country, frankly hardly bears thinking about. Yet this is precisely what can be done to people with HIV if they are not seen as human. Recent events in Europe should force us to remember that history does not necessarily move 'forwards'. The stakes here are extremely high—nothing less than our lives, and the lives of our friends and loved ones. How do you suppose being thought a monster might affect your treatment, and your care?

28. Political Funerals

On the stormy, rain-sodden afternoon of Sunday, 11 October, a small but determined group of mourners/activists managed to dodge the attentions of the Washington police in order to deposit the ashes of friends and loved ones onto the lawns of the White House—a 'political funeral'—just a few hundred yards away from where the celebrated AIDS Quilt had been unfurled on the previous day.

The Quilt has become the acceptable face of American Aids mortality statistics, rather like the annual Candlelit Vigil in Trafalgar Square. Both The Quilt and the Vigil provide opportunities of sorts to register private losses in public. Yet neither are able to articulate anything about the epidemic beyond a picture of individual deaths.

On an average day two or three people will die from AIDS in Britain, compared to an average of no less than 123 in the United States. The US epidemic is approaching what epidemiologists term 'steady state'. That is, the annual rate of AIDS-related deaths is fast catching up with the annual rate of new cases of HIV infection, currently estimated at 50,000 per annum. There are already well over one million people thought to be HIV positive in the United States; and as elsewhere, unless an affordable, effective anti-retroviral drug becomes available in the immediate future, few are likely to survive.

Yet the epidemic didn't have to be like this. It didn't have to be this terrible. In America, as in most other countries, it is demonstrably effective, community-based HIV education which has been prevented rather than HIV transmission. Because the overwhelming majority of cases have been amongst gay and bisexual men, injecting drug users, and poor black and Hispanic women, it is widely accepted that the US government has been reluctant to act, from indifference, and the wish not to 'offend' Christian fundamentalist voters. A massacre wasn't planned. But without systematic neglect throughout the entire American governmental, legal, political and intellectual world, many hundreds of thousands of cases of HIV might have been avoided, by means of needle-exchange facilities, and proper funding and support for HIV prevention strategies amongst gay men.

In such circumstances, AIDS deaths are necessarily political, whatever else they may also be in terms of individual and collective grief and trauma. Suffering has been made far worse than it need be as the result both of governmental action and inaction. We cannot blame governments for not coming up with a cure. We can justifiably blame them for just about everything else that is currently going badly wrong. Thus every AIDS death is also a political event, a life which governments of all political persuasions, from the Right in America to the Left in France, have effectively disallowed.

Hence the call earlier this year by veteran activist John S. James in *Aids Treatment News* for political funerals, understood as an institution which could help establish what is really going on in this epidemic to the rest of the population which has little opportunity to understand AIDS except on the degraded terms of the mass media.

From their myopic perspective, AIDS is 'old news', and thus of little interest. Hence the question of how to explain the fundamental political dimension of the epidemic, including the complex relation between the pharmaceutical industry and government research, becomes ever more pressing.

Political funerals draw attention to the relations between individual deaths on a fast growing scale, and the political circumstances which have all along contributed so much to the overall mortality rates. It is of vital importance that we establish AIDS as a national issue, rather than merely regarding it as a problem for discrete 'minorities' or individuals.

In times of tragedy we look to our national leaders above the crude lines of party politics, to articulate the necessary national rituals of shared losses, regret and mourning, as recently demonstrated by the Queen of Holland and the Mayor of Amsterdam after the tragic El Al plane disaster. Yet less than 200 people perished in that accident. We face losses in the tens and hundreds of thousands, and nobody with such powerful symbolic authority is speaking out on our behalf. Princess Diana's evident concern for the sick and dying is of course an admirable exception, yet she is most unlikely to speak out on questions of murderous social policies which lead directly to the avoidable tragedy of overflowing hospices, and the relentless toll of death in our communities.

Neither under Reagan and Bush, or Thatcher and Major, has AIDS been properly acknowledged as a national issue. In the first of the televised Presidential election debates, Mr Bush hypocritically attacked AIDS activists, rather than those actively responsible for preventing proper education, care, and research. In such circumstances, it should be recognised that the frankly political funeral is a strategic fusion of grief with basic democratic ethical principles. It also speaks of the will to survive in the worst-affected communities, together with the recognition that there is no way round the larger losses yet to come.

That it should have come to the spectacle of distraught mourners, scattering the remains of their loved ones on the White House lawns, is enough to suggest something of how desperate the American situation has become. Whilst the latest display of The Quilt made it onto prime-time network television, the political funeral was almost entirely ignored in the US media. This tells us more perhaps than we would like to know about the degree and extent to which the US is currently willing to recognise and respond to AIDS, understood as it should be, as an American tragedy.

29. Gay Teenagers and Gay Politics

Most of the gay men who first got involved in British AIDS work early on in the history of the epidemic had previously been involved in lesbian and gay organisations such as the Switchboard movement in the 1970s and early 1980s. For many of us, AIDS took over our lives. Many of us are still full-time AIDS workers, struggling against institutional and personal forms of homophobia which continue to prevent the provision of proper HIV education to those in greatest need.

We have worked very hard indeed for many long years to try to establish a model of non-directive, supportive safer sex education for British gay and bisexual men. The entire complex world of AIDS work is however largely invisible to most lesbians and gay men, who have little idea how community-based AIDS organisations work, let alone how they were started, or by whom. One of my principal aims has always been to try to stimulate wider debate in our communities about the methods and aims of HIV/AIDS work, but I am constantly surprised by how little many lesbians and gay men still know about the epidemic, and especially about medical treatment issues.

At the end of October the *National Aids Manual* published the first issue of its new monthly *AIDS Treatment Update,* edited by Edward King. As Peter Scott explains, intelligent and energetic treatment activism has already had important consequences, in making clinical trials of potential treatment drugs faster, fairer, and more efficient; improving general standards of care; and making accessible information available to people living with HIV as a basis for well-informed choices about their treatment options.

Such initiatives do not simply come into being magically. They are the result of prodigious amounts of research, planning, and organisation, in order to produce reliable, community-based information and other materials. Nobody does this for us, or pays for it directly out of State funds. Companies have to be set up, staff employed and trained, funds raised. I am however concerned that this 'AIDS community' is not really understood very well by the wider communities of lesbians and gay men whom it does its best to service.

There is also the added complication that the world of lesbian and gay rights organisations is of course sadly very impoverished. Yet surely the result of this should not be resentment against paid AIDS workers, as is sometimes unfortunately the case. In reality, there are disproportionately few jobs in the field of specialised HIV/AIDS education for gay men, and I remain stubbornly convinced that the neglect of gay men's HIV education should be recognised as the most pressing single issue in contemporary gay politics.

Yet this is not, I fear, a very widely shared opinion amongst British gay men and lesbians, who often seem far more concerned about the rhetoric of 'pretend families', rather than the mortal losses the epidemic is increasingly inflicting. Many lesbians and gay men regard the scenario of deathbeds as the single 'authentic' image of AIDS, and seem unable to look beyond to the wider political circumstances surrounding HIV prevention work for gay men in Britain. For example HIV is the single most important reason why we should continue to campaign energetically for reform of the age of consent laws. Yet this is almost never the context in which reform is called for. Yet why should we want to target gay teenagers at all? In last month's *Gay Times,* Mark Simpson has quoted researchers who question the very idea of younger men's 'vulnerability' to HIV.

Several years ago Peter Aggleton and Ian Warwick published a series of important strategic articles in which they argued strongly against the widespread sociological tendency in HIV/AIDS research to pathologise and patronise teenagers as 'adolescents'. Yet this was precisely in order to draw attention to teenagers' real, rather than imagined needs. Some researchers however, seem far more agitated about the need to avoid patronising language than about the need to target gay teenagers at all. We should not ignore the results of the *Gay Times* readers' survey published alongside last month's article, which showed that 42 per cent of the under 25s in the study had had unsafe sex before learning about safer sex!

Peter Weatherburn, a member of the Project Sigma, was quoted in the *Independent* on 3 November, pointing out that the high age of consent 'prevents young gay men getting the sexual education they need at school'. Three days later the same paper noted a significant rise in teenage pregnancies, from 58.7 per thousand in 1980 to 69 per thousand girls in 1990. If a 13-year-old girl can become pregnant in 1992 when she believes she's too young to have a baby, how much can we expect a 13-year-old queer teenage boy to understand about HIV transmission?

I genuinely cannot understand the opposition to talking about 'risk groups' in relation to HIV. Between January 1982 and July 1992, 3,304 of the 3,708 men who have died from AIDS in Britain were gay or bisexual. And, as Jamie Taylor from MESMAC pointed out: 'It makes sense to reach people at the beginning of their sex lives, before they develop unsafe habits, so that they need never have unsafe sex'.[1]

The *Gay Times* survey suggested that only 41 per cent of the 16–25 year olds thought that their gay friends are having safer sex most of the time. Some of us never abandoned the concept of risk groups, because we could see so clearly that gay men have all along been at vastly greater risk from HIV than anyone else. To question the need for properly researched HIV education for gay teenagers is to passively collude with their decimation.

30. Powers of Observation:
AIDS and the writing of history

In a permanently transitional age we must expect unevenness, contradictory outcomes, disjunctures, delays, contingencies,
uncompleted projects, overlapping emergent ones.—Stuart Hall,
Marxism Today, October 1988

Detachment is itself a moral position.—Isaiah Berlin, Four Essays on
Liberty

For those actively involved in HIV/AIDS work, the time has not yet
arrived for the writing of history. We have other priorities. Our writing tends to be strategic, and often directly instrumental; it provides
information; it counters lies; it adapts its voice to its audience; it is as
up-to-date as we can make it; it aims to provide the reassurance of re-
liability; it affirms values and experience that are elsewhere denigrated
or denied. It strives to convince and it is almost entirely contingent, on
a day-by-day, week-by-week basis. Because we are not observers, but
closely engaged participants, we are also aware that our writings constitute their own form of historiography: we cannot however be expected
to provide cool appraisal of the constantly changing and unpredictable
circumstances in which we find ourselves. We are not dispassionate, and
we are not seduced by fantasies about neutrality. As Isaiah Berlin has
pointed out:

> The very use of normal language cannot avoid conveying what the
> author regards as commonplace or monstrous, decisive or trivial,
> exhilarating or depressing . . . I can say that so many million men
> were brutally done to death; or alternatively, that they perished;
> laid down their lives; were massacred; or simply, that the popula-
> tion of Europe was reduced, or that its average age was lowered;
> or that many men lost their lives. None of these descriptions . . .

is wholly neutral: all carry moral implications. What the historian says will, however careful he may be to use purely descriptive language, sooner or later convey his attitude. Detachment is itself a moral position. The use of neutral language ('Himmler caused many persons to be asphyxiated') conveys its own ethical tone.[1]

Moreover, AIDS has already been narrated many times, in many different genres. We possess an extensive testimonial literature in the form of books written by people living with HIV and AIDS; books written by and about their doctors and leading biomedical researchers; collections of poetry; AIDS fiction; collections of essays; historical accounts, and so on. There is also a vast periodical literature, which may be subdivided in different ways. For example, it is helpful and indeed necessary to contrast the national daily and weekly heterosexual press to the gay press. It is also helpful and necessary to note how, from early on in the history of the epidemic, community-based publications have played a vital role in translating the specialist scientific literature into more accessible and practically useful newsletters. These publications do not however stand on an equal social or economic footing with the *Lancet* or the *New England Journal of Medicine*. In no health crisis in history has the written word played such a central, extensive and heavily contested role. Hence the significance in this context of Isaiah Berlin's insistence that:

> History is not an ancillary activity; it seeks to provide as complete an account as it can of what men do and suffer; to call them men is to ascribe to them values that we must be able to recognise as such, otherwise they are not men for us. Historians cannot therefore (whether they moralise or not) escape from having some position about what matters and how much (even if they do not ask why it matters). This alone is enough to render the notion of a 'value-free' history, as the transcriber *rebus ipsis dictantibus,* an illusion.[2]

Indeed, it is precisely because so many people affected most directly by HIV are not widely regarded as fellow human beings that the question of the historiography of AIDS acquires such significance. AIDS is an especially contested subject because it focuses attention simultaneously on many of the most controversial topics of our times: abortion, reproductive sexual technology, homosexuality, bisexuality, 'the family', 'the nation', race, and so on. The wider public discursive formation surrounding AIDS is thus always heavily over-determined by this attendant litany of contingent issues.

The history and management of the British AIDS epidemic has, unsurprisingly, been largely determined by and in response to the wider disposition of power that we now know as Thatcherism. Considering the cultural roots and terrain of Thatcherism, Stuart Hall has noted how:

> Areas of contestation which may appear, to a more orthodox or conventional reading, to be 'marginal' to the main question, acquire in the perspective of an analysis of 'hegemony', an absolute centrality: questions about moral conduct, about gender and sexuality, about race and ethnicity, about ecological and environmental issues, about cultural and national identity. Thatcherism's search for the enemies within'; its construction of the respectable, patriarchal, entrepreneurial subject with 'his' orthodox tastes, inclinations, preferences, opinions and prejudice . . . its rooting of itself inside a particularly narrow, ethnocentric and exclusivist conception of 'national identity'; and its constant attempts to expel symbolically one sector of society after another from the imaginary community of the nation—these are as central to Thatcherism's hegemonic project as the privatisation programme or the assault on local democracy.[3]

Yet rather than relating AIDS to its specific, conjunctural national circumstances, the dominant historiographic tendency on the contrary locates it within a discrete 'history of epidemics' which is itself one tributary of an equally abstracted 'history of medicine'. Thus, for example, Professor Robert M. Swenson concludes a lengthy article on 'Plagues, history and AIDS' with the observation that:

> Although our advanced biotechnology has allowed us to apply sophisticated solutions to the biological problems of AIDS, our human responses have changed little from previous epidemics and hinder us from dealing effectively with many of the social problems that are part of the AIDS epidemic.[4]

In much the same vein, Elizabeth Fee and Professor Daniel M. Fox prefaced their influential anthology *AIDS: The Burdens Of History* with a quotation from Dr Frederick C. Tilney, on the polio epidemic: 'We have learned very little that is new about the disease, but much that is old about ourselves.'[5] The discursive and institutional pressure to articulate AIDS from within a continuous history of epidemics, understood to reflect a uniformly flawed human nature manifested in prejudice and discrimination, thus tends to displace any concrete consideration of the irreducible specificities of HIV and its multiple collisions with the late twentieth century.

In fact, Tilney's quote could hardly be less appropriate to our understanding of this epidemic. For we demonstrably now know far more about the microchemistry and natural history of HIV, than we do about the infinitely complex, unpredictable political, social, and psychological consequences of the epidemic, both in the lives of individuals and entire societies. Rather than inviting us to locate our understanding of the epidemic in the context of the political present and its recent history, Tilney's quotation is used to anchor the epidemic to the type of narrative which contrasts scientific progress to universal and invariant human frailties. Such an approach reveals the stance of the supposedly neutral observer, standing outside the epidemic, surveying its natural history.

Yet the international HIV pandemic is at least as much a socio-political phenomenon as it is biological or medical. AIDS has no 'natural history', at least in the sense of an inevitable, irreversible, biologically driven necessity. On the contrary, it is demonstrably amenable to prevention strategies.[6] Many of these problems seem to point back towards the constitutive metaphor of AIDS as a plague in the early years of the epidemic, a metaphor which many medical historians seem to have followed far too literally. David Black's early popular account of the epidemic, 'The Plague Years', first published in two parts in *Rolling Stone* early in 1985, opens with two quotations. The first, from Proust, depicts homosexual love derived 'not from an ideal of beauty . . . but from an incurable disease'.[7] The second cites Charles Creighton's *History of Epidemics in Britain:*

> The period from 1348 to 1352 [the time of the Black Death in England] is an absolute blank. . . . Most of the monastic chronicles are interrupted at the same point; if there is an entry at all under the year 1349 it is for the most part merely the words *magna mortalitas.*[8]

Thus, on the one hand AIDS is interpreted in the context of a pathological model of homosexuality, and on the other in relation to visions of pre-modern medical catastrophe. Such framing repeats and reinforces the initial mass-media presentation of the epidemic in the early 1980s as a 'gay plague', together with the implication that it is some kind of judgement, like the Biblical plagues of Egypt. Yet plague metaphors are singularly misleading and inappropriate in relation to AIDS for the simple reason that unlike the Black Death or cholera, HIV is *not* contagious. On the contrary, there is copious evidence concerning how infection may be prevented, by the introduction of needle-exchanges, and an energetic commitment to safer sex education, especially for risk groups—education that recognises and respects people's differing sexual needs and pleasures. Moreover, plague metaphors ignore the plain fact that, with few exceptions, the response to AIDS has not consisted of draconian quarantine measures, mandatory HIV testing, and so on, in spite of the fact that such practices have been widely implemented this century in relation both to contagious diseases such as tuberculosis, and sexually transmitted diseases such as syphilis.

This in itself fuels the suspicion that plague metaphors represent a form of cultural displacement away from other more appropriate interpretive models. In other words, it may be easier, and more convenient, to continue to think of AIDS in relation to the concept of plague, than to institutionalised homophobia and racism for example. The widespread acceptance of plague metaphors of AIDS as the central model for historical analysis only serves to encourage spurious analogies with the history of contagious disease. In this manner historians run the risk of introjecting a profoundly prejudiced model of the epidemic into the very heart of their work. Plague metaphors are not accidental. They embody a particular kind of ideological operation. To take just one example, in 1985 the *Sun* was already able to refute opposition to 'gay plague' interpretations of AIDS, on the grounds that people living with AIDS:

> have only themselves to blame for their terrible plight. But now gay campaigners are trying to turn the argument the other way round and make the whole community bear some of the guilt. This is nonsense. The term Gay Plague upsets some people, but that effectively is exactly what it is. . . . Homosexual intercourse spreads a killer disease. Lay off it before it's too late.[9]

We may initially respond to such crude assertions in many different ways. We may refute their claims rationally, pointing out that HIV does not target gay men specifically; or any other social constituency. We may point to the great social diversity of the epidemic as it affects different nations and continents. We may argue that most people with AIDS were infected by HIV before anyone knew the virus even existed. We may insist that gay sex does not 'cause' AIDS, and that HIV can only be sexually transmitted by *unprotected* sex, whether anal or vaginal. Yet such rational responses do not begin to come to grips with the *unconscious* of such pronouncements: the wish to blame; the articulation of guilt; the more or less hysterically defensive tone; the imputation of conspiracy to gay men; the drawing of rigid boundaries between licit and illicit sex; the absence of any trace or vestige of concern, or sorrow, or sympathy, or urgency, or any sense whatsoever of AIDS as a vast and terrible human tragedy. The unconscious logic is clear: if AIDS is 'caused' by gay sex, only gay men are at risk, and if gay sex 'causes' AIDS, there is no reason for anyone else to be at all concerned. In this manner HIV is dismissed as a deadly by-product of homosexuality *per se,* and the 'solution' to the epidemic lies in the extinction of gay men. In this context it is also vital to note that homosexuality is imagined as a voluntary desire, a 'deadly choice' which amounts to suicide. It is the fact of sexual diversity which is the real target of such pronouncements, not HIV. From the perspective of homophobic fantasy, gay men must cease to exist. The only tolerable option is heterosexuality or death. When AIDS is depicted in this manner, as an essentially retributive spectacle, questions of government policy, the direction of medical research, or the provision of safer sex education, can all be equally *dismissed as irrelevant.*[9]

Such attitudes are by no means confined to the easily criticised tabloid press. After Elizabeth Taylor recommended the use of condoms at the memorial concert for the singer Freddie Mercury, the *Daily Telegraph* dismissed her advice as 'shamelessly immoral', whilst the *Independent* saw Mercury's death as 'a powerful and distressing cautionary tale'.[10] But a tale cautionary of what? The neglect of gay men's health education in Britain in the 1980s? The homophobia of the British press? It is sometimes assumed that press coverage of the epidemic has 'improved'. Any such opinion ignores the continued widespread confusion surrounding almost every aspect of HIV education, treatment, and degrees of relative risk. If the cultural response to AIDS is interpreted only from the point of view of a larger, general history of epidemics, such issues can be easily neglected, with renewed recourse to the familiar sorrowful note of disapproval concerning the supposed continuities of human 'folly'. Such an approach merely sustains the discursive construction of AIDS as plague by other means. In this manner the distancing, brutal prejudice of the UK press may be directly translated into articulate, scholarly, homophobic evasions on the part of the historian.

The history of medicine has much to teach us in this epidemic, but it has nothing to say about what is most specific to it, namely, the homophobic neglect of gay men's needs as those at greatest risk of infection. This is hardly surprising since the history of medicine has hitherto only acknowledged gay men as individual 'deviants', rather than as a social constituency. This is wholly in keeping with the wider discursive obliteration of gay men throughout the sociology of medicine, and in most modern epidemiology. Policies have thus been determined within a field of overlapping specialist disciplines that are homophobic. If gay men's needs have been consistently neglected throughout the epidemic, this needs to be interpreted in relation to the fact that we are not generally regarded as part of the general 'humanity' which is the subject of the social sciences, and medicine. It is this massive indifference to our lives that historians should attempt to explain, rather than emulate.

For it is precisely the discourse of 'History' that is so frequently employed in order to legitimate homophobic evasions in accounts of the epidemic written outside the domain of academic studies. Thus, writing in *Newsweek* in 1988, Matt Clark published an article in the Society and Medicine section, entitled 'Plagues, Man and History', with the sub-heading 'Lessons about AIDS from the Black Death', where we are quickly reassured that: 'the epidemics of the past hold medical lessons that can keep the AIDS threat in perspective'.[11]

According to Clark:

> To historians there's really nothing new about AIDS. Epidemics have changed the course of human events just as readily as wars, religious movements, royal houses and the imperatives of trade between nations.[12]

We are then treated to lengthy descriptions of the 1918–19 influenza epidemic, and the 'upsurge' of syphilis in the sixteenth century, which end with the pious conclusion that:

> If history remains a reliable guide, this epidemic too will run its vicious course, spreading acute misery. Then it will take its place in the background of the ecosystem, alongside the organisms that cause influenza, syphilis, measles and a host of other infections.[13]

In this manner, misleading and, at most, picturesque historical analogies are used to displace away any sense of social or political forces in conflict, or indeed any political dimension whatever. Instead, the epidemic is casually naturalised, made to seem *inevitable,* and all sense of human agency, or injustice, or ethical responsibilities, neatly and conveniently disappears.

Hence the inadequacy of accounts of the epidemic which do not address the central and indispensable role of the gay press in defining debate and information for gay men, and which choose to ignore the basic level of gay community experience, values, and institutions. The metaphor of plague naturalises homophobia, and makes it appear inevitable. It also naturalises the *impact* of HIV amongst gay men, and displaces attention away from the direct consequences of homophobic denial of safer sex education to those in greatest need—a denial which may be accurately tallied in our mounting mortality statistics. All too often the whole complexity and richness of gay culture can be ignored, with perhaps at most a largely misleading footnote reference to the work of Randy Shilts.[14] Indeed, the tendency to refer to *And The Band Played On* as if it were an oracular text, explaining all gay men's responses to AIDS, is itself a typical example. Historical accounts of AIDS that overlook the achievements of the non-government AIDS service organisations, or treatment activism, or the role of gay men in the statutory sector, amount to nothing more than strategic disinformation.

Similar problems also afflict the other principal canonical text of AIDS criticism, Susan Sontag's *AIDS And Its Metaphors*.[15] For Sontag, what is 'new' about AIDS are metaphors of mutability and contemporaneity, as in the discourse of 'computer viruses'.[16] So homophobic is her text that, though writing in Manhattan in the late 1980s she does not even *mention* the word 'gay'. Furthermore, her complete embargo on war metaphors makes it difficult to convey the enormity of the consequences of government policies and government neglect in most countries. As the American AIDS activist group, Gran Fury, asked in a poster concerning HIV education for gay men: 'When a government turns its back on its people, is it civil war?' Plague metaphors for AIDS did not simply appear spontaneously in popular consciousness, carried over at some level of innate cultural memory from the distant past. On the contrary, they were mobilised by homophobic institutions in order to articulate their specific ideological and political vision of the epidemic. To accept historical analogies between people with AIDS and medieval plague victims, is to miss the point that whilst the plagues of history struck with arbitrary venom, demonstrably effective safer sex campaigns for those most at risk (gay men) have been almost everywhere either neglected, or subjected to many different forms of direct censorship and harassment. *This epidemic is unique in so far as its prevention has been prevented, rather than transmission.* Resources and education campaigns have been targeted at those at least risk of contracting HIV, as if the priority of preventing an epidemic amongst heterosexuals had been established at the expense of halting the epidemics that are actually raging throughout the developed world. One need only consider the paradoxical British response, which has successfully slowed down transmission amongst injecting drug users through the sharing of needles by introducing needle-exchanges. Yet almost nothing has been done for gay men, who are at much greater risk; in France, both groups are left to what is evidently thought of as their 'fate'.

If gay men have been regarded as expendable, and fundamental policies have been determined by homophobia, the historian can hardly sustain a neutral pose. For what she is 'observing' is, in effect, an ongoing massacre, quietly overseen and tacitly approved by the entire cultural and political system of the first world. Nobody may have set out with the intention that huge numbers of gay men should contract HIV, but that has been the inevitable consequence of government action, and inaction, all around the world, with only a handful of exceptions—Denmark, Australia and the Netherlands. In such circumstances, neutrality amounts to collusion. If we seek a historical model in the twentieth century it is not to the history of epidemics that we should initially turn, but to the history of medical atrocities, especially when these have been committed with state supervision and support.

What has happened is unprecedented, for the simple reason that the diaspora of gay identity is of very recent origin. Since we have not been widely accepted as a legitimate social constituency, our deaths are as unreal to most heterosexuals as our lives. Our situation is the more intolerable since we are not yet admitted into most notions of the common 'humanity' against which crimes may be said to be committed in such extraordinary and terrible circumstances. However, the history of medical atrocities directs us immediately to situations when specific groups of people have been treated inhumanely, in the wider name of 'care', or the advancement of science, because they themselves were not officially regarded as fully or properly 'human' in the first place.[17] When HIV is regarded as an agent of 'natural' extermination, it may be ignored in specific population groups where its effects will be taken for granted. This is not extermination by conscious policy, but by default, and the long-term consequences are not dissimilar.

We need to consider what happens in countries such as Britain, France and the US, where national identities are increasingly played out and defined in relation to demonised others—whose 'otherness' could hardly be made more apparent than in the spectacle of their suffering an epidemic, their dying like flies, like the non-humans they are thought to be. That gay men deserve to die from AIDS has never been challenged by heterosexuals, but has retained widespread legitimacy, as homophobic fanatics have successfully influenced governments of the left and the right alike. As an activist, I write from a position which has seen bad policies translated into inadequate actions. I have become extremely intolerant of those who have made no attempt whatsoever to educate themselves about HIV or AIDS. Their indifference to the epidemic is evidence of their wider indifference to whether gay men live or die. All around the world gay men have struggled to secure services for everyone affected by HIV, especially for those who are also marginalised as the result of their race, or gender, or class, or whatever. By so doing, however, we have frequently neglected 'our own'. Whilst vast sums of money have been squandered on generally dreadful AIDS education aimed at the 'general public', horribly little has been done on behalf of gay men, for whom nobody else will speak up. Hence the responsibility of historians to properly analyse this epidemic in its correct narrative contexts, which are overwhelmingly political. We cannot afford the luxurious delusion of some ultimate recognition of the scale of injustice perpetrated at all levels of the management of the epidemic, because we don't have time. Too many lives are still at stake. It is the historian's responsibility to narrate, and not to further legitimate the vast, ongoing atrocity that is AIDS.

Conclusion: The Horses of Achilles—an allegory

In Book Seventeen of *The Iliad*, we read of the immortal horses sent by Zeus to Achilles, which weep for the untimely death of their brave young charioteer, Achilles's beloved, Patroclus. They weep at the news of his treacherous murder by Hector, Prince of Troy:

> Firm as a gravestone planted on the barrow of a dead man or woman, they stood motionless in front of their beautiful chariot with their heads bowed down to the earth. Hot tears ran from their eyes to the ground as they mourned for their lost driver, and their luxuriant manes were soiled.[18]

The immortal horses weep because they have been touched by mortal, human tragedy. Homer is very clear about this. They mourn an avoidable loss.

Eventually Zeus intervenes, and the horses recover their equilibrium. They gallop off to save Patroclus's squire, Automedon, who is in danger. After all, there was still everything to play for. The death of Patroclus had no direct effect on the course of the siege, save to harden Achaean resolve.

Notes

Preface: My project

1 For example see Gay Left Collective (eds), *Homosexuality: Power And Politics,* Allison and Busby, London, 1980.

2 Simon Watney, *Policing Desire: Pornography AIDS and the Media,* Comedia/Methuen, London, 1987. US edition from University of Minnesota Press, 1987 and 1989.

3 Simon Watney and Sunil Gupta, 'The Rhetoric of AIDS', *Screen,* vol. 27, no. 1, Jan–Feb 1986, pp. 72–86.

4 Anon, 'The Talk of the Town', *New Yorker,* 10 February 1992, pp. 25–6.

5 See Peter Aggleton, et al., *Aids: Scientific and social issues, a resource for health educators,* Churchill Livingstone, Edinburgh, 1989.

6 Simon Watney, 'Lesbian and Gay Studies in the Age of AIDS', *NYQ,* no. 21, 22 March 1992, p. 42.

7 See Simon Watney, 'Short-Term Companions: AIDS and popular entertainment', in this collection.

8 Douglas Crimp, 'Mourning and Militancy', *October,* no. 51, MIT, Winter, 1989, pp. 8–9.

9 Lynn Barber, '*The Oldie* picks up an unpleasant virus', *Independent on Sunday,* London, 8 March 1992, p. 23. I should like to thank Keith Alcorn for drawing this article to my attention.

10 For example, Simon Watney, 'AIDS USA', *Square Peg,* no. 17, London, 1987, pp. 28–31; Simon Watney, 'AIDS USA 1988', *Square Peg,* no. 21, 1988, pp. 14–17; etc.

11 For example, John Seabrook, 'Letter from London', *Vanity Fair,* vol. 53, no. 12, December 1990, pp. 94–111; and Simon Watney, 'Silence Equals Death', *Elle,* London, November 1990, pp. 99–106 (reprinted in this collection).

12 Watney, *Policing Desire,* op. cit.

13 Erica Carter and Simon Watney (eds), *Taking Liberties: AIDS and Cultural Politics,* Serpent's Tail, London, 1989. Winner of the Words Project for AIDS, WPA/Gregory Kolovakos Award, Lambda Literary Awards, USA, 1990.

14 Neil Bartlett, *Who Was That Man? A Present for Mr Oscar Wilde,* Serpent's Tail, London, 1988, pp. 229–30.

1. AIDS, 'Moral Panic' Theory, and Homophobia

This article was written for the first UK Social Aspects of AIDS conference, held at Bristol Polytechnic in October 1986. It was published in Peter Aggleton and Hilary Homans (eds), *Social Aspects of AIDS*, Falmer Press, London, 1988, pp. 52–65.

1   J. Owen, and C. Rosen, 'Put AIDS victims in holiday camps: Doctor's shock remedy', *People*, 28 September 1986.
2   J. Ferry, 'AIDS: The chilling last-chance warning for Britain', *Mail on Sunday*, 12 October 1986.
3   C. Doyle, 'AIDS: It does affect us all', *Daily Telegraph*, 15 September 1986.
4   *Daily Telegraph*, 2 December 1986.
5   R. Goldstein, 'Heartsick: Fear and loving in the gay community', *Village Voice*, 28 June 1983.
6   S. Cohen, *Folk Devils and Moral Panics: The Creation of the Mods and Rockers*, Martin Robertson, Oxford, 1972.
7   S. Hall, et al., *Policing The Crisis*, Macmillan, London, 1978.
8   J. Weeks, *Sex, Politics and Society: The Regulation of Sexuality Since 1800*, Longman, Harlow, 1981.
9   J. Weeks, *Sexuality*, Ellis Horwood, Chichester, 1986.
10   G. Rubin, 'Thinking sex: Notes for a radical theory of the politics of sexuality', in C. Vance (ed.), *Pleasure and Danger: Exploring Female Sexuality*, Routledge & Kegan Paul, London, 1984.
11   A. Giudici Fettner, 'Is the CDC dying of AIDS?', *Village Voice*, 21, 40, 7 October 1986.
12   M. Foucault, 'On governmentality', *Ideology and Consciousness*, no. 6, 1979, pp. 5–21.
13   D. Henke, 'Boyson condemns "evil" single parents', *Guardian*, 10 October 1986.
14   J. Donzelot, *The Policing of Families: Welfare versus the State*, Hutchinson, London, 1979.
15   G. Weinberg, *Society and the Healthy Homosexual*, Doubleday, New York, 1973.
16   S. Watney, *Policing Desire: Pornography, AIDS and the media*, Comedia/Methuen, London, 1987.
17   L. Bersani, *Baudelaire and Freud*, University of California Press, Los Angeles, CA, 1977.

2. Visual AIDS: Advertising ignorance

This article first appeared in *New Socialist*, March 1987. It was reprinted in *Radical America*, vol. 20, no. 6, 1987; and in Peter Aggleton and Hilary Homans (eds), *Social Aspects of AIDS*, Falmer Press, London, 1988, pp. 177–82.

3. The Subject of AIDS

This article was first published in *Copyright*, no. 1, Harvard University, USA, 1987, pp. 125–33. It was reprinted in Peter Aggleton, et al. (eds), *AIDS: Social Representations, Social Practices*, Falmer Press, London, 1988, pp. 64–74. It was based on a talk which I gave at the *Homosexuality, Which Homosexuality?* conference, held at the Free University, Amsterdam.

1   Michel Foucault, *The Birth of the Clinic: An Archeology of Medical Perception*, Vintage Books, 1975, p. 171.

2 Gayle Rubin, 'Thinking Sex: Notes for a radical theory of the politics of sexuality', in Carol S. Vance (ed.), *Pleasure and Danger: Exploring female sexuality*, Routledge & Kegan Paul, London, 1984, p. 271.

3 Sylvia Moreno, '40% think AIDS can be caught by giving blood', *Newsday*, 16 June 1987.

4 Richard Goldstein, 'States of emergency', *Village Voice*, 30 June 1987.

5 Michel Foucault, 'On governmentality', *Ideology and Consciousness*, no. 6, Autumn 1979.

6 Jacqueline Rose, *The Case of Peter Pan, or The Impossibility of Children's Fiction*, Macmillan, Basingstoke, 1984, p. 16.

7 *Ibid.*

8 See Simon Watney, 'AIDS: how big did it have to get?', *New Socialist*, March 1987.

9 See Simon Watney, 'The banality of gender', *Oxford Literary Review*, vol. 8, 1986.

10 See Simon Watney, 'AIDS, "Moral Panic" Theory, and Homophobia' (in this volume).

11 See Simon Watney, 'AIDS USA', *Square Peg*, no. 17, 1987.

12 *Ibid.*

4. The Politics of AIDS

This article was published in *City Limits*, London, March 1987.

5. Talking to the Future: Gay rights in Britain and the USA

This article appeared in *Gay Times*, London, February 1988, pp. 37–9.

1 *Independent*, 8 December 1987.

2 Senator Jesse Helms, letter to the *New York Times*, 12 November 1987.

3 Jesse Helms quoting Monsignor Eugene Clark, Congressional Record—Senate, 14 October 1987.

4 *New York Native*, Issue 238, 9 November 1987, p. 11.

5 Patrick J. Buchanan, 'AIDS And Moral Bankruptcy', *New York Post*, 2 December 1987.

6 David Lister, *Independent*, 12 December 1987.

6. The Spectacle of AIDS

First published in *October*, no. 43, MIT, Cambridge MA, 1987, pp. 71–87.

1 Zbigniew Herbert, 'Mr. Cogito on the Need for Precision', in *Report From the Besieged City*, Oxford University Press, New York and Oxford, 1987, p. 67.

2 See Simon Watney, 'The Subject of AIDS', *Copyright*, vol. 1, no. 1, Fall 1987.

3 Andrew Veitch, 'AIDS Cases Exceed 1,000', *Guardian*, 8 September 1987; Anthony Smith, 'AIDS Death Toll Hits 1,000', *Star*, 8 September 1987.

4 Andrew Veitch, ' "Up to 10 Million" Have AIDS Virus', *Guardian*, 24 June 1986.

5 See Simon Watney, 'AIDS: How Big Did It Have To Get?', *New Socialist*, March 1987.

6 See Dennis Altman, *AIDS in the Mind of America*, New York, Doubleday, 1986, p. 33; published as *AIDS and the New Puritanism*, Pluto Press, London, 1986.

7 See Simon Watney, 'AIDS USA', *Square Peg*, no. 17, Autumn 1987.

8 See Patrick Wright, *On Living in an Old County*, Verso, London, 1985.

9   See for example, Mary Douglas, *Risk Acceptability According to the Social Sciences*, Routledge & Kegan Paul, London, 1986.

10 David Green, 'Veins of Resemblance: Photography and Eugenics', in Holland, Spence, and Watney (eds), *Photography/Politics: Two*, Comedia/Methuen, London, 1987, p. 13.

11 See Robert Jay Lifton, *The Nazi Doctors: Medical Killing and the Psychology of Genocide*, Basic Books, New York, 1986, p. 25. This book should be read by anyone interested in the archaeology of AIDS commentary.

12 For an example, see William E. Dannemeyer, 'AIDS Infection Must Be Reportable', *Los Angeles Times*, 12 June 1987.

13 Michel Foucault, 'On Governmentality', *Ideology and Consciousness*, no. 6, Autumn 1979, p. 17.

14 Simon Watney, 'AIDS: The Cultural Agenda', paper presented at the conference 'Homosexuality, Which Homosexuality?' at the Free University, Amsterdam, December 1987.

15 Oscar Wilde, *The Portrait of Dorian Gray* (1891), Oxford University Press, New York and Oxford, 1974, p. 224.

16 J. Laplanche and J.-B. Pontalis, *The Language of Psycho-Analysis*, The Hogarth Press, London, 1983, p. 205.

17 Parveen Adams, 'Versions of the Body', *m/f*, nos.11–12 (1986), p. 29.

18 Leo Bersani, *Baudelaire and Freud*, University of California Press, Berkeley, 1977, p. 129.

19 *Ibid.*, pp. 41, 42.

20 Meyrick Horton, 'General Practices', paper presented at the second annual 'Social Meanings of AIDS conference', South Bank Polytechnic, London, November 1987.

21 Jacques Donzelot, *The Policing of Families: Welfare versus the State*, Hutchinson, London, 1979, p. xxvi.

22 See Simon Watney, *Policing Desire: Pornography, AIDS, and the Media*, Comedia/Methuen, London 1987; University of Minnesota Press, Minneapolis, 1987, Chapter 4.

23 Kaye Wellings, 'Sickness and Sin: The Case of Genital Herpes', paper presented to the British Sociological Association, Medical Sociology Group, 1983, p. 10.

24 Ernesto Laclau and Chantal Mouffe, *Hegemony and Socialist Strategy: Towards a Radical Democratic Politics*, Verso, London, 1985, p. 181.

7. *Photography and AIDS*

This article first appeared in *Ten.8*, no. 26, Birmingham, 1987. The version included here was updated for republication in Carol Squiers (ed.), *The Critical Image: Essays On Contemporary Photography*, Bay Press, Seattle, 1990, pp. 173–93.

1   Michel Foucault, *The Birth of the Clinic, An Archaeology of Medical Perception*, Vintage, New York, 1975, p.171.

2   *Ibid.*, p. 196.

3   See Allan M. Brandt, *No Magic Bullet: A Social History of Venereal Diseases in the United States Since 1880*, Oxford University Press, Oxford, 1987.

4   Gayle Rubin, 'Thinking Sex: Notes for a Radical Theory of the Politics of Sexuality', in Carol S. Vance (ed.), *Pleasure and Danger: Exploring Female Sexuality*, Routledge & Kegan Paul, London, 1984, p. 282.

5   *Sunday Times,* London, 21 June 1987.
6   Mary Douglas and Aaron Wildavsky, *Risk and Culture,* University of California Press, Berkeley, 1983, p. 37.
7   See Brandt, *No Magic Bullet,* op. cit.
8   'Panic', *The Face,* May 1985.
9   David Schonauer, *A Way of Life,* Introduction to Bob Mahoney, 'Looking Death in the Face', *American Photographer,* April 1986, p. 97.
10 Kevin Kelly on Matt Herron, *Whole Earth Review,* Fall 1985, p. 34.
11 For example, see the special issue of *Scientific American,* 259, 4 October 1988.
12 See Simon Watney, 'Introduction', in Erica Carter and Simon Watney (eds), *Taking Liberties: AIDS and Cultural Politics,* Serpent's Tail, London, 1989.
13 Tim Radford, 'Estimated incubation period for AIDS rises to 10 years', *Guardian,* London, 17 March 1989.
14 Philip M. Boffey, 'Campaign to Find Drugs for Fighting AIDS Is Intensified', *New York Times,* 15 February 1988, p.A14.
15 George Whitmore, 'Bearing Witness', *New York Times Magazine,* 31 January 1988. See also more recently, Dena Kleiman, 'Gay Men Find Sadness Colors Life as They Make the Most of Their Days', *New York Times,* 7 February 1989.
16 See Simon Watney, 'The Spectacle of AIDS', in D. Crimp (ed.), *AIDS: Cultural Analysis, Cultural Activism,* MIT Press, Cambridge MA, 1988.
17 Cindy Patton, 'Safer Sex and Lesbians', *The Pink Paper,* London, Issue 14, 25 February 1988, p. 2.
18 Michael Callen, 'Not Everyone Dies of AIDS', *Village Voice,* 3 May 1988, p. 31.
19 James Baldwin, *The Evidence of Things Not Seen,* Henry Holt, New York, 1985, p. 52.
20 See *Famine and Photojournalism,* special issue of *Ten.8,* 19, Birmingham, 1985.
21 See Susan Scott-Parker, *They Aren't in the Brief: Advertising People with Disabilities,* The King's Fund, London, 1989.
22 For example, Crimp, *AIDS: Cultural Analysis, Cultural Activism;* and Jan Zita Grover, *Introduction to AIDS: The Artists' Response,* Hoyt L. Sherman Gallery, Columbus, Ohio, 1989; and *Bearing Witness: Artists Respond to AIDS,* curated by Kristen Engberg and Mary Ann Nilson, Mobius/ICA, Boston, 1988.
23 Susan Sontag, *AIDS and Its Metaphors,* London, Allen Lane, 1989. See also Simon Watney, 'Guru of AIDS', *Guardian,* London, 10 March 1989, p. 30.
24 For example, Sontag, *AIDS and Its Metaphors,* op. cit., and Elizabeth Fee and Daniel M. Fox, 'Introduction: Public Policy and Historical Enquiry', in *AIDS: The Burdens of History,* University of California Press, Berkeley, 1988.
25 Jo Spence, 'Questioning Documentary Practice?', paper given at the first National Conference on Photography, organised by the Arts Council of Great Britain, Salford, Lancashire, April 1987.

8. 'AIDS' or 'HIV Disease'?

This article appeared in *Capital Gay,* October 1988. Reprinted as 'Let's stop talking about AIDS', in *Rites,* April 1989, Toronto.

1   Steve Connor and Sharon Kingman, *The Search for the Virus,* London, Penguin, 1988, provides the clearest available account of this history.

9. 'The Day After Hiroshima'

Text of a talk given at Vasteras, Sweden, 7 October 1988. An edited version subsequently appeared in a Swedish newspaper.

1   Oliver Gillie, 'Antenatal care "has stagnated for 30 years in many areas" ', *Independent*, London, 8 December 1987, p. 8.
2   Aileen Ballantyne, 'Doctors blame shortages for 2,000 baby deaths', *Guardian*, London, 29 September 1988, p. 4.
3   David Brindle and David Hencke, 'MP's warn of health service patients at risk', *Guardian*, London, 23 September 1989, p. 28.
4   Hanif Kureishi, 'England, bloody England', *Guardian*, London, 15 January 1988, p. 19.
5   Allan M. Brandt, 'AIDS in Historical Perspective: Four Lessons from the History of Sexually Transmitted Diseases', *American Journal of Public Health*, vol. 78, no. 4, April 1988, p. 371.
6   World Health Organisation, 'Report Of The Consultation On International Travel And HIV Infection', Geneva, April 1987.
7   June E. Osborn, 'AIDS politics and Science', *The New England Journal of Medicine*, 18 February 1988, p. 445.
8   Simon Watney, 'Missionary Positions: AIDS, "Africa" and Race', *Differences: A Journal of Feminist Cultural Studies*, vol. 1, no. 1, University of Indiana Press, 1988 (in this volume).
9   Cindy Patton, 'Safer sex and lesbians', *The Pink Paper*, London, 14, 25 February 1988, p. 2.
10   Simon Watney, *Policing Desire, Pornography, AIDS, and the Media*, Comedia/Methuen, London, 1987, p. 132.
11   Susan Jacoby, 'Risky Business', *The New York Times Magazine*, Section 6, 24 April 1988, p. 28.
12   See Martin Breum and Aart Hendriks, *AIDS And Human Rights: An International Perspective*, Akademic Forlag, Copenhagen, 1988.
13   See Dr Robin Weiss and Dr Samuel O. Thier, 'HIV Testing Is The Answer—What's The Question?', *New England Journal of Medicine*, 13 October 1988.

10. Cross-Over

Published as *Cross-Over, En film av Staffan Hildebrand*, in *Lambda Nordica*, no. 1, 1989, pp. 206–17, Stockholm, Sweden. *Cross-Over* was screened at the opening ceremony of the Fifth International AIDS Conference, in Montreal.

1   Simon Watney 'Missionary Positions; AIDS, "Africa", Race', *Differences: A Journal of Feminist Cultural Studies*, vol. 1, no. 1, University of Indiana Press, 1988.
2   See Simon Watney 'The Day After Hiroshima: Some Reflections on Official British and Swedish AIDS Education Materials and Government Policies', 1988 (in this volume).
3   See D. Allan and M. Brandt, 'AIDS in Historical Perspective: Four Lessons from the History of Sexually Transmitted Diseases', *American Journal of Public Health*, vol. 78, no. 4, April, 1988.

11. *Politics, People and the AIDS Epidemic:* And the Band Played On

Published in *Gay Scotland,* May/June, 1988; reprinted in Swedish in *Lambda Nordica,* nos.3–4, 1989; a shorter version appeared in *New Scientist,* 7 April 1988.

12. Missionary Positions: AIDS, 'Africa', and race

First published in *Differences,* vol. 1, no. 1, Brown University, Providence RI, Winter 1988, pp. 83–101. The version printed here was updated for republication in *Critical Quarterly,* vol. 31, Autumn 1989, pp. 45–78, University of Manchester Press; and in Russell Ferguson, et al. (eds), *Out There: Marginalisation and Contemporary Cultures,* The New Museum of Contemporary Art/MIT, Cambridge MA, 1990, pp. 89–107.

1   I am indebted to Cindy Patton for the concept of 'African AIDS', which she has elaborated in 'Inventing African AIDS', *City Limits,* 363, 15–22 September, 1988.

2   Rod Nordland, et al., 'Africa in the plague years', *Newsweek,* 1 December 1986, p. 44.

3   Peter Murtagh, 'AIDS in Africa: a present from Buffalo Bill', *Guardian,* 3 February 1987.

4   Nordland, et al., 'Africa in the plague years', op. cit., p.46.

5   Thomson Prentice, 'Africa's new agony: dark future', *The Times,* 29 October 1986.

6   Alex Shoumatoff, 'In search of the source of AIDS', *Vanity Fair,* 51 (7), July 1988, p. 105.

7   Thomson Prentice, 'Africa's new agony: a continent under siege', *The Times,* 27 October 1986.

8   Joseph Conrad, *Heart of Darkness,* 1899, Oxford, Oxford Paperbacks, 1984.

9   *Ibid.,* p. 67.

10   Simon Watney, *Policing Desire: Pornography, AIDS, and the Media,* Comedia/Methuen, London and University of Minnesota Press, Minneapolis, 1987 and 1989, p. 4.

11   Murtagh, 'AIDS in Africa', op. cit.

12   Peter Murtagh, 'Highlanders get all clear after Kenya AIDS alarm', *Guardian,* 25 March 1987.

13   Conrad, *Heart of Darkness,* op. cit., p. 66.

14   *Ibid.,* p. 67.

15   Lawrence K. Altman, 'AIDS in Africa: a pattern of mystery', *New York Times,* 8 November 1985, p. A8.

16   See Renee Sabatier, 'Blaming others: prejudice, race and worldwide AIDS', The Panos Institute, London, 1988, p. 54.

17   Nordland, et al., 'Africa in the plague years', p. 46.

18   Andrew Veitch, 'The cruel march of AIDS', *Guardian,* 16 February 1988, p. 32.

19   See World Health Organisation, 'Report Of The Consultation On International Travel And HIV Infection', Geneva, April 1987.

20   See Simon Watney, *Policing Desire: Pornography, AIDS, and the Media,* op. cit.

21   Patrick Brantlinger, 'Victorians and Africans: the genealogy of the myth of the Dark Continent', *Critical Inquiry,* 12 (1), Autumn 1985, p. 181.

22   Nordland, et al., 'Africa in the plague years', op. cit., p.45.

23   Shoumatoff, 'In search of the source of AIDS', op. cit., p.95.

24   Robin McKie, 'Straight sex link with AIDS epidemic', *Observer,* 10 November 1985, p. 15.

25 Nicholas Timmins, 'Old people are getting AIDS, doctors reveal', *Independent*, 16 September 1988, p. 1.
26 Brantlinger, 'Victorians and Africans', op. cit., p. 194.
27 *Ibid.*
28 Conrad, *Heart of Darkness*, op. cit., p. 116.
29 *Ibid.*, p. 144.
30 *Ibid.*, p. 135.
31 Stephen Jay Gould, *The Mismeasure of Man*, Penguin, Harmondsworth, 1981, p. 35.
32 See Michel Foucault, 'On governmentality', *Ideology and Consciousness*, 6 Autumn 1979, pp. 5–23.
33 The notion of 'leakage' has been a central term in British and American discussion concerning the epidemiology of HIV.
34 Ronald Hyams, 'Empire and sexual opportunity', *Journal of Imperial and Commonwealth History*, 14 (2), January 1986, p. 75. I would like to thank Michael Budd for drawing this article to my attention.
35 For example, see Susan Sontag, *AIDS and its Metaphors*, Allen Lane, London, 1989; and Elizabeth Fee and Daniel M. Fox (eds), *AIDS: The Burdens of History*, University of California Press, Berkeley, 1989. I would except the work of Paula A. Treichler and Allan M. Brandt from my judgement of the latter book.
36 Altman, 'AIDS in Africa', op. cit., p. A14.
37 Steven Connor and Sharon Kingman, *The Search for the Virus: the Scientific Discovery of AIDS and the Quest for a Cure*, Penguin, London, 1988, p. 204.
38 *Ibid.*, p. 196.
39 Patton, 'Inventing African AIDS', op. cit., p. 85.
40 Sander Gilman, *Disease and Representation: Images of Illness from Madness to AIDS*, Cornell University Press, New York, 1988, p. 262.
41 See Richard C. Chirimuuta and Rosalind I. Chirimuuta, *AIDS, Africa and Racism*, R. Chirimuuta, Burton-on-Trent, 1987.
42 See Simon Watney, 'Psychoanalysis, sexuality and AIDS', in M. Wallis and S. Shepherd (eds), *Coming on Strong: Gay Politics and Culture*, Unwin-Hyman, London, 1989.
43 Andrew Brown, 'Africans attack "sin of homosexuality"', *Independent*, 5 August 1988.
44 Subsection 2A of Section 28 of the 1988 Local Government Act states that 'A local authority shall not—(a) intentionally promote homosexuality or publish material with the intention of promoting homosexuality; (b) promote the teaching in any maintained school of the acceptability of homosexuality as a pretended family relationship.'
45 Cindy Patton, 'Safer sex and lesbians', *The Pink Paper*, 14, 25 February 1988, p. 2.
46 Conrad, *Heart of Darkness*, op. cit., p. 49.
47 See Alex Brazier, *A Double Deficiency?: A Report On The Social Security Act 1986 And People With Acquired Immune Deficiency Syndrome (AIDS), AIDS Related Complex (ARC), And HIV Infection*, The Terrence Higgins Trust, London, 1989; see also Erica Carter and Simon Watney (eds), *Taking Liberties: AIDS and Cultural Politics*, Serpent's Tail, London, 1989.

13. Young People and AIDS

First published in *Gay Times*, July 1989.

1 *The Sun*, 13 May 1989.

2   *Guardian,* 22 March 1989.
3   *Guardian,* 28 April 1989.
4   *Equal Time,* Issue 181, 15 March 1989, Minneapolis.
5   *The Listener,* 24 October 1985.
6   *Guardian,* 17 May 1989.
7   *Guardian,* 7 January, 1989.

14. Community Responsibilities

First published in *Gay Times,* November 1989.

1   *British Medical Journal,* 3 June 1989, p. 1521.
2   *Outweek,* 26 June 1989.

15. Safer Sex as Community Practice

This is an extended version of a presentation given on 7 June 1989 as part of the 'Eroticism, Safer Sex and Behaviour Change' panel at the Fifth International Conference on AIDS, Montreal, Canada. It develops ideas originally presented in a paper, 'Theorising Rumour in Relation to Perceptions of Risk', at the Third Conference on Social Aspects of AIDS, February 1989 and published in Peter Aggleton, et al. (eds), *AIDS: Individual, Cultural and Policy Dimensions,* Falmer Press, London, 1990, pp. 19–35.

1   D. Altman, et al., *Which Homosexuality?* London, Gay Men's Press, 1989; Simon Watney, *Policing Desire: Pornography, AIDS, and the Media,* Comedia/Methuen, London, 1987, etc.
2   Michel Foucault, 'The Return of Morality', in S. Lotringer (ed.), *Foucault Live,* Semiotext(e), New York, 1989.
3   Douglas Crimp, 'How to Have Promiscuity in an Epidemic', in D. Crimp (ed.), *AIDS: Cultural Analysis, Cultural Activism,* MIT Press, Cambridge MA, 1988, p. 253.
4   M. Callen, *How to Have Sex in an Epidemic,* News From The Front Publications, New York, 1983.
5   See 'Ins and Outs', *Time Out,* 977, 1900; P. Aggleton, T. Coxon and P. Weatherburn, *Aids Health Promotion Activities Directed towards Gay and Bisexual Men in London,* NKJ: A Briefing Document Prepared for the World Health Organisation Global Programme on AIDS, WHO/EPA, Geneva.
6   A. Evans, et al., 'Trends in Sexual Behaviour and Risk Factors among Homosexual Men, 1980–87', *British Medical Journal,* 298, pp. 215–18.
7   R. Stall, 'Implications of Relapse from Safer Sex', *Focus,* 4, 3, University of California, 1989, p. 3.
8   B. Schatz, 'Coverage of Selected Drugs under State Medical Assistance (Medicaid) Programs in the USA', paper presented at the Fifth International Conference on AIDS, Montreal, Canada, 1989.
9   Cindy Patton, Resistance and the Erotic', *Radical America,* vol. 20, no. 6, 1986, pp. 28–39.
10 Simon Watney, 'A Common Tragedy: The Politics of AIDS', *Gay Times,* 130, 1989, pp. 42–5.
11 Cindy Patton, 'Resistance and the Erotic', *Radical America,* vol. 20, no. 6, 1986, pp. 28–39.
12 J. D'Eramo, 'New Sex—Building a Gay Renaissance', *Mandate,* 14, 4, p. 72.

13   H. Stipp and D. Karp, 'Determinants of Public Opinion about AIDS', paper presented at the annual meeting of the American Association for Public Opinion Research, Toronto, Canada, 1988.

14   *Ibid.*

15   *Ibid.*

16   I am not aware of any such research in the UK. The current ESRC-funded work of the Glasgow Media Group has no such specific aims.

17   The *Denver Principles* on the treatment and reporting of people living with AIDS date from 1983 and are reprinted in M. Callen (ed.), *Surviving and Thriving with AIDS: Collected Wisdom,* vol. 2, People with AIDS Coalition, New York, 1988. The forty-first World Health Assembly adopted a clear set of anti-discriminatory resolutions as WHA 41.24 in Geneva on 13 May 1988.

18   A. Brandt, 'AIDS in Historical Perspective: Four Lessons from the History of Sexually Transmitted Diseases', *American Journal of Public Health,* 78, 4, 1988, pp. 369–92.

19   See the *British Medical Journal,* 297, 1197.

20   A. Evans, et al., 'Trends in Sexual Behaviour and Risk Factors among Homosexual Men, 1980–87', *British Medical Journal,* 298, pp. 215–18.

21   A. Karpf, *Doctoring the Media: The Reporting of Health and Medicine,* Routledge, London, 1988, pp. 16, 17.

22   See Ellen Herman's article 'Getting to Serendipity: Do Addiction Programs Sap Our Political Vitality?', *Outlook,* Summer 1988, pp. 1–22.

23   Personal communication.

24   M. Breum and A. Hendriks, *AIDS and Human Rights: An International Perspective,* Akademisk Forlag, Copenhagen, 1988.

25   M. Helquist, 'The Helquist Report', *The Advocate,* 519, 1989, p. 30.

26   Personal communication.

27   Michel Foucault, 'The Return of Morality', in S. Lotringer (ed.), *Foucault Live,* Semiotext(e), New York, 1989.

28   Simon Watney, 'Introduction', in E. Carter and S. Watney (eds), *Taking Liberties: AIDS and Cultural Politics,* Serpent's Tail, London, 1989.

16. Re-gaying AIDS

Gay Times, March 1992. This related closely to a longer speech I gave in Copenhagen in February 1990 at the First European Conference on Homosexuality and HIV.

17. Practices of Freedom

This article was first published in a longer version in Jonathan Rutherford (ed.), *Identity: Community, Culture, Difference,* Lawrence & Wishart, London, 1990, pp. 157–87. The version included here was published in Geoff Andrews (ed.), *Citizenship,* Lawrence & Wishart, London 1991, pp. 164–83.

1   Douglas Crimp, 'Mourning and Militancy', *October,* no. 51, Winter 1989, MIT, pp. 3–19.

2   Medical Research Council, AIDS Directed Programme, Programme Plan and Research Opportunities, London, July 1988.

3   See Simon Watney, 'Tasks in AIDS Research', *Gay Times,* May 1989.

4   *Daily Mirror,* 4 October 1988.
5   See Simon Watney, 'The Possibilities of Permutation: Pleasure, Proliferation and the Politics of Gay Identity in the Age of AIDS', in James Miller (ed.), *AIDS: Crisis and Criticism,* University of Toronto Press, Toronto, 1990.
6   See Simon Watney, 'Safer Sex as Community Practice', in Peter Aggleton, et al. (eds), *AIDS: Individual, Cultural and Policy Dimensions,* Falmer Press, London, 1990.
7   'Frontliners disassociation from ACT UP', *Frontiers,* no. 4, 1 June 1989.
8   Michel Foucault, 'The Ethic of Care for the Self as a Practice of Freedom', in James Bernauer and David Rasmussen (eds), *The Final Foucault,* MIT Press, Cambridge MA, 1988, 1:4.
9   Michel Foucault, 'Truth, Power, Self: An Interview', in Luther H. Martin, et al. (eds), *Technologies of the Self: A Seminar with Michel Foucault,* Tavistock, London, 1988.
10 *Ibid.,* p. 11.
11 A. Silvestre, et al., "Factors related to seroconversion among homosexual and bisexual men after attending a risk reduction education session," *AIDS,* vol. 3, 1989, pp. 647–50.
12 Michel Foucault, 'The Social Triumph of the Sexual Will', *Christopher Street,* Issue 64, vol. 6, no. 4, New York, 1982, p.38.
13 Michel Foucault, 'The Return of Morality', in Sylvère Lotringer (ed.), *Foucault Live,* Semiotext(e), New York, 1989, p. 330.
14 Agnes Heller and Ferenc Feher, *The Postmodern Political Condition,* Polity Press, Oxford, 1989, p. 97.
15 *Ibid.,* p. 89.

18. AIDS, The Second Decade

This article was an expanded version of the Keynote Speech I gave at the fourth annual Social Aspects of AIDS conference, March 1990. It was published in Peter Aggleton, et al. (eds), *AIDS: Responses, Interventions And Care,* Falmer Press, London, 1991, pp. 1–19.

1   *Outweek,* 59, 15 August 1990, p. 5.
2   'Sharp Rise in AIDS Infection is Reported in Third World', *New York Times,* 2 August 1990, p. A18.
3   S. Hall, 'Cultural Identity and Diaspora', in J. Rutherford (ed.), *Identity: Community, Culture, Difference,* Lawrence & Wishart, London, 1990.
4   *Ibid.*
5   S. Watney, 'Safer Sex as Community Practice', in P. Aggleton, et al. (eds), *AIDS: Individual, Cultural and Policy Dimensions,* Falmer Press, London, 1990.
6   H. Moerkerk, 'AIDS Prevention in Europe: The Gay Response', paper given at the First European Conference on HIV and Homosexuality, Copenhagen, 1990.
7   H. Moerkerk and P. Aggleton, 'AIDS Prevention Strategies in Europe', in P. Aggleton, et al. (eds), *AIDS: Individual, Cultural and Policy Dimensions,* op. cit.
8   S. Watney, Foreword to L. Kramer, *Reports from the Holocaust: The Making of An AIDS Activist,* Penguin, Harmondsworth, 1990.
9   S. Watney, Introduction to E. Carter and S. Watney (eds), *Taking Liberties: AIDS and Cultural Politics,* Serpents Tail, London, 1989.
10 Moerkerk and Aggleton, 'Aids Prevention Strategies in Europe', op. cit., p. 7.
11 Silvestre, et al., op. cit., 647–50.

12   H. Kinnell, 'Prostitute's Perceptions of Risk and Factors Related to Risk-Taking', in P. Aggleton, G. Hart, and P. Davies (eds), *AIDS: Responses, Interventions and Care,* Falmer Press, London, 1991, pp. 79–94.

13   J.B. Cohen, 'Overstating the Risk of AIDS: Scapegoating Prostitutes', *Focus,* University of California Regents, 4, 2, pp. 2–3, 1989.

14   'Prostitute with AIDS Sent to Jail', *The Times,* 21 April 1990; see also, 'You Deserve to Die If You Go with a Hooker', *Star,* 21 April 1990.

15   The modern locus classicus for this debate remains Michel Foucault, *The History of Sexuality: An Introduction,* vol. 1, Vintage Books, New York, 1980.

16   The Social Aspects of the prevention of AIDS Project is located at Macquarie University, New South Wales 2109, Australia.

17   R.W. Connell, et al., 'Unsafe Anal Sexual Practice Among Homosexual and Bisexual Men', *Social Aspects of the Prevention of AIDS, Study A,* Report 7, Macquarie University, School of Behavioural Sciences, Sydney, 1989, pp. 19–20.

18   *Ibid.,* p. 21.

19   S. Kippax, et al., 'The Importance of Gay Community in the Prevention of HIV Transmission', mimeo, University of Macquarie, School of Behavioural Sciences, Sydney, 1990, p. 44.

20   Jack O'Sullivan, 'Young Homosexuals "Giving Up Safe Sex" in Setback on AIDS', *Independent,* 20 April 1990.

21   For one such typical article, see R. Fitzpatrick, et al., 'High Risk Sexual Behaviour and Condom Use in a Sample of Homosexual and Bisexual Men', *Health Trends,* 21, 1989, pp. 76–9. However, for an important and rare critique of orthodox epidemiological methods in relation to HIV/AIDS, see J.P. Vandenbroucke, 'An Autopsy of Epidemiological Methods: The Case of "Poppers" in the Early Epidemic of the Acquired Immune Deficiency Syndrome (AIDS)', *American Journal of Epidemiology,* 129, 3, 1989, pp. 455–7.

22   A. Prieur, et al., 'Gay Men: Reasons for Continued Practice of Unsafe Sex', paper presented at the First European Conference on HIV and Homosexuality, Copenhagen, 1990, p. 12.

23   Z. Bauman, *Modernity and the Holocaust,* Polity Press, 1989, Cambridge, p. 104.

24   See, for example, Hannah Arendt, *Eichman in Jerusalem: A Report on the Banality of Evil,* Penguin, Harmondsworth, 1963.

19. Silence Equals Death

This article appeared in *Elle,* UK, London, November 1990, pp. 99–106.

20. State of Emergency

This article appeared in *Gay Times,* April 1991.

21. Perspectives on Testing

This article appeared in *Gay Times,* April 1991.

1   Martin Delaney, *The Advocate,* no. 519, p. 32.

2   David Miller and Tony Pinching, *AIDS,* 1989, 3, pp. 187–93.

22. Perspectives on Treatment

This article appeared in *Gay Times*, June 1991.

1   See Bruce Nussbaum, 'Good Intentions: How Big Business and the Medical Establishment Are Corrupting The Fight Against AIDS', *Atlantic Monthly Press*, USA, 1990.

23. Short-Term Companions: AIDS and 'popular' entertainment

This article was originally written for a projected but subsequently abandoned anthology
of articles on AIDS and cinema from the BFI. A shorter version was included in *Leap
In The Dark: AIDS, Art & Contemporary Cultures*, edited by Allan Klusacek and Ken
Morrison, Vehicule Press, Montreal, 1992, pp. 152–66.

In memory of Vito Russo.

1   Judith Williamson, 'Every virus tells a story', in E. Carter and S. Watney (eds), *Taking
Liberties: AIDS and Cultural Politics*, Serpent's Tail, London, 1989, pp. 69–70.

2   See Simon Watney, *Policing Desire: Pornography, AIDS, and the Media*, Comedia/
Methuen, London, 1987, University of Minnesota Press, Minneapolis, 1987 and 1989.

3   The work of Mary Douglas remains very useful in relation to such questions as the
drawing of symbolic social boundaries around definitions of disease or disability,
although she herself has not analysed the role of sexual difference in the drawing
of such boundaries in modern societies. This is a major task for queer theory in the
years ahead.

4   See Simon Watney, 'Missionary Positions: AIDS, "Africa" and Race' (in this volume);
also Cindy Patton, 'Inventing African AIDS', in *Inventing AIDS*, Routledge, New York,
1990; also Paula Treichler, 'AIDS and HIV infection in the Third World: A First
World Chronicle', in B. Kruger and P. Mariani (eds), *Remaking History*, Bay Press,
Seattle, 1989.

5   See Hilary Kinnell, 'Prostitutes' perceptions of risk and factors related to risk-taking',
in P. Aggleton, et al. (eds), *AIDS: Responses, Interventions and Care*, Falmer Press,
London, 1991, pp. 19–65.

6   See interviews with Cindy Patton, Douglas Crimp, *Gran Fury*, Ellen Spiro and Ray
Navarro, Jean Carlomusto and Greg Bordowitz in S. Watney (ed.), 'ART AIDS NYC',
Art and Text, no. 38, January 1991, Sydney, Australia; see also, Timothy Landers,
'Bodies and Anti-Bodies: A Crisis in Representation', *Independent*, New York, Jan–
Feb. 1988, pp. 18–24.

7   'AIDS chief killer of NY women', *Guardian*, London 9 July 1987; and Andrew Veitch,
'AIDS cases exceed 1000', *Guardian*, London, 8 September 1987. See also Timothy
Landers, 'Bodies and antibodies: a crisis in representation', *Independent*, New York,
Jan–Feb., 1988, pp. 18–24.

8   Deborah Rogers, 'AIDS spreads to the soaps, sort of', *New York Times*, Sunday
28 August, 1988. I'd like to thank Charles Barber for drawing this article to my
attention.

9   Vito Russo, *The Celluloid Closet: Homosexuality in the Movies* (Revised Edition),
Harper & Row, New York, 1987, p. 277.

10 See Simon Watney, 'The AIDS Community: An Interview with Dennis Altman', *Gay
Times*, London, February 1990, pp. 47–8.

11 See Simon Watney, 'Foreword: the persistence of memory', to Larry Kramer, *Reports*

from the Holocaust: The Making of an AIDS Activist, Penguin Books, Harmondsworth, 1990, pp. XIII–XXX.

12   Quoted from Walt Odets, 'The Secret Epidemic', *Outlook,* Issue 14, Fall 1991, San Francisco, p. 49.

13   Simon Watney, sleeve-notes, *Red Hot & Blue,* Chrysalis Records, 1990.

14   Julie Burchill, 'An HIV hit squad carries out the Porter Slaughter', *Mail on Sunday,* 16 September 1990. For a very different view of *Red Hot & Blue,* see Ethan Mordden, 'Rock and Cole', *The New Yorker,* 29 October 1991, pp. 91–100; see also Victoria Starr, 'Too darn hot; how ABC is muzzling the message', *Outweek,* no. 75, New York, 1990, pp. 38–41.

15   Quoted from The Media Show, *Red Hot & Blue,* Channel Four, 11 November, 1990.

16   *Ibid.*

17   *Ibid.*

18   *Ibid.*

19   *Ibid.*

20   See Simon Watney, 'Rights and responsibilities', *Gay Times,* November 1991, London, p. 12.

21   The films of Stuart Marshall since *Bright Eyes* (1984) have all explored the relations between lesbian and gay experience, and our exclusion from the dominant notions of national identity, whether in relation to 'official' accounts of the Second World War, or to AIDS. Marshall's concern is always with questions of popular historical memory—and the power of institutions such as film and television play in privileging some sets that cultural memories, whilst systematically underprivileging or even erasing others.

24. AIDS and Social Science

This article was published in two parts in *NYQ,* nos. 11 and 12, 12 and 19 January 1992, New York. A slightly shorter version also appeared in *The Trust: The Newsletter of The Terrence Higgins Trust,* no. 18, 1992. Both versions were evaluative report-backs from the Seventh International AIDS Conference in Florence in June 1991.

25. Muddling Through: The UK responses to AIDS

First published as 'Le "fighting spirit" des gays anglais', *Le Journal du SIDA,* nos.38–9, Avril–Mai, 1992, Paris, pp. 1822.

1   Chris Mihill, 'Inner London rates highest in HIV tests', *Guardian,* 18 May 1991, p. 2.

2   *Ibid.*

3   See Simon Watney, 'Safer Sex as Community Practice' in P. Aggleton, et al. (eds), *AIDS: Individual, Cultural And Policy Dimensions,* Falmer Press, London, 1990, pp. 19–35.

4   See Simon Watney, 'School's Out', in D. Fuss (ed.), *Inside/Out: Lesbian Theories, Gay Theories,* Routledge, New York and London, 1991, pp. 387–405.

5   Michel Foucault, 'Sexual Choice, Sexual Act', in S. Lotringer (ed.), *Foucault Live,* Semiotext(e), New York, 1989, pp. 211–33. See also Simon Watney, 'Troubleshooters, *Artforum,* November 1991, New York, pp. 16–18.

6   See Hans Moerkerk with Peter Aggleton, 'AIDS prevention strategies in Europe: a comparison and critical analysis', in P. Aggleton, et al. (eds), *AIDS: Responses, Interventions and Care,* Falmer Press, London, 1991, pp. 1–19.

7   Daniel Defert, '*L'enjeu des gais: L'homosexualisation du SIDA',* Gai Pied, no. 446, 29 November 1990, Paris, pp. 60–3.

8   I believe this construction was first used by Cindy Patton, whom I heard lead a seminar on the topic at the US National Lesbian and Gay Health Conference, in Boston, in 1988. See Cindy Patton, *Inventing AIDS,* Routledge, New York and London, 1990.

9   See Simon Watney, 'Introduction', in E. Carter and S. Watney (eds), *Taking Liberties: AIDS and Cultural Politics,* Serpent's Tail, London, 1989, p. 11–57.

10   Martin Newland, 'AIDS charity "should lose public grant"', *Daily Telegraph,* 7 May 1991, p. 3.

11   Eve Kosofsky Sedgwick, *Epistemology of the Closet,* University of California Press, Berkeley CA, 1990, p. 159.

12   See interview with Lindsay Neil in *Le Journal Du SIDA,* English edition, August 1992, p. 64–5.

13   For example, the four volumes of social science research that Aggleton has co-edited for the Falmer Press in Britain since 1988, and many other publications.

14   Liz Hunt, 'Heterosexual AIDS cases rise by 50 per cent', *Independent,* 30 January 1992.

15   Judy Jones, 'Study showing African AIDS link criticised', *Independent,* 8 February 1992.

16   James Le Fanu, 'Pointless panic on AIDS', *The Times,* 11 February 1992.

26. Duesberg's Dangerous Dogma

This article appeared in *Gay Times,* July 1992.

27. Bad, Mad and Dangerous

This article appeared in *Gay Times,* October 1992.

28. Political Funerals

First published in *Gay Times,* November 1992. A slightly different version of this article also appeared in the *Village Voice,* New York, 20 October 1992, p. 18.

29. Gay Teenagers and Gay Politics

First published in *Gay Times,* December 1992.

1   Jamie Taylor, cited in Mark Simpson, 'Birth of a Legend', *Gay Times,* November 1992.

30. Powers of Observation: AIDS and the writing of history

Previously unpublished and written as a Conclusion to this book.

1   Isaiah Berlin, 'Introduction', *Four Essays on Liberty,* Oxford, 1982, p. XXIX.

2 *Ibid.*, p. XXX.
3 Stuart Hall, 'Introduction', *The Hard Road to Renewal,* Verso, London, 1988, p. 8.
4 Robert M. Swenson, 'Plagues, History, and AIDS', *The American Scholar,* vol. 57, no. 2, Spring, 1988, p. 200. Much the same universalist conclusion is also reached by Charles E. Rosenberg, in 'What is an epidemic? AIDS in historical perspective', *Daedalus* vol. 18, no. 2, Spring 1989, Cambridge MA, pp. 1–17.
5 Elizabeth Fee and Daniel M. Fox, *AIDS: The Burdens of History,* University of California Press, Berkeley and London, 1988, n.p.
6 See Simon Watney, 'Safer Sex as Community Practice' (in this volume).
7 David Black, 'The Plague Years', Parts One & Two', *Rolling Stone,* 28 March 1985, pp. 48–125; and *Rolling Stone,* 25 April 1985, pp. 35–62. Published in book form by Picador, London, 1986.
8 *Ibid.*
9 *Sun,* 11 April 1986.
10 'The life and death of a star', *Independent,* 22 April 1992, p. 16.
11 Matt Clark, 'Plagues, Man and History: Lessons about AIDS from the Black Death', *Newsweek,* 9 May 1988, p. 65.
12 *Ibid.*
13 *Ibid.*, p. 67.
14 See Simon Watney, 'Politics, People and the AIDS Epidemic' (in this volume). See also Douglas Crimp, 'How to Have Promiscuity in an Epidemic', in D. Crimp (ed.), *AIDS: Cultural Analysis, Cultural Activism,* MIT, Cambridge MA, 1988, pp. 237–70.
15 Susan Sontag, *AIDS and Its Metaphors,* Allen Lane/The Penguin Press, London, 1988. See also Simon Watney, 'Guru of AIDS', *Guardian,* 10 March 1989; and David Miller, 'Sontag's Urbanity', *October,* no. 49, MIT, Cambridge MA, Summer 1989, pp. 91–102.
16 *Ibid.*, pp. 70–1.
17 See Hannah Arendt, *Eichmann In Jerusalem: A Report On The Banality Of Evil,* Penguin Books, Harmondsworth, 1977; also Robert Jay Lifton, *The Nazi Doctors: Medical Killing and the Psychology of Genocide,* Basic Books, New York, 1986; also Robert N. Proctor, *Racial Hygiene: Medicine Under The Nazis,* Harvard University Press, Cambridge MA, 1988; also Zygmunt Bauman, *Modernity and the Holocaust,* Polity Press, Oxford, 1989.
18 Homer, *The Iliad,* trans. E.V. Rieu, Penguin Books, Harmondsworth, 1976, pp. 327–8.

Index

Simon Watney is Director of the Red Hot AIDS Charitable
Trust. He is the author of *Policing Desire: Pornography, AIDS,
and the Media* and co-editor of *Taking Liberties: AIDS and
Cultural Politics*. He lives in London.
Library of Congress Cataloging-in-Publication Data
Watney, Simon.
Practices of freedom: selected writings on HIV/AIDS by
Simon Watney.—1st U.S. ed.
(Series Q)   Includes index
ISBN 0-8223-1553-X (cl.) —ISBN0-8223-1564-5 (pa)
1. AIDS (Disease)—Social aspects. I. Title. II. Series.
RC607.A26W373   1994   362. 1'969792—dc20   94-11033 CIP